VOLUME TWO

Textbook of Diagnostic Ultrasonography

VOLUME TWO

*T*extbook *of* *D*iagnostic *U*ltrasonography

fifth edition

with 2538 illustrations

SANDRA L. HAGEN-ANSERT, M.S., RDMS, RDCS
Ultrasound Consultant and Educational Specialist
Former Program Director and Clinical Sonographer
Baptist College of Health Sciences, Memphis, Tennessee
University of California, San Diego Medical Center, San Diego, California

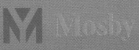

An Affiliate of Elsevier Science
St. Louis   London   Philadelphia   Sydney   Toronto

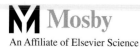

An Affiliate of Elsevier Science

Executive Editor: Jeanne Wilke
Senior Developmental Editor: Carolyn Kruse
Developmental Editor: Linda Woodard
Project Manager: John Rogers
Project Specialist: Beth Hayes
Designer: Kathi Gosche
Medical Illustrator: Jeanne Robertson

FIFTH EDITION

Mosby, Inc.
An Affiliate of Elsevier Science
11830 Westline Industrial Drive
St. Louis, Missouri 63146

Printed in the United States of America

Library of Congress Cataloging in Publication Data

Hagen-Ansert, Sandra L.
    Textbook of diagnostic ultrasonography / Sandra L. Hagen-Ansert.– 5th ed.
      p. ; cm.
    Includes bibliographical references and index.
    ISBN 0-323-01009-1
    1. Diagnosis, Ultrasonic. 2. Echocardiography. I. Title: Diagnostic ultrasonography. II. Title.
    [DNLM: 1. Ultrasonography. WN 208 H143t 2001]
    RC78.7.U4 H33 2001
    616.07'543–dc21

                                          00-064720

02 03 04 05 GW/KPT 9 8 7 6 5 4 3 2

CONTRIBUTORS

FRANK CHERVENAK, MD
Professor of Obstetrics and Gynecology
Director of Obstetrics
Director, Maternal-Fetal Medicine
New York Hospital, Cornell Medical Center
New York, New York

DAWN GANGLOFF, BS, RDMS, RT(R)
Staff Sonographer, Ultrasound Department
St. Francis Hospital
Peoria, Illinois

M. ELIZABETH GLENN, MD
Women's Health Center at Baptist East
Memphis, Tennessee

CHARLOTTE HENNINGSEN, MS, RDMS
Program Director, Diagnostic Medical Sonography
Florida College of Health Science
Orlando, Florida

MIRA L. KATZ, PhD, RVT
Research Technologist
Radiology Department
The Children's Hospital of Philadelphia
Philadelphia, Pennsylvania

LAURENCE B. McCULLOUGH, PhD
Professor of Medicine and Medical Ethics
Center for Medical Ethics and Health Policy
Baylor College of Medicine
Houston, Texas

TRACI PARKER, RDMS
Department of Radiology/Ultrasound
Boulder, Colorado

KERRY WEINBERG, MPA, RT(R), RDMS, RDCS
Program Director, Diagnostic Medical Sonography
New York University
New York, New York

REVIEWERS

KEVIN P. BARRY, MEd, RDMS, RDCS, RT(R)
Professor/Department Head
Diagnostic Medical Imaging
New Hampshire Technical Institute
Concord, New Hampshire

JAN D. BRYANT, MS, RDMS, RT(R)
Program Director
Diagnostic Medical Sonography Program
El Centro College
Dallas, Texas

CASEY CLARKE, BSRT, RT(R), RDMS, RDCS
Program Director
Diagnostic Medical Sonography
South Suburban College
South Holland, Illinois

JOAN CLASBY, BvE, RT, RDMS, RDCS
Director and Professor
Diagnostic Medical Sonographer
Orange Coast College
Costa Mesa, California

DALE E. COLLINS, MS, RT(R) (M) (QM), RDMS
Instructor
Medical Radiography
State University of New York–HSC–Syracuse
Syracuse, New York

STEVEN M. CURRIER, MS, RT, RDMS, RVT
Director
Medical Imaging
Lake Wales Medical Center
Lake Wales, Florida

JANICE D. DOLK, MA, RT(R), RDMS
Director
Diagnostic Medical Sonography Program
University of Maryland, Baltimore
Baltimore, Maryland

JANET M. FELDMEIER, BSRT, RDMS
Staff Ultrasonographer
Cardinal Glennon Children's Hospital
St. Louis, Missouri

KATHLEEN KURSHINSKY, RT(R)M, RDMS
Clinical Instructor
Chippewa Valley Technical College
Eau Claire, Wisconsin

THOMAS F. WALSH, MA, RDMS
Program Director
Middlesex Community College
Bedford, Massachusetts

KIMBERLEE B. WATTS
Director of Sonography
Caldwell Community College & Technical Institute
Hudson, North Carolina

CHERYL L. ZELINSKY, BA, RT(R), RDMS
Director
Diagnostic Medical Sonography Program
Oregon Institute of Technology
Klamath Falls, Oregon

To our own little sonic boomers:
Rebecca, Alyssa, and Katrina,
who are growing up to make their own waves.

FOREWORD

I am pleased to offer a foreword for this prestigious Silver Anniversary Edition of *Textbook of Diagnostic Ultrasonography*.

Continuing growth in the field of sonography certainly has warranted this new edition and Sandra Hagen-Ansert and her colleagues have proved more than equal to the task. New in this edition are chapters on the *foundations of sonography, scanning techniques and protocols, the vascular system, the liver, the genitourinary system, the retroperitoneal cavity, the scrotum, the breast, and the thyroid,* complementing existing chapters on general sonography. Special attention to neonates has resulted in specific chapters on cranial, abdominal, and renal sonography. Obstetric and gynecologic sonography have also been enhanced by revised offerings in normal anatomy and physiology, as well as embryosonology, congenital anomalies, and fetal echocardiography. The vascular chapters have been completely updated to include the latest techniques in vascular imaging. The cardiology section offers introductory material on anatomy and physiology, in addition to the normal echocardiographic protocol and images required to perform a complete examination. A brief overview of pathology the cardiac sonographer may encounter during an echocardiographic procedure is found in the echocardiographic pathology chapter. As with previous editions the quality of the text and illustrations remains very high. The authors are to be commended for their efforts in making a very readable textbook.

The focus of this text has always been on the sonographer actually performing studies. Those who assume this role have a unique relationship with physicians responsible for interpreting sonographic studies. Real-time sonography provides the sonographer with vast amounts of information, most of which is discarded. Final images reaching the physician are a distillation of this information. In a very real sense the sonographer performs diagnosis during the study. Nowhere else in medicine does this relationship exist. Perhaps the closest analogy is in gastrointestinal fluoroscopy, in which spot films are made of real-time images, often sacrificing functional information. Technologists perform these studies in virtually no institutions. Yet curiously, in these same institutions, sonographers daily churn out complex studies of the heart, abdomen, and pelvis—in my view a far more complex task.

This unique role as a physician's assistant clearly deserves recognition. It requires high-quality instruction, of which this book is an excellent example. It also requires outstanding and dedicated individuals, of which the book's principal author is an excellent example. She and her co-authors are to be congratulated on their success in advancing our knowledge in this discipline.

It is hard to overestimate the number of individuals who have benefited from previous editions of this text. Although this text was initially conceived for sonographers, I frequently see it used by sonologists as well. It is my belief that this usage typifies the close relationship between these groups, which is essential for top-quality sonography. In this edition, Sandra Hagen-Ansert and her colleagues have once again shown us that through prodigious effort it is still possible to produce a text benefiting all who labor in this vineyard.

George R. Leopold, MD

PREFACE

A LOOK BACK

Medicine has always been a fascinating field to me. I was introduced to it by Dr. Charles Henkelmann in 1963, who provided me with the opportunity to learn radiography. Although x-ray technology was interesting, it did not provide the opportunity to evaluate patient history or to follow through interesting cases, which seemed to be the most intriguing aspect of medicine and my primary concern.

Shortly after I finished my radiographic training in 1968, I was assigned to the radiation therapy department, where I was introduced to a very quiet, young, dedicated radiologist, whom I would later grow to admire and respect as one of the foremost authorities in diagnostic ultrasound. Convincing George Leopold that he needed another hand to assist him was difficult in the beginning, and it was through the efforts of his resident, Dan MacDonald, that I was able to learn what has eventually developed into a challenging and exciting new medical modality.

Using high-frequency sound waves, diagnostic ultrasound provides a unique method for visualization of soft tissue anatomic structures. Identifying such structures and correlating the results with clinical symptoms and patient data offers an ongoing challenge to the sonographer. The state of the art demands expertise in scanning techniques and maneuvers to demonstrate the internal structures; without quality scans, limited diagnostic sonographic information can be provided to the physician.

Our initial experience in ultrasound took us through the era of A-mode techniques, identifying aortic aneurysms through pulsatile reflections, trying to separate splenic reflections from upper-pole left renal masses, and, in general, attempting to echo every patient with a probable abdominal or pelvic mass. Of course, the one-dimensional A-mode techniques were difficult for me to conceptualize, let alone trust. However, with repeated successes and experience gained from mistakes, I began to believe in this method. The conviction that Dr. Leopold had about this technique was a strong indicator of its success in our laboratory.

In 1969, when our first two-dimensional ultrasound unit arrived in the laboratory, the "skeptics" started to believe a little more in this modality. I must admit that those early images looked like weather maps to me for several months. The repeated times I asked, "What is that?" were enough to try anyone's patience.

I can recall when Siemens installed our real-time unit and we saw our first obstetric case. It was such a thrill for us to see the fetus move, wave his hand, and show us fetal heart pulsations!

We scouted the clinics and various departments in the hospital for interesting cases to scan. With our success rate surpassing our failures, the case load increased, so that soon we were involved in all aspects of ultrasound. There was not enough material for us to read to see the new developments. It was for this reason that excitement in clinical research soared, attracting young physicians throughout the country to develop techniques in diagnostic ultrasound.

Because Dr. Leopold was so intensely interested in ultrasound, it became the diagnostic method of choice for our patients. It was not long before conferences were incomplete without the mention of the technique. Later, local medical meetings and eventually national meetings grew to include discussion of this new modality. A number of visitors were attracted to our laboratory to learn the technique, and thus we became swamped with a continual flow of new physicians, some eager to work with ultrasound and others skeptical at first but believers in the end.

In 1970, the beginning of education progressed slowly, with many laboratories offering a one-on-one teaching experience. Commercial companies thought the only way to push the field was to develop their own national training programs, and thus several of the leading manufacturers were the first to put a dedicated effort into the development of ultrasound.

It was through the combined efforts of our laboratory and commercial interests that I became interested in furthering ultrasound education. Seminars, weekly sessions, local and national meetings, and consultations became a vital part of the growth of ultrasound.

Thus, as ultrasound grew in popularity, more intensified training was desperately needed to maintain the initial quality that the pioneers strived for. Through working with one of the commercial ultrasound companies conducting national short-term training programs, I became acquainted with Barry Goldberg and his enthusiasm for quality education in ultrasound. His organizational efforts and pioneer spirit led me to the east coast to further develop more intensive educational programs in ultrasound. The challenge grew of establishing new programs and continuing education in diagnostic medical sonography in the years to follow as we ventured across the United States and Canada.

INTRODUCING THE NEW FIFTH EDITION

Welcome to the Silver Anniversary Edition of the *Textbook of Diagnostic Ultrasonography*. This fifth edition continues the tradition of excellence begun when the first edition was published in the 1970s. Of course, the textbook has been vastly updated and reorganized over the years. The field of diagnostic ultrasound has changed so dramatically in the past 40 years that the approach to many procedures has been altered significantly. Phenomenal strides in transducer design, instrumentation, and color flow Doppler have provided increased resolution in the ultrasound image. The introduction of contrast media is becoming more clinically accepted to image the gastrointestinal tract, the female reproductive system, and the multiple vascular pathways in the body. Three-dimensional imaging has provided additional information on the fetus to help the clinician obtain a clearer definition of fine detail.

The primary goal of this textbook continues: to provide an in depth resource for students studying sonography, as well as practitioners in hospitals, clinics, and private radiology, cardiology, and obstetric settings. This new, fifth edition strives to keep up with this fast-moving field, giving students and practitioners not only complete, but also up-to-date information in sonography.

ORGANIZATION

Textbook of Diagnostic Ultrasonography remains divided into two volumes to compensate for its expanded coverage and to make the book more convenient and easier to use. The content has been completely reorganized to provide better flow for the reader. The first volume covers general ultrasound applications, that is, abdominal and retroperitoneal cavities, superficial structures, and pediatrics. Also included in this volume are four chapters on cerebrovascular and peripheral vascular Doppler imaging, as well as two chapters focusing on an introduction to echocardiography with an overview of cardiac pathology. The second volume has been reorganized to primarily focus on obstetrics and gynecology.

Each chapter begins with a list of key terms and definitions to aid the reader. Sonographic concepts continue to be presented in a logical and consistent manner in each chapter. To help the student and the sonographer understand the patient's total clinical picture before the sonographic examination, discussions on anatomy, physiology, laboratory data, clinical signs and symptoms, pathology, and sonographic findings are found within each specific chapter. References cited in the text are listed at the end of each chapter. In addition, review questions are included at the end of each chapter to help the reader measure comprehension of the material.

ILLUSTRATIONS AND VISUALS

The reader will notice colorful illustrations throughout and color within the layout of the chapters. Focus charts highlight important areas throughout both volumes.

To keep up with the continually changing field of ultrasound, hundreds of new images have been incorporated, including many new color Doppler images. *Out of more than 3000 images, approximately 70% are new.* In addition, the multitude of anatomic illustrations have been completely redrawn in color to demonstrate many of the relevant landmarks the sonographer should look for when performing an ultrasound examination.

Ultrasound findings for particular pathologies and conditions are now preceded by the following special head:

Ultrasound findings.

This makes location of these sections easier for both the student and the practicing sonographer.

NEW TO THE FIFTH EDITION

This edition has been completely revised and expanded to offer a comprehensive textbook for the student in general ultrasound. The peripheral vascular chapters are appropriate for the student to understand vascular applications within a general ultrasound department. New chapters have been added on the foundations of sonography; the breast, thyroid, and scrotum and prostate; renal and retroperitoneal areas; high-risk pregnancy; congenital anomalies; fetal head and neural tube defects; and ethics and legal issues in obstetric ultrasound.

Particularly noteworthy is the section on obstetrics and gynecology, which has been completely updated from the excellent work of Kara Mayden Argo and her collegues in the fourth edition, with several excellent new contributors. The pediatric ultrasound section written by Suzanne Devine and her colleagues from Children's Hospital in Chicago in the last edition has been updated as well. The cerebrovascular and peripheral vascular chapters have been completely revised by Mira Katz. Dr. Elizabeth Glenn has extensively rewritten the chapter on the breast from the focus of a sonographer working within a women's health center.

It is my hope that this textbook will not only introduce the reader to the field of ultrasound, but also go a step beyond to what I have found to be a very stimulating and challenging experience in diagnostic patient care.

Sandra Hagen-Ansert

ACKNOWLEDGMENTS

The author would like to recognize the work of the following individuals on the fourth edition, which allowed a building block to continue for this fifth edition: Kara Mayden Argo, BS, RDMS, RDCS, RTR (obstetrics); Kathleen Bauman, RDMS (neonatal head); Dale Cyr, BS, RDMS (first trimester); Suzanne Devine, RT, RDMS (pediatrics); Kate A. Feinstein, MD (pediatrics); Deborah Levine, MD (gynecologic pathology); Holly D. Lloyd, BS, RDMS (gynecology); Arnold Shkolnik, MD (pediatrics); Laura J. Zuidema, MD; and William J. Zwiebel, MD (liver physiology).

I would like to acknowledge the individual who contributed most to my early interest in diagnostic ultrasound, Dr. George R. Leopold, for his personal perseverance and instruction, as well as for his outstanding clinical research. My thanks also go to the following:

Dr. Sam Halpern, who encouraged me to publish

Dr. Barry Goldberg, for the opportunity to develop training programs in an independent fashion and for his encouragement to stay with it

Drs. Dolores Pretorius, Nancy Budorick, Wanda Miller-Hance, and David Sahn, for their encouragement throughout the years at the UCSD Medical Center

Dr. Daniel Yellon, for his early hour anatomy dissection and instruction in clinical cardiology

Dr. Carson Schneck, for his excellent instruction in gross anatomy and sections of "Geraldine"

Dr. Jacob Zatuchni, for the interest, enthusiasm, and understanding he showed me while at Episcopal Hospital

Dr. Fred Sample, whose quest for the anatomic ultrasound demonstration of the abdomen and pelvis was an inspiration to us all

Dr. Bill Sobotor, for his perserverance for quality and teamwork in the Allied Health curriculum at Baptist College of Health Science

Dr. Thomas Tabb, for his enthusiam and quest for quality imaging in high-risk obstetrics

Darlene Bak, RDMS, for her support in supplying high-risk obstetric images

Cindy Owen, RDMS, for her support in supplying abdominal and vascular images

Phil Thompson, RDMS, for his support in supplying general ultrasound images

Dr. James Machin, for his support for education in the Diagnostic Medical Sonography program

GE Medical Systems for providing sonograms

For their support, I would like to thank the students I have taught in Diagnostic Ultrasound from the various medical institutions I have been involved with: Episcopal Hospital, Thomas Jefferson University Medical Center, University of Wisconsin, Madison Medical Center, UCSD Medical Center, Baptist College of Health Science, and Trident Technical College, who continually work toward the development of quality ultrasound techniques and instruction.

I would also like to acknowledge and thank the excellent staff at Harcourt Health Sciences, especially Carolyn Kruse, Linda Woodard, Jeanne Robertson, and Jeanne Wilke, all of whom were most patient and enduring for the entire preparation of the manuscript during tornados, multiple relocation moves, and reviewer comments. A special thank you to my production editor, Beth Hayes, whose eye for accuracy and detail has been outstanding in the production of this textbook.

Very special recognition goes to my patient and understanding family, Art, Rebecca, Alyssa, and Katrina, who were usually very tolerant of the hours upon hours of preparation and writing this edition bestowed upon all of our lives. The girls have grown up with these five editions and have volunteered their tiny hearts, and now abdominal vessels, for various illustrations throughout the book. They have vowed never to volunteer again.

CONTENTS

*T*extbook *of D*iagnostic *U*ltrasonography

PART VII

Foundations of Obstetric Sonography

CHAPTER *25*

The Role of Ultrasound in Obstetrics

Sandra L. Hagen-Ansert

abruptio placenta - bleeding from a normally situated placenta causing its complete or partial detachment after the twentieth week of gestation

amniocentesis - aspiration of a sample of amniotic fluid through the mother's abdomen for diagnosis of fetal maturity and/or disease by assay of the constituents of the fluid

amnion - smooth membrane enclosing the fetus and amniotic fluid; it is loosely fused with the outer chorionic membrane

anencephaly - absence of the brain; the cerebellum and basal ganglia may be present

cervix - inferior segment of the uterus; more that 3.5 cm long during normal pregnancy, decreases in length during labor

chorion - cellular, outermost extraembryonic membrane, composed of trophoblast lined with mesoderm; it develops villi about 2 weeks after fertilization, is vascularized by allantoic vessels a week later, gives rise to the placenta, and persists until birth

corpus luteum - yellow body formed from the Graafian follicle after ovulation that produces estrogen and progesterone

ductus venosus - fetal vein that connects the umbilical vein to the inferior vena cava and runs at an oblique axis through the liver

embryo - conceptus to the end of the ninth week of gestation

gestational age - gestational age since the date of conception

gestational sac - structure that is normally within the uterus that contains the developing embryo

hydatidiform mole - condition in which there is partial or complete conversion of the chorionic villi into grapelike vesicles; villia are avascular and there is trophoblastic proliferation; condition may result in malignant trophoblastic disease

incompetent cervix - cervix dilates silently during the second trimester with the result that the membranes bulge and rupture and the fetus drops out

intrauterine growth restriction (IUGR) - abnormal growth pattern of the fetus; usually small abdomen compared with other growth parameters

lower uterine segment - thin expanded lower portion of the uterus that forms in the last trimester of pregnancy

macrosomia - exceptionally large infant with fat deposition in the subcutaneous tissues; seen in fetuses of diabetic mothers

oligohydramnios - insufficient amount of amniotic fluid

placenta - organ of communication (nutrition and products of metabolism) between the fetus and the mother; forms from the chorion frondosum with a maternal decidual contribution

placenta previa - placental implantation encroaches upon the lower uterine segment; the placenta comes first and bleeding is inevitable

polyhydramnios - excessive amount of amniotic fluid (>20 cm)

trimester - pregnancy is divided into three 13-week periods

umbilical cord - connecting lifeline between the fetus and placenta; it contains two umbilical arteries and one umbilical vein encased in Wharton's jelly

yolk sac - circular structure seen between 4 and 10 weeks that supplies nutrition to the fetal pole (the developing embryo); it lies within the chorion outside the amnion

---

Ultrasound has become one of the primary tools used by the obstetrician to evaluate the developing fetus during pregnancy. Obstetric ultrasound allows the clinician to assess the development, growth, and well-being of the fetus. When an abnormal condition is recognized prenatally, obstetric management may be altered to provide the best care for the fetus and child.

The sonographer performing fetal studies should understand both sonographic and obstetric principles. This allows the sonographer to accurately and thoroughly compile pertinent information to provide a complete assessment of the fetus. This profile includes anatomic and biometric analyses.

This chapter describes the medical indications for obstetric ultrasound examinations; reviews guidelines for scanning as outlined by the American College of Radiology (ACR), the American Institute of Ultrasound in Medicine (AIUM), and the American College of Obstetricians and Gynecologists (ACOG); and describes the risk factors associated with congenital fetal anomalies.*

RECOMMENDATIONS FOR OBSTETRIC AND GYNECOLOGIC ULTRASOUND

There are recommended indications for obstetric ultrasound examinations. The sonographer should be aware of the indications for ultrasound and should understand the medical complications associated with maternal disease states during pregnancy. This knowledge helps determine appropriate scanning techniques based on the specific indication for the study and the clinical history of the mother.

The indications for obstetric and gynecologic studies as detailed by the National Institute of Child Health and Human Development and National Institutes of Health Consensus Report on Safety of Ultrasound are as follows[6]:

1. Estimation of **gestational age** for patients with uncertain clinical dates or verification of dates for patients who are to undergo scheduled elective repeat cesarean delivery, indicated induction of labor, or other elective termination of pregnancy. Ultrasonographic confirmation of dating permits proper timing of cesarean delivery or labor induction to avoid premature delivery.

2. Evaluation of fetal growth, for example, when the patient has an identified etiology for uteroplacental insufficiency, such as severe preeclampsia, chronic hypertension, chronic renal disease, or severe diabetes mellitus, or for other medical complications of pregnancy in which fetal malnutrition (e.g., **intrauterine growth restriction [IUGR]** or **macrosomia**) is suspected. Following fetal growth permits assessment of the impact of a complicating condition of the fetus and guides pregnancy management.

3. Vaginal bleeding of undetermined etiology in pregnancy. Ultrasound often allows determination of the source of bleeding and status of the fetus.

4. Determination of fetal presentation when the presenting part cannot be adequately determined in labor or the fetal presentation is variable in late pregnancy. Accurate knowledge of presentation guides management of delivery.

5. Suspected multiple gestation based on detection of more than one fetal heart beat pattern, fundal height larger than expected for dates, or prior use of fertility drugs. Pregnancy management may be altered in multiple gestation.

6. Adjunct to **amniocentesis**. Ultrasound permits guidance of the needle to avoid the **placenta** and fetus, to increase the chance of obtaining amniotic fluid and to decrease the chance of fetal loss.

7. Significant discrepancy between uterine size and clinical dates. Ultrasound permits accurate dating and detection of such conditions as oligohydramnios and polyhydramnios, as well as multiple gestation, IUGR, and anomalies.

8. Pelvic mass detected clinically. Ultrasound can detect the location and nature of the mass and aid in the diagnosis.

9. Suspected **hydatidiform mole** on the basis of clinical signs of hypertension, proteinuria, or the presence of ovarian cysts felt on pelvic examination or failure to detect fetal heart tones with a Doppler ultrasound device after 12 weeks. Ultrasound permits accurate diagnosis and differentiation of this neoplasm from fetal death.

10. Adjunct to cervical cerclage placement. Ultrasound aids in timing and proper placement of the cerclage for patients with **incompetent cervix.**

11. Suspected ectopic pregnancy or when pregnancy occurs after tuboplasty or prior ectopic gestation. Ultrasound is a valuable diagnostic aid for this complication.

12. Adjunct to special procedures such as cordocentesis, intrauterine transfusion, shunt placement, in vitro fertilization, embryo transfer, or chorionic villi sampling. Ultrasound aids instrument guidance that increases the safety of these procedures.

---

*ACR: www.ACR.org; AIUM: www.AIUM.org; ACOG: www.ACOG.org.

13. Suspected fetal death. Rapid diagnosis enhances optimal management.
14. Suspected uterine abnormality (e.g., clinically significant leiomyomata, congenital structural abnormalities such as bicornuate uterus or uteri didelphys). Serial surveillance of fetal growth and state enhances fetal outcome.
15. Intrauterine contraceptive device (IUD) localization. Ultrasound guidance facilitates removal, reducing chances of IUD-related complications.
16. Ovarian follicle development surveillance. This facilitates treatment of infertility.
17. Biophysical evaluation for fetal well-being after 28 weeks of gestation. Assessment of amniotic fluid, fetal tone, body movements, breathing movements, and heart rate patterns assists in management of high-risk pregnancies.
18. Observation of intrapartum events (e.g., version or extraction of second twin, manual removal of placenta). These procedures may be done more safely with the visualization provided by ultrasound.
19. Suspected **polyhydramnios** or **oligohydramnios.** Confirmation of the diagnosis is permitted, as well as identification of the cause of the condition in certain pregnancies.
20. Suspected **abruptio placentae.** Confirmation of diagnosis and extent assists in clinical management.
21. Adjunct to external version from breech to vertex presentation. The visualization provided by ultrasound facilitates performance of this procedure.
22. Estimation of fetal weight and presentation in premature rupture of the membranes or premature labor. Information provided by ultrasound guides management decisions on timing and method of delivery.
23. Abnormal maternal serum alpha-fetoprotein (MSAFP) value for clinical gestational age when drawn. Ultrasound provides an accurate assessment of gestational age for the MSAFP comparison standard and indicates several conditions (e.g., twins, **anencephaly**) that may cause elevated AFP values.
24. Follow-up observation of identified fetal anomaly. Ultrasound assessment of progression or lack of change assists in clinical decision making.
25. Follow-up evaluation of placenta location for identified **placenta previa.**
26. History of previous congenital anomaly. Detection of recurrence may be permitted, or psychologic benefit to patients may result from reassurance of no recurrence.
27. Serial evaluation of fetal growth in multiple gestation. Ultrasound permits recognition of discordant growth, guiding patient management and timing of delivery.
28. Evaluation of fetal condition in late registrants for prenatal care. Accurate knowledge of gestational age assists in pregnancy management decisions for this group.

MATERNAL RISK FACTORS

Maternal risk factors that increase the chances of producing a fetus with congenital anomalies include the maternal age, abnormal alpha-fetoprotein values, maternal disease (e.g., diabetes mellitus, systemic lupus erythematosus), and a pregnant uterus that is either too small or too large for dates. Other risk factors include a previous child born with a chromosomal disorder or exposure to a known teratogenic drug or infectious agent known to cause birth defects.

PATIENT HISTORY

There are several important questions the sonographer should ask the patient before beginning the obstetric ultrasound evaluation. The date of the last menstrual period is necessary to correlate the obstetric measurements with the expected gestational age. The sonographer also needs to know if the patient is currently taking any medication or has experienced any clinical problems with the pregnancy such as bleeding, decreased fetal movement, or pelvic pain. If the patient has had problems with previous pregnancies, that is, congenital or chromosomal, this also should be documented on the preliminary record.

THE SAFETY OF ULTRASOUND

It has been estimated that more than one half of all pregnant women in the United States are examined with ultrasound.[10] A number of experiments have been conducted to study the safety of ultrasound. In both animal experiments and therapeutic applications that use very-high-intensity levels of ultrasound, modification of biologic structures and functions does occur.[10] However, no confirmed ultrasonically induced adverse effects in humans have been reported when diagnostic levels of ultrasound are used.[9,10] Furthermore, the acoustic outputs, carrier frequencies, and pulse lengths of diagnostic ultrasound are all significantly less than those used for the reviewed experiments.[10]

The major biologic effects of ultrasonography are believed to be thermal (a rise in temperature) and cavitation (production and collapse of gas-filled bubbles).[7,9] Although it has been shown that a rise in temperature of less than one degree Celsius may occur during diagnostic ultrasound evaluation, this is unlikely to have any clinical impact in humans.[3,11] Likewise, cavitation (which requires the preexistence of stable gas-filled nuclei) may occur with in vitro experiments but is also unlikely to occur in humans.[5]

The major difficulties with the studies investigating a possible deleterious effect of diagnostic ultrasound evaluation are threefold:

1. Experimental ultrasound exposure levels often far exceeded those that are normally used diagnostically.
2. The systems used to show ultrasound effect (plants, cell culture, laboratory animals) may not be applicable to humans.
3. Many studies that have demonstrated adverse effects in vitro have not been reproducible.[9]

A review of the safety of ultrasound with respect to the fetus has concluded that "current data indicate that there are no confirmed biologic effects on patients and their fetuses from the use of diagnostic ultrasound evaluation and that the benefits to patients exposed to the prudent use of this modality outweigh the risks, if any."[9] The sonographer should perform the ultrasound evaluation only when there are clear clinical indications.

SAFETY OF DOPPLER IN THE OBSTETRIC PATIENT

Doppler ultrasound provides a safe, noninvasive, and expedient method to assess the physiology and pathophysiology of the fetal and maternal circulations. In most cases, pulsed wave Doppler (requires less power) is used in the fetus rather than continuous wave Doppler. Doppler may be used to detect flow in the maternal vessels, the fetal vessels (umbilical artery and vein, aorta and inferior vena cava, renal arteries, and cerebral vessels), the fetal **ductus venosus,** the fetal heart, and the placenta. Specific applications of Doppler are presented in the respective chapters.

The AIUM's position statement on the use of Doppler ultrasound is as follows[4]:

> AIUM feels there is currently sufficient information to justify clinical use of continuous wave, pulsed, and color flow Doppler ultrasound to evaluate blood flow in uterine, umbilical, and fetal vessels, the fetal cardiovascular system, and to image flow in these structures using color flow imaging technology.

GUIDELINES FOR ANTEPARTUM OBSTETRIC ULTRASOUND EXAMINATION

The ACR introduced scanning guidelines for obstetric ultrasound examinations.[2] The purpose of the guidelines are (1) to standardize obstetric studies, (2) to optimize the detection of fetal growth abnormalities, and (3) to detect fetal anomalies. Fetal ultrasound should be performed only when there is a valid medical reason, and the lowest possible ultrasonic exposure settings should be used to obtain the necessary diagnostic information.[2]

The guidelines outline the qualifications of personnel performing the examination, specifications of the examination, documentation, equipment specification, and quality assurance. Real-time ultrasound allows the confirmation of fetal life and permits the examiner to view fetal anatomy and to obtain biometric parameters used to determine fetal age and growth.

The guidelines further describe the appropriate selection of transducers according to the type of examination and body habitus of the patient. Obstetric studies should incorporate the highest-frequency transducers possible to obtain the best resolution. Most obstetric examinations may be performed with the 5-MHz curved array transducer in the first and second **trimester.** Most equipment is capable of multifrequency ranges on the transducer, and thus the image quality is improved as the sonographer incorporates the various frequencies throughout the examination; structures closer to the transducer require a higher frequency, whereas those located deep in the uterus may require a lower frequency or adjustment of the gain con-

trol to adequately image the fetus. The patient with a thicker abdominal wall will of course require a lower-frequency transducer to adequately image the fetus.

The sonographer should also understand the overall knobology of the particular equipment to produce a high-quality image. Utilization of transmitter gain, TGC controls, depth, and proper focus controls will aid in producing a high-quality image. The focal zone is usually placed at or slightly below the area of interest to provide the highest resolution.

A combination of abdominal and/or transvaginal transducers should be used when appropriate. Most laboratories will use both the abdominal and transvaginal transducer for the examination of the first-trimester fetus. The abdominal transducer provides an overview of the entire pelvic cavity, enables the sonographer to image the uterus from the **cervix** to the fundus, evaluate the ovaries and adnexal areas for abnormal collections of fluid or a mass, and look for the presence of free fluid. The transvaginal transducer provides a limited view of the pelvic cavity but allows excellent visualization of the **embryo,** yolk sac, **amnion, chorion,** and **gestational sac.** The transvaginal view of the embryo is the best method to measure the crown-rump length.

The permanent documentation of both biometric and anatomic profiles of the fetus is essential for quality care. Images should be appropriately labeled with the patient's name, date, and image orientation. Fetal echocardiography is often stored on a real-time format for future reference and review. A written ultrasound report by the physician should outline the findings of the study.

FIRST TRIMESTER

Indications for first-trimester sonography are shown in Box 25-1. The first-trimester guidelines should include ultrasound evaluation by the transabdominal or transvaginal approach. If the transabdominal examination fails to provide definitive information concerning any of the following, a transvaginal scan should be done if possible.

Sample Protocol
1. The uterus and adnexa should be evaluated for the presence of a gestational sac.
   • If a gestational sac is seen, its location should be documented (intrauterine or extrauterine).

BOX 25-1 INDICATIONS FOR FIRST-TRIMESTER SONOGRAPHY

• Confirm presence of intrauterine pregnancy
• Evaluate for suspected ectopic pregnancy
• Define cause of vaginal bleeding
• Determine gestational age
• Confirm suspected multiple gestations
• Confirm embryonic life
• Aid in invasive procedures (chorionic villi sampling, amniocentesis, embryo transfer, IUCD removal)
• Evaluate pelvic masses
• Detect uterine abnormalities

- The presence or absence of an embryo should be noted and the crown-rump length recorded.
- The earliest structure seen within the gestational sac is the yolk sac (the yolk sac will indicate the presence of an intrauterine pregnancy).
- The embryo is seen at 4 weeks as a echogenic curved structure adjacent to the yolk sac.
- The blood tests (hCG levels) should be positive 7 to 10 days after conception.
- The placenta is seen as a thickened density (trophoblastic reaction) along part of the margin of the gestational sac.
- The bowel herniates out from the fetal abdomen at 8 to 11 weeks, then returns back into the abdominal cavity.
- The crown-rump length is the most accurate measurement for gestational age.

2. Absence of fetal cardiac activity should be reported.
- Remember that the fetal heart rate is much faster than the mother's heart rate. The fetal heart rate changes according to fetal development stages; early in embryologic development the heart rate is slow (90 beats per minute). The rate may go up to 170 beats per minute in the middle of the first trimester, before returning to 120 to 140 beats per minute throughout the remainder of the pregnancy.

3. Fetal number should be documented.
- Remember to count only the embryo and yolk sac to determine the number.

4. Evaluation of the uterus, adnexal structures, and cul-de-sac should be performed.
- It is important to document the texture of the ovaries (rule out the presence of **corpus luteum** or other ovarian cyst development); look for abnormal uterine texture patterns that may represent leiomyomatous growth that may be stimulated by the hormonal changes of pregnancy.

SECOND AND THIRD TRIMESTERS

The indications for second- and third-trimester sonography are shown in Box 25-2. The guidelines for the second- and third-trimester ultrasound examination include a biometric and anatomic survey of the fetus. The guidelines suggest the following[8]:

1. Fetal life, number, presentation, and activity should be documented.
- In multiple gestations, the following individual studies should be performed on each fetus: placental number, sac number, comparison of fetal size, presence or absence of an interposed membrane, amount of amniotic fluid (increased, decreased, or normal) on each side of the membrane, and fetal genitalia (when visualized).

2. Estimation of the quantity of amniotic fluid. Abnormal fluid amounts should be described.
- In the first trimester, amniotic fluid is produced by the placenta; in the second trimester, the fetal kidneys begin to produce urine and contribute to the production of amniotic fluid as the fetus swallows and urinates. The fluid increases in volume until the 34th week of gestation.
- The fetus gains one third of its weight during the first two thirds of pregnancy and gains two thirds of its weight during the last third of pregnancy. The volume of the amniotic fluid is calculated through the amniotic fluid index (AFI).
- Too much fluid is termed *hydramnios (polyhydramnios);* too little fluid is called *oligohydramnios.*

3. Placental localization, appearance, and relationship to the internal cervical os should be recorded. The **umbilical cord** and the number of vessels should be recorded.
- The cervical os is normally 3 to 4 cm long. The maternal bladder must be adequately filled to see the cervical os well in the lower **uterine segment.** Make sure the lower end of the placenta is well away from the cervical os to rule out placenta previa.
- An overdistended maternal urinary bladder or a contraction in the lower uterine cavity can give a false impression of placenta previa.

4. In assessment of fetal age at least two dating parameters should be evaluated. Fetal growth studies include a serial growth analysis when multiple examinations are performed. Biometric parameters that may be used include the following:
- Biparietal diameter (BPD) (measure in axial plane that includes thalamus and cavum septum pellucidum)
- Head circumference (measure at same level as BPD, around outer perimeter of the calvarium)
- Femur length (measured after 14th week of gestation)
- Abdominal circumference (measure on transverse view at level of the junction of the umbilical vein and portal sinus)
- Head circumference to abdominal circumference ratio (used in cases in which head to abdomen disproportion is suspected or unusual head or body contours are observed)

5. Uterine, adnexal, and cervical evaluation should be performed to exclude masses that may complicate obstetric management.

6. Anatomic survey of fetal anatomy to exclude major congenital malformations. Comprehensive studies may be necessary when a fetal anomaly is suspected.

Basic ultrasound examinations should evaluate the anatomic areas listed below. More detailed studies may be performed. Documentation of the required anatomy should be completed. Anatomic areas include the following:

1. Cerebral ventricles (exclusion of ventriculomegaly)
2. Choroid plexus
3. Posterior fossa (including cerebellar hemisphere and cisterna magna)

BOX 25-2   INDICATIONS FOR SECOND- AND THIRD-TRIMESTER SONOGRAPHY

- Estimate gestational age for patients with uncertain dates
- Evaluate uterine size and clinical date discrepancies
- Evaluate fetal growth
- Estimate fetal weight
- Determine fetal presentation
- Evaluate fetal life
- Provide adjunct to amniocentesis, percutaneous umbilical blood sampling procedure, or cerclage placement
- Evaluate uterine abnormality
- Evaluate abnormal maternal serum alpha-fetoprotein values
- Evaluate abnormal amniotic fluid
- Evaluate placenta
- Evaluate for vaginal bleeding or fluid leakage
- Evaluate and follow up fetal anomalies
- Evaluate high-risk patients with history of previous congenital anomalies
- Provide biophysical profile analysis

4. Spine (long and transverse; exclusion of large spinal defects)
5. Stomach (exclusion of gastrointestinal obstruction); determine situs
6. Urinary bladder (exclusion of severe renal disease)
7. Fetal insertion of umbilical cord (exclusion of an anterior abdominal wall defect); cord insertion at placental site; three vessels in the cord
8. Renal regions (exclusion of severe renal malformations)
9. Anterior abdominal wall
10. Heart (four-chamber view; many laboratories have added the right ventricular and left ventricular outflow views)

The ACOG further elaborated on obstetric scanning guidelines.[1] This bulletin suggests two types of fetal ultrasound studies: basic and targeted examinations. The basic study includes all aspects of the preceding ACR and AIUM recommendations, with several additions to the anatomy survey. These include evaluation of the skull contour, falx cerebri and midline structures, frontal bone configuration, and cerebellum; a four-chamber cardiac view; and a survey of the long bones. The cavum septum pellucidi, cisterna magna, orbital distances, lungs and diaphragm, liver, bowel, and umbilical cord should also be studied. This basic study is appropriate for the majority of patients referred for fetal ultrasound.

The targeted study is reserved for the patient who requires a more in-depth investigation of fetal anatomy or condition based on a clinical history of a fetal anomaly, physiologic problem, chromosomal disorder or syndrome, or an inherited condition that may be detected by prenatal ultrasound. The targeted study is best performed by sonographers and sonologists with considerable expertise and experience in recognizing fetal anomalies and in understanding the complexities of birth defects.

In accordance with the recommended guidelines the sonographer should establish a systematic scanning protocol encompassing all criteria of the guidelines. An organized approach to scanning ensures completeness and reduces the risk of missing a birth defect.

ACKNOWLEDGMENT

The author would like to acknowledge the contribution of Kara L. Mayden Argo to this chapter in the fourth edition of this book.

REVIEW QUESTIONS

1. What is the purpose of obstetric scanning guidelines as outlined by the ACR, AIUM, and ACOG?
2. Which anatomic and biometric parameters should be included in a basic fetal study?
3. How does a targeted ultrasound study differ from a basic obstetric examination?
4. Why is it important to recognize normal fetal anatomy?
5. Why is determination of fetal presentation clinically important?
6. List at least seven reasons why ultrasound may be helpful during pregnancy.
7. Name the risk factors associated with producing a fetus with congenital anomalies.
8. If ultrasound is recommended, at what gestational age would the most information be obtained?
9. At what level should the biparietal diameter be taken?
10. At what level should the abdominal circumference be measured?
11. List the guidelines for defining the first-trimester embryo.
12. List the guidelines for defining the second- and third-trimester fetus.
13. Name the risk factors the sonographer should be aware of in an obstetric study.
14. Why is the day of the last menstrual period important for the sonographic evaluation?

REFERENCES

1. American College of Obstetrics and Gynecology: *Ultrasound in pregnancy*, Tech Bull 116, Washington, DC, May 1988, The College.
2. American College of Radiology: *ACR Standard for the performance of antepartum obstetrical ultrasound*, Richmond, Va 1995, The College.
3. American Institute of Ultrasound in Medicine: Bioeffects consideration for the safety of diagnostic ultrasound, *J Ultrasound Med*, 7(suppl):53, 1998.
4. Callen PW, editor: *Ultrasonography in obstetrics and gynecology*, ed 3, Philadelphia, 1994, WB Saunders.
5. Carstensen EL: Acoustic cavitation and the safety of diagnostic ultrasound, *Ultrasound Med Biol* 13:597, 1987.
6. Consensus Development Conference: *Diagnostic ultrasound imaging in pregnancy*, Pub No 84-667, Washington, DC, 1984, United States Department of Health and Human Services.
7. Kremkau WF: Biologic effects and possible hazards, *Clin Obstet Gynecol* 10:395, 1983.
8. Leopold GR: Obstetrical ultrasound examination guidelines, *J Ultrasound Med* 5:241, 1986 (editorial).
9. Reece EA et al: The safety of obstetric ultrasonography concern for the fetus, *Obstet Gynecol* 76:139, 1990.
10. Reece EA, Goldstein I, Hobbins JC: *Fundamentals of obstetric & gynecologic ultrasound*, Norwalk, Conn, 1994, Appleton & Lange.
11. Wells PNT: The safety of diagnostic ultrasound: report of a British Institute of Radiology Working Group, *Br J Radiolol* 20(suppl):1, 1987.

CHAPTER 26

The Normal First Trimester

Sandra L. Hagen-Ansert

amniotic cavity - cavity in which the fetus exists; forms early in gestation; fills with amniotic fluid to protect the fetus

chorionic cavity - surrounds the amniotic cavity; the yolk sac is between the chorion and amnion

crown-rump length (CRL) - most accurate measurement of the embryo in the first trimester

decidua basalis - the villi on the maternal side of the placenta or embryo; unites with the chorion to form the placenta

decidua capsularis - the villi surrounding the chorionic sac

diamniotic - multiple pregnancy with two amniotic sacs

dichorionic - multiple pregnancy with two chorionic sacs

double decidual sac sign - interface between the decidua capsularis and the echogenic, highly vascular endometrium

embryologic age (conceptual age) - date from when conception occurs

embryonic period - time between 6 and 12 weeks of gestation

human chorionic gonadotropin (hCG) - human chorionic gonadotropin; laboratory test indicates pregnancy when values are elevated.

IUP - intrauterine pregnancy

menstrual age (gestational age) - length of time calculated from the first day of the last normal menstrual period (LMP) to the point at which the pregnancy is being assessed

monoamniotic - multiple pregnancy with one amniotic sac

monochorionic - multiple pregnancy with one chorionic sac

MSD - mean sac diameter

primary yolk sac - first site of formation of red blood cells that will nourish the embryo

secondary yolk sac - formed at 23 days when the primary yolk sac is pinched off by the extra embryonic coelom.

transvaginal transducer - high-frequency transducer that is inserted into the vaginal canal to obtain better definition of first-trimester pregnancy

yolk stalk - the umbilical duct connecting the yolk sac with the embryo

zygote - fertilized ovum resulting from union of male and female gametes

Ultrasonography has become an important component in evaluating obstetric patients in the first trimester. Sonography during the first trimester offers the clinician a wealth of information that may affect clinical management or aid in diagnosis of conditions that require emergent treatment. Although the ability to image the first-trimester pregnancy with ultrasound may seem routine, the potential for false-positive and false-negative diagnoses for any given pathology is substantial. Extreme care should always be taken when sonographically evaluating the first-trimester pregnancy.

EARLY DEVELOPMENT

EMBRYONIC DEVELOPMENT

All embryonic dates in this chapter reflect menstrual age rather than embryologic age. **Menstrual age** (also known as **gestational age**) is calculated by adding 2 weeks (14 days) to **embryologic age.**[24] During a 28-day menstrual cycle, a mature ovum is released at day 14. The ovum is swept into the distal fallopian tube via fimbria; fertilization occurs within this region 1 to 2 days after ovulation. Meanwhile the follicle that released the mature ovum hemorrhages and collapses to form the corpus luteum, which begins to secrete progesterone and some estrogen (Figure 26-1).

The fertilized ovum, which should now be referred to as a **zygote,** undergoes rapid cellular division to form the 16-cell morula. Further cell proliferation brings the morula to the blastocyst stage, which contains trophoblastic cells and the "inner cell mass," which forms the embryo. The blastocyst typically enters the uterus 4 to 5 days after fertilization, with implantation occurring 7 to 9 days after ovulation. During implantation, proteolytic enzymes produced by the trophoblasts erode endometrial mucosa and maternal capillaries, resulting in a primitive blood exchange network between mother and conceptus.

When implantation is completed the trophoblast goes on to form primary villi, which initially circumvent the early gestational sac. Within the conceptus the inner cell mass matures into the bilaminar embryonic disc, the future embryo, and the primary yolk sac. At approximately 23 days menstrual age the **primary yolk sac** is pinched off by the extra embryonic coelom, forming the **secondary yolk sac.** The secondary yolk sac is the yolk sac seen sonographically throughout the first trimester. The amniotic and chorionic cavities also develop and evolve during this period of gestation.[21,22]

LABORATORY VALUES IN EARLY PREGNANCY

The laboratory values particular to pregnancy can be very useful in sonographic evaluation of the first trimester. An intimate relationship between the sonographic findings and quantitative serum **human chorionic gonadotropin (hCG)** levels normally exists during early pregnancy. Gestational sac size and hCG levels increase proportionately until 8 menstrual weeks, at which time the gestational sac is approximately 25 mm mean sac diameter **(MSD)** and an embryo should be easily detected by either transabdominal or transvaginal sonography.[5] After 8 weeks, hCG levels plateau and subsequently decline while the gestational sac continues to grow.[5]

Because the quantitative hCG levels correlate with the gestational sac size in normal pregnancies, the sonographer or clinician is able to use this objective assessment to establish if the pregnancy is normal or abnormal when the embryo is too small to be imaged with ultrasound. A normal gestational sac can be consistently demonstrated when the hCG level is 1800 mIU/ml (Second International Standard) or greater when using transabdominal sonography.[5] This detection threshold is significantly reduced by transvaginal

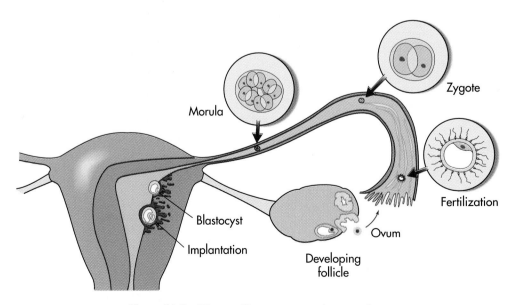

Figure 26-1 Diagram illustrates normal conception.

sonography and may be as low as 500 mIU/ml.[5] Many laboratories will use hCG levels of 1000 to 1200 mIU/mL as the number to indicate a normal pregnancy.

Abnormal pregnancies demonstrate a low hCG level relative to gestational sac development, and it has been shown that hCG levels fall before spontaneous expulsion of nonviable gestations.[5] The sonographer must be aware when the hCG level is elevated and the gestational sac is not seen within the uterus, an ectopic pregnancy should be considered.

The best method for assessment of the early gestation is to use the hCG levels along with the gestational sac measurement to determine if the pregnancy correlates with the normal levels for the particular gestational age

SONOGRAPHIC TECHNIQUE AND EVALUATION OF THE FIRST TRIMESTER

Imaging the first-trimester pregnancy with ultrasound has rapidly progressed over the past decade with the development of **transvaginal transducers,** which allow the gravid uterus and adnexa to be visualized with greater detail than transabdominal techniques by allowing higher frequencies to be used (5 to 7.5 MHz) and the placement of the transducer closer to anatomic structures. With transvaginal

transducers the pelvic anatomy is imaged in both sagittal and coronal/semicoronal planes. Such coronal imaging of the pelvis is unique within sonography, and the images should not be misconstrued as transverse sections (Figure 26-2).

Although transvaginal sonography has gained overall acceptance within the ultrasound community because of improved image quality, transabdominal and transvesical sonography should not be overlooked. The transabdominal-transvesical approach allows visualization of a larger field of anatomy, which is important when specific anatomic relationships are in question. For instance, the size, extent, and anatomic relationships of a large pelvic mass with surrounding structures can only be determined with transabdominal techniques.[2,18,23]

The following goals have been outline for sonography in the first-trimester pregnancy[2]:

- Visualization and localization of the gestational sac (intrauterine or ectopic pregnancy) (Figure 26-3)
- Identification of embryonic demise or living embryonic gestation
- Identification of embryos that are still alive but at increased risk for embryonic or fetal demise
- Determination of the number of embryos and the chorionicity and amnionicity in multifetal pregnancies

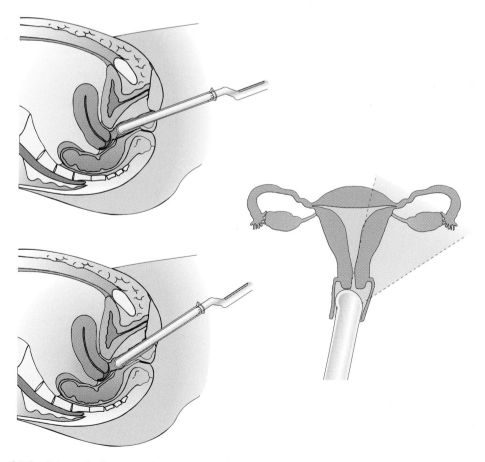

Figure 26-2 Schematic demonstrating transvaginal transducer techniques of sagittal and coronal-semicoronal anatomic planes.

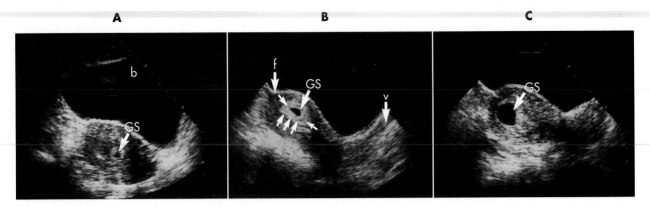

Figure 26-3 Sagittal transabdominal scans demonstrating the appearance of the gestational sac from 4 to 6 weeks gestation. **A,** A 4-week gestational sac *(GS)* noted within the fundus of the uterus. *b,* Maternal bladder. **B,** A 5-week gestational sac *(GS)* with the characteristic trophoblastic ring *(arrows).* *f,* Fundus of uterus; *v,* vagina. **C,** A 6-week gestational sac *(GS)* within the fundus of the uterus.

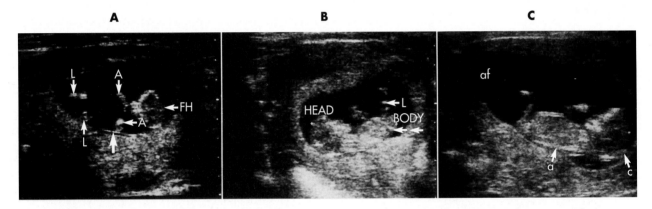

Figure. 26-4 **A,** Transverse transabdominal scan of an 11-week gestation with cross-sections through the upper and lower limbs *(L);* fetal head *(FH);* and amnion, *(A).* **B,** A fetus at 11.5 weeks of gestation. *Arrows,* Body; *L,* Leg. **C,** A fetus at 12 weeks of gestation. Note the fetal arm and leg in this profile view. *a,* Abdomen; *af,* amniotic fluid; *c,* cranium.

- Estimation of the duration or menstrual age of the pregnancy (Figure 26-4)
- Early diagnosis of fetal anomalies, including identification of embryos that are more likely to be abnormal based on secondary criteria (abnormal yolk sac)

SONOGRAPHIC VISUALIZATION OF THE EARLY GESTATION

During the 5th week of embryonic development the **intrauterine pregnancy (IUP)** can be visualized sonographically. It appears as a 1- to 2-mm sac with an echogenic ring having a sonolucent center. The anechoic center represents the chorionic cavity. The circumferential echogenic rim seen surrounding the gestational sac represents trophoblastic tissue and associated decidual reaction. The echogenic ring around the gestational sac can be divided embryologically into several components. The villi on the myometrial or burrowing side of the conceptus villi are known as the **decidua basalis.** The villi covering the rest of the developing embryo are referred to as the **decidua capsularis** (Figure 26-5). The interface between the decidua capsularis and the echogenic, highly vascularized endometrium forms the **double decidual sac sign,** which has

been reported to be a reliable sign of a viable gestation. The gestational sac is eccentrically placed in relation to the endometrial cavity, secondary to its implantation. Typically, a fundal location is noted (Figure 26-6).

The normal sonographic features of a gestational sac include a round or oval shape; a fundal position in the uterus, or an eccentrically placed position in the middle portion of the uterus; smooth contours; a decidua wall thickness greater than 3 mm; and a yolk sac with an MSD greater than 10 mm and an embryo with an MSD greater than 18 mm (see Box 26-1).[30] Once the gestational sac is sonographically imaged, rapid growth and development occur. The gestational sac size grows at a predictable rate of 1 mm per day in early pregnancy.

Often the first intragestational sac anatomy seen is the sonographic yolk sac (secondary yolk sac), which is routinely visualized between 5 and 5.5 weeks gestation. Invariably, the observer sees the yolk sac before the beating embryonic heart, which may be normal because embryonic heart motion begins between 5.3 and 5.5 weeks. The yolk sac may be used as a landmark to image the embryo, given the connection between yolk sac and embryo.

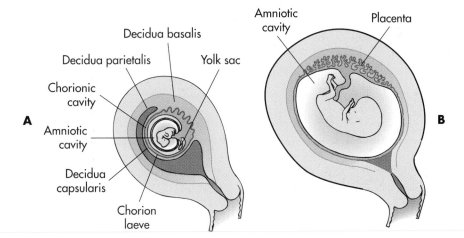

Figure. 26-5 Schema showing the relation of the fetal membranes and the wall of the uterus. **A,** End of the second month. Note the yolk sac in the chorionic cavity between the amnion and chorion. At the abembryonic pole the villi have disappeared (chorion leave). **B,** End of the third month. The amnion and chorion have fused and the uterine cavity is obliterated by fusion of the chorion leave and the decidua parietalis.

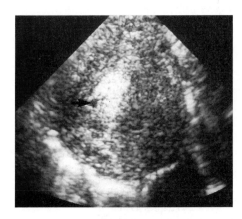

Figure 26-6 Sagittal transvaginal sonogram demonstrating a very early gestational sac, approximately 5 weeks of gestation *(arrow)*. Note the fluid center, which at this time represents chorionic cavity and the eccentric placement in relation to the very echogenic endometrial cavity.

BOX 26-1 SONOGRAPHIC FEATURES OF A NORMAL GESTATIONAL SAC

- *Shape:* Round or oval
- *Position:* Fundal or middle portion of uterus; a center position relative to endometrium (double decidua sac or intradecidua finding)
- *Contour:* Smooth
- *Wall (trophoblastic reaction):* Echogenic; 3 mm or more in thickness
- *Internal landmarks:* Yolk sac present when gestational sac is larger than 10 mm; embryo present when gestational sac is larger than 18 mm
- *Growth:* 1 mm per day (range: 0.7 mm to 1.5 mm per day)

From Nyberg DA, Hill LM: Normal early intrauterine pregnancy: sonographic development and hCG correlation. In Nyberg DA and others, editors: *Transvaginal ultrasound,* St Louis, 1992, Mosby.

At this point in gestation, rapid embryonic development increases gestational sac size, leading to better-defined intragestational sac anatomy. Between 5.5 and 6 weeks of gestation, the amniotic cavity and membrane, chorionic cavity, yolk sac, and embryo should be seen.

Yolk Sac. As stated, the yolk sac is routinely the earliest intragestational sac anatomy seen, routinely from 5 weeks of gestation. The secondary or sonographic yolk sac has essential functions in embryonic development, including: (1) provision of nutrients to the developing embryo, (2) hematopoiesis, and (3) development of embryonic endoderm, which forms the primitive gut.

Initially the yolk sac is attached to the embryo via the yolk stalk, but with amniotic cavity expansion, the yolk sac, which lies between the amniotic and chorionic cavities, detaches from the yolk stalk at approximately 8 weeks of gestation. (Figure 26-7).

Typically, the yolk sac resorbs and is no longer seen sonographically by 12 weeks. Persistent yolk sac does occur and may be visualized at the placental umbilical cord insertion where the amniotic and chorionic membranes are fused.[24]

Embryo. At the beginning of the 5th week the bilaminar embryonic disc undergoes gastrulation and is converted into the trilaminar (three-germ-layer) embryonic disc. It is at this point that organogenesis begins.

Sonographically, the early embryo is usually not identified until heart motion is detected at approximately 5.5 weeks when the **crown-rump length (CRL)** is approximately 2 mm. At this stage the embryo is seen between the secondary yolk sac and the immediate gestational sac wall. Because the amniotic cavity is still relatively small, it appears that no space lies between the yolk sac and embryo (Figure 26-8).

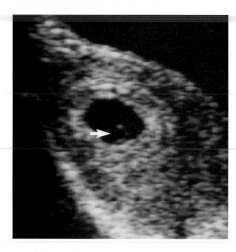

Figure 26-7 Sonogram demonstrating an approximate 6-week gestational sac with normal-appearing secondary or sonographic yolk sac *(arrow)*.

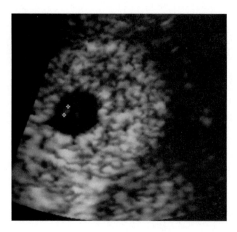

Figure 26-8 Sonogram at approximately 5.5 weeks of gestation with calipers placed on embryo with positive fetal heart motion. The crown-rump length of this trilaminar embryonic disc is approximately 2 mm. Although yolk sac was present, it is not demonstrated in this image.

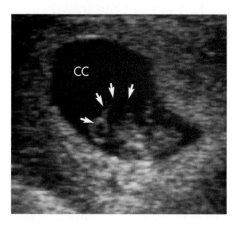

Figure 26-9 Sonogram demonstrating a 7.5-week gestation with surrounding amniotic membrane *(arrows)*. *Arrows,* Yolk sac; *CC,* chorionic cavity.

Between the 5th and 6th weeks of gestation, identification of the amniotic membrane may not be possible using transabdominal techniques. Using transvaginal transducers the amniotic membrane that separates the **amniotic** and **chorionic cavities** is routinely seen after 5.5 weeks. Although with normal gain settings the chorionic cavity (extraembryonic coelom) may appear sonolucent, increased overall gain settings may fill the fluid with low-level echoes, which correspond to a thicker consistency of the chorionic cavity in relation to the amniotic cavity. Later the amniotic cavity expands and the chorionic cavity decreases in size, with eventual chorioamniotic fusion occurring at approximately 16 to 17 weeks.[24] (Figure 26-9)

General Embryology and Sonographic Appearances: 6 to 12 Weeks. The time between 6 and 12 weeks of gestation is often considered the **embryonic period.** Although controversial, it is generally believed that the fetal period begins after 10 weeks of gestation.[24] A distinct embryologic pattern of development occurs through the embryologic and fetal periods and is outlined in Table 26-1.

At the beginning of the 6th week of gestation the trilaminar embryonic disc folds into a C-shaped embryo (Figure 26-10). While embryonic folding continues, the embryonic head, caudal portions, and lateral folds form, resulting in a constriction or narrowing between embryo and yolk sac, creating the **yolk stalk.** While embryonic folding occurs, the dorsal aspect of the yolk sac is incorporated into the embryo, developing the foregut, midgut, and hindgut, and forming the entire gastrointestinal tract, liver, biliary tract, and pancreas. At the same time, the yolk stalk, connecting stalk, and allantois are brought together by the expanding amnion, which acts as an epithelial covering, forming the umbilical cord (Figure 26-11).

The limb buds are embryologically recognizable during the 6th week of gestation, as is the embryonic tail, which is not unlike that of a tadpole (Figure 26-12). The spine is also developing during the embryonic period, particularly in the 5th through 7th weeks of gestation. The spine, which develops from ectoderm, initially evolves from the primitive neural tube, which is closed about the 6th week of gestation; sonographically parallel echogenic lines can be demonstrated at 7 to 8 weeks of gestation (Figure 26-13).[10,24]

Throughout the first trimester the sonographer or sonologist should be able to observe general differences in embryonic appearances. For example, the linear trilaminar disc seen at 5.5 weeks rapidly changes through the 7th week of gestation, when the cranial neural folds and closure of the neural pore are completed, forming a cranial vault that is recognizable sonographically (Figure 26-14).[24,37]

The skeletal system begins to develop during the 6th week, with the upper limbs forming first, followed by the lower extremities. The hands and feet develop later in the first trimester and are completed by the end of the 10th

TABLE 26-1	NORMAL EMBRYONIC DEVELOPMENT
Menstrual age	**Embryonic observations**
WEEK 5	Prominent neural folds and neural groove are recognizable.
Day 36	Heart begins to beat.
WEEK 6	Anterior and posterior neuropores close and neural tube forms.
Day 41	Upper and lower limb buds are present.
Day 42	Crown-rump length is 4.0 mm.
Day 46	Paddle-shaped hand plates are present.
	Lens pits and optic cups have formed.
Day 48	Cerebral vesicles are distinct.
Day 50	Oral and nasal cavities are confluent.
Day 52	Upper lip is formed.
Day 54	Digital rays are distinct.
Day 56	Crown-rump length is 16.0 mm.
WEEK 9	Cardiac ventricular septum is closed.
	Truncus arteriosus divides into aorta and pulmonary trunk.
	Kidney collecting tubules develop.
Day 58	Eyelids develop.
Day 64	Upper limbs bend at elbows.
	Fingers are distinct.
WEEK 10	Glomeruli form in metanephros
Day 73	Genitalia show some female characteristics but are still easily confused with male.
Day 80	Face has human appearance.
Day 82	Genitalia have male and female characteristics but are still not fully formed.
Day 84	Crown-rump length is 55 mm.
MONTH 7	Ossification is complete throughout vertebral column.
MONTH 8	Ossification centers appear in distal femoral epiphysis.

From Neiman HL: Sonoembryology. In Nyberg DA and others, editors: *Transvaginal ultrasound,* St Louis, 1990, Mosby.

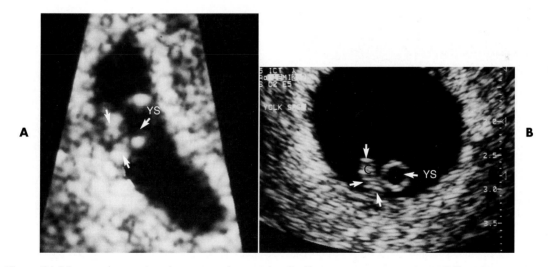

Figure 26-10   A, A 5.5-week embryo. Note the straight, disclike appearance *(arrows); YS,* Yolk sac. **B,** A 6.2-week gestation is seen at the beginning stages of embryonic "curling." *C,* Embryonic cranium; *YS,* Yolk sac.

week of gestation. Sonographically, limb buds can be detected, generally from the 7th week on; the fingers and toes are recognizable at 11 weeks using transvaginal sonography.[10,26]

The embryonic face undergoes significant evolution starting in the 5th week of gestation, with palate fusion beginning around the 12th week of gestation.[37] Sonographically, the embryonic face cannot presently be seen with diagnostic detail. By the 9th week, the maxilla and mandible

are noted as brightly echogenic structures; further bony palate development is often visualized from the 10th week (Figure 26-15).[27]

Physiologic Herniation of Bowel. The anterior abdominal wall is developed by 6 weeks of gestation from the fusion of four ectomesodermal body folds. Simultaneously, the primitive gut is formed as a result of the incorporation of the dorsal yolk sac into the embryo. The

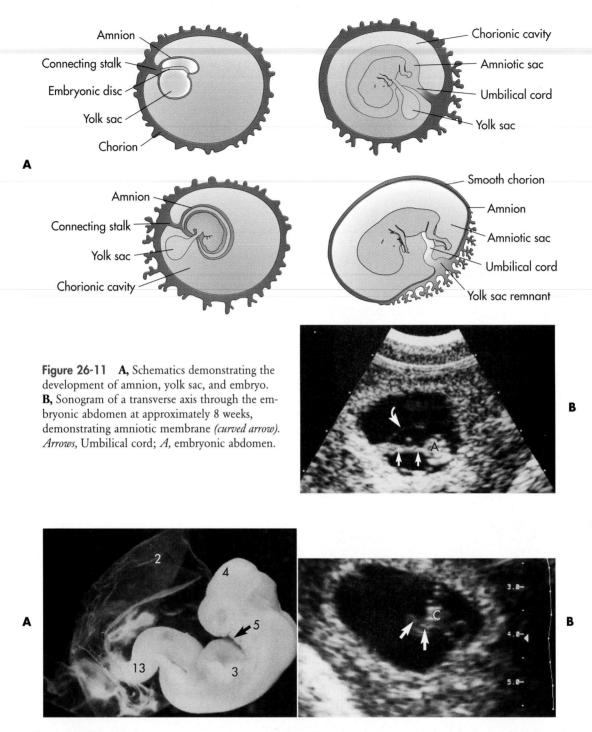

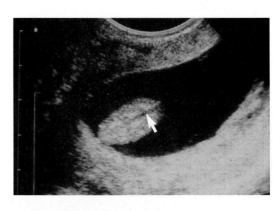

Figure 26-11 **A,** Schematics demonstrating the development of amnion, yolk sac, and embryo. **B,** Sonogram of a transverse axis through the embryonic abdomen at approximately 8 weeks, demonstrating amniotic membrane *(curved arrow). Arrows,* Umbilical cord; *A,* embryonic abdomen.

Figure 26-12 **A,** Embryo at approximately 6 weeks of gestation, demonstrating early limb buds *(3)* and embryonic tail *(13). 2,* Amnion; *4,* cranium; *5,* heart. (From England MA: *Color atlas of life before birth,* St Louis, 1983, Mosby.) **B,** Corresponding sonogram of a 6-week gestation, demonstrating embryonic tail *(arrows). C,* Embryonic cranium.

Figure 26-13 Sonogram of an 8-week embryo demonstrating parallel echogenic lines with the sonolucent center representing spine *(arrow).*

midgut, derived from the primitive gut, develops and forms the majority of the small bowel, cecum, ascending colon, and proximal transverse colon. Because the midgut is in direct communication with the yolk sac, amniotic cavity expansion pulls the yolk sac away from the embryo forming the yolk stalk.

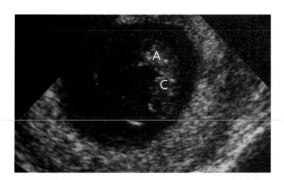

Figure 26-14   Sonogram demonstrating a 7- to 7.5-week gestation. Note morphologic distinction between embryonic cranium *(C)* and embryonic abdomen *(A)*.

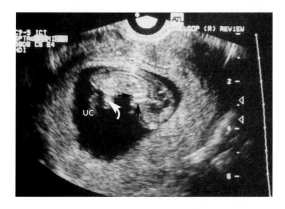

Figure 26-15   Sonogram of a 10-week embryo, demonstrating echogenic structures representing maxilla and mandible *(arrow)*. Also note limb bud *(curved arrows)*. *UC,* Umbilical cord.

While amniotic expansion occurs, the midgut elongates faster than the embryo is growing, causing the midgut to herniate into the base of the umbilical cord. Until approximately 10 weeks of gestation, the midgut loop continues to grow and rotate before it descends into the fetal abdomen at about the 11th week.

Sonographically, this transition of bowel within the base of the umbilical cord can readily be visualized.[8] The small bowel appears as an echogenic mass within the base of the umbilical cord; little echogenic bowel is seen within the embryonic or fetal abdomen. After 12 weeks of gestation, the echogenic umbilical cord mass is no longer visualized and echogenic bowel is seen within the fetal abdomen.[40] Recent data suggest that normally the echogenic umbilical cord mass should not exceed 7 mm at any gestational age and never measure less than 4 mm.[3] It is important that this normal embryologic event not be confused with pathologic processes such as omphalocele or gastroschisis (Figure 26-16).

Embryonic Cranium. Although the embryonic cranium undergoes dramatic changes from the 6th to 11th week of gestation, specific anatomy can be sonographically visualized. Around the 6th week of gestation, three primary brain vesicles develop: the prosencephalon, the mesencephalon, and the rhombencephalon (Figure 26-17). Because of rapid cell proliferation in relation to cranial vault space, flexures of the developing brain occur.

The rhombencephalon divides into two segments: the cephalic portion or metencephalon and the caudal component or myelencephalon. Once the rhombencephalon divides with its corresponding flexure, the cystic rhomboid fossa forms. The cystic rhomboid fossa can sonographically be imaged routinely from the 8th to 11th week of gestation (Figure 26-18). With increasing gestational age, further evolution of the cerebellum, medulla, and medulla oblongata encloses the rhomboid fossa to

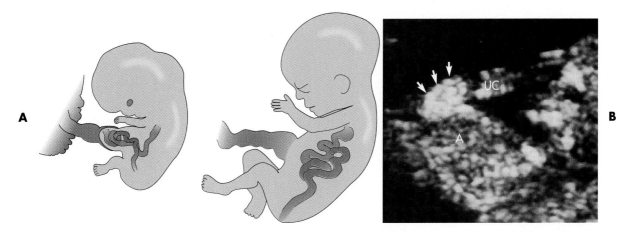

Figure 26-16   **A,** Schematic demonstrating normal gut migration. The bowel normally migrates into the base of the umbilical cord between 8 and 12 menstrual weeks (6 to 10 embryonic weeks). The bowel returns to the abdominal cavity by 12 menstrual weeks. **B,** Sonogram of a 9-week gestation demonstrating echogenic "mass" at the base of the umbilical cord *(arrows)*. Note that there is no echogenic material within embryonic abdomen. *A,* Embryonic abdomen; *UC,* umbilical cord.

form the primitive fourth ventricle and part of the cerebral aqueduct of Sylvius.[7,19] This cystic structure, seen within the posterior aspect of the embryonic cranium, should not be confused with pathology, such as Dandy-Walker deformity.

The cerebral hemispheres may be seen at around 9 weeks gestation. The echogenic choroid plexus, which fills the lateral cerebral ventricles, can be visualized. Sonolucent cerebral spinal fluid can be demarcated around the choroid plexus. It is important to note that the lateral ventricles completely fill the cerebral vault at this time in gestation. The cerebral hemispheres are relatively small compared with the rest of the brain, although this relationship rapidly changes at the beginning of the second trimester. The cerebral falx and midline may also be seen in axial views of the embryonic brain (Figure 26-19). [6,26]

Embryonic Heart. The heart is the first organ to function within the embryo. The embryonic heart starts beating at approximately 35 days (5.3 to 5.5 weeks) when the endocardial heart tubes fuse to form a single heart tube. Complex embryonic evolution occurs so that by the end of the 8th week of gestation, the heart has obtained its adult configuration.[24,37]

Embryonic cardiac activity should always be seen by 46 menstrual days.[33,38] Embryonic cardiac rates vary with gestational age. Rates of 90 beats per minute at 6 weeks increase to rates of 170 beats per minute at 9 weeks, with rates of approximately 140 beats per minute through the remainder of the first and second trimesters (Figure 26-20). [38,39]

Although with present technology, detailed morphologic anatomy of the first-trimester heart cannot be seen,

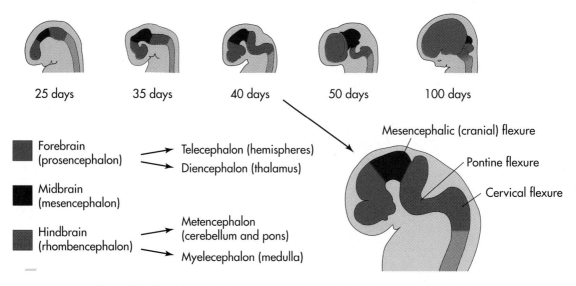

Figure 26-17 Schematic demonstrating embryonic development of the brain.

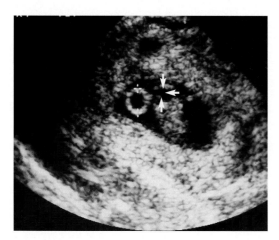

Figure 26-18 Sonogram of an 8.5-week gestation demonstrating the cystic rhombencephalon within the fetal cranium *(arrows)*. Note yolk sac between calipers.

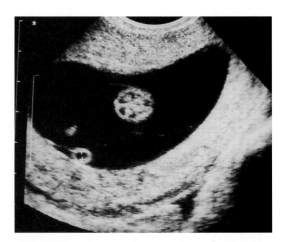

Figure 26-19 Sonogram demonstrating an axial plane of a 10-week embryo demonstrating cerebral falx and choroid plexus. Note the lateral ventricles and choroid plexus occupy the entire cranial vault at this gestation.

further development of high-frequency transducers and ultrasound technology may allow more anatomy to be described in the future.

DETERMINATION OF GESTATIONAL AGE

It is widely accepted that the most accurate gestational dating during pregnancy is the use of ultrasound within the first trimester.[13,36] Two parameters for sonographic gestational dating may be used: (1) CRL and (2) gestational sac size.

CROWN-RUMP LENGTH

Determination of first-trimester gestational dates by direct measurement of the embryo using the CRL was first reported in 1975.[36] This produced gestational dating standard deviations of plus or minus 5 to 7 days, by far the most accurate dating parameters within obstetric biometry. Another study[13] recently reevaluated CRL data using modern equipment and determined gestational age standard deviation to be plus or minus 8% throughout the first

trimester, essentially unchanged from the original data[36] (Figure 26-21).

CRL measurements can be obtained as early as 5.5 weeks using transvaginal sonography. The main sonographic observation of implementing direct embryonic measurement is the visualization of embryonic heart motion, which is crucial because CRL measurement at this gestational age would be less than 1 mm.

CRLs should be used until approximately 12 weeks of gestation, when the fetus begins to "curl" into the fetal position, making measurement of length more difficult (Figure 26-22).

GESTATIONAL SAC SIZE

Several studies have shown that mean gestational sac size correlates closely with menstrual age during early pregnancy (Figure 26-23). As a rule, the gestational sac size remains accurate through the first 8 weeks of gestation.[30,35] Sonographically the gestational sac size or mean sac diameter is determined by the average sum of the length, width, and height of the gestational sac. These measurements are ob-

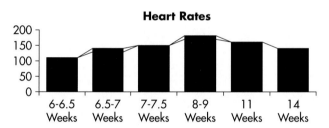

Figure 26-20   Graph demonstration embryonic heart rates in relation to gestational weeks. (From Cyr DR: *Embryosonography,* paper presented at 37th annual convention of the American Institute of Ultrasound in Medicine, Honolulu, Hawaii, 1993.)

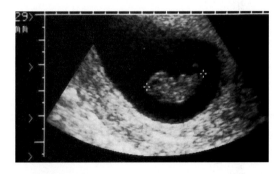

Figure 26-22   Sonogram demonstrating crown-rump length measurement on an 8-week embryo.

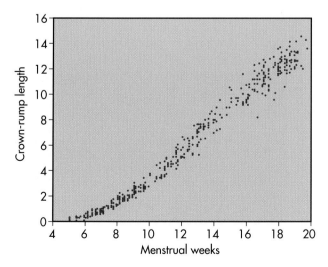

Figure 26-21   Graph demonstrating crown-rump length versus menstrual age. (From Nyberg DA and others: *J Ultrasound Med* 6:23, 1987.)

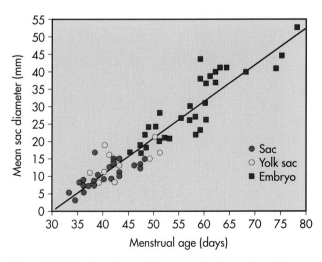

Figure 26-23   Graph correlating growth of sac size, yolk sac size, and embryo length in relation to mean sac diameter and menstrual days. (Redrawn from Hadlock FP, Shah YP, Lindsey JV: *Radiology* 182:501, 1992.)

tained in both sagittal and coronal/semicoronal sonographic planes. When measuring the mean sac diameter, the sonographer should only measure gestational sac fluid space, not including the echogenic decidua (Figure 26-24).[30]

To calculate mean sac diameter (MSD), the following formula should be used[30]:

Length (mm) + Width (mm) + Height (mm)/3 = MSD

MSD (mm) + 30 = Menstrual age (days)

Menstrual age (days) divided by 7 = Menstrual age (weeks)

It is important to note that precise standard deviations for gestational sac size have not been determined, although linear regression analysis demonstrates excellent correlation of mean sac diameter and menstrual age.[30]

YOLK SAC SIZE

Visualization of the yolk sac predicts a viable pregnancy in over 90% of cases.[31] Conversely, failure to visualize the yolk sac, with a minimum of 8 mm MSD, using transvaginal sonography, should provoke suspicion of abnormal pregnancy. Transabdominal studies have shown that the yolk sac should be seen within mean sac diameters of 10 to 15 mm and should always be visualized with a mean sac diameter of 20 mm.[22]

The growth rate of the yolk sac has been reported to be approximately 0.1 mm per millimeter of growth of the MSD when the MSD is less than 15 mm, and 0.03 mm per mm of growth of the MSD through the first trimester.[22] The normal diameter of the yolk sac should never exceed 5.6 mm. Enlarged yolk sacs have ominous outcomes (Figure 26-25).

MULTIPLE GESTATIONS

The sonographic diagnosis of multiple gestations within the first trimester is valuable information for the obstetrician. A multiple-gestation pregnancy is, by definition, high risk, with significant increases in morbidity and mortality rates in relation to singleton pregnancies. Overall, twin gestations have a 7 to 10 times greater mortality rate than singletons.[20]

Using transvaginal sonography, multiple gestations can readily be diagnosed at very early stages, between 5.5 and 6.5 weeks. Sonographic identification of multiple gestational sacs with incorporated yolk sacs, amniotic membranes, and, ideally, embryos with cardiac motion allows definitive diagnosis. The literature contains data concerning the identification of chorionicity and amnionicity in twin pregnancies.

Fortunately, dizygotic (two ova) twin pregnancies, which comprise 70% of all twins, are by definition **dichorionic** and **diamniotic.**[25]

Ultrasound findings. Sonographically, dichorionic and diamniotic twins appear as two separate gestational sacs with individual trophoblastic tissue, which allows the appearance of a thick dividing membrane. As pregnancy pro-

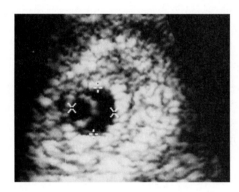

Figure 26-24 Sagittal sonogram of an approximate 6-week gestational sac demonstrating caliper placement for appropriate mean sac diameter measurement. Coronal images would also be taken for a third dimension.

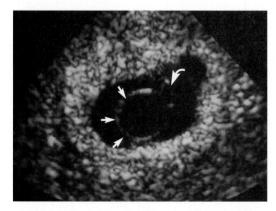

Figure 26-25 Sonogram demonstrating an enlarged yolk sac, measuring approximately 9-mm *(arrows).* Also note enlarged or hydropic amniotic sac *(curved arrow).* Although embryonic heart motion was initially detected follow-up studies diagnosed embryonic demise at 8.5 weeks gestation.

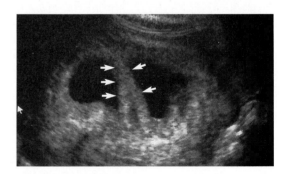

Figure 26-26 Sonogram demonstrating a diamniotic-dichorionic pregnancy. Note the thick membrane separating the two gestational sacs *(arrows).*

gresses, this membrane becomes thinner secondary to the diminished space between the two sacs, so this diagnosis may be more difficult later in gestation. In a dichorionic-diamniotic pregnancy, each sac has an individual yolk sac, amniotic membrane, and embryo (Figure 26-26).

Monochorionic-diamniotic twins appear to be contained within one chorionic sac; two amnions, two yolk sacs, and two embryos are identified (Figure 26-27). The most crucial diagnosis for the sonographic observer to make is that of the monozygotic, **monoamniotic-monochorionic** twin gestation. This type of twinning has a mortality rate of approximately 50%. Sonographically, one would identify one gestational sac with one amniotic membrane, which may contain one or two yolk sacs and two embryos within the single amniotic membrane (Figure 26-28). [5,41]

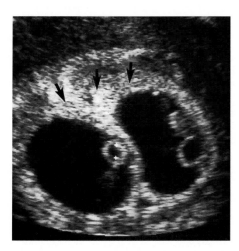

Figure 26-27 Sonogram demonstrating early monochorionic-diamniotic pregnancy. Note two yolk sacs and two embryos with single chorion-placenta (arrows).

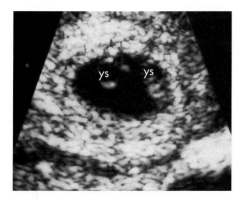

Figure 26-28 Sonogram demonstrating monoamniotic-monochorionic pregnancy. Note two yolk sacs (ys) with no separating amniotic membrane.

ACKNOWLEDGMENT

The author acknowledges the previous work from the fourth edition of this book of Dale R. Cyr, Hahn Vu Nghiem, and Laurence A. Mack.

REVIEW QUESTIONS

1. What is the difference between menstrual age and embryologic age?
2. Describe fertilization from the point at which the ovum is swept into the tube to the development of the yolk sac.
3. Describe the relationship between the sonographic findings and quantitative serum hCG levels in early pregnancy.
4. What level does the hCG need to be to demonstrate a normal gestational sac?
5. Descibe the sonographic appearance of an early intrauterine pregnancy.
6. Name the embryologic components of the echogenic ring around the gestational sac.
7. At what gestational age is the yolk sac routinely visualized?
8. What is the purpose of the secondary yolk sac?
9. At what gestational age is the embryo identifiable on ultrasound?
10. When is the amniotic and chorionic cavities routinely imaged with transvaginal ultrasound?
11. When does the fetal skeletal system begin to develop?
12. Describe what happens to the bowel migration in the first trimester.
13. Name the three primary brain vesicles that develop after the sixth week of gestation.
14. Describe the development of the rhombencephalon in the first trimester.
15. Describe the development of the choroid plexus and cerebral ventricles in the later part of the first trimester.
16. What is the first organ to function in the embryo?
17. Describe the normal early cardiac activity.
18. Name the two parameters for sonographic gestational dating in the first trimester.
19. How is the mean sac diameter determined?
20. How closely does visualizaion of the yolk sac predict a viable pregnancy?
21. What is the morbidity and mortality rate of a multiple pregnancy in relation to a singleton pregnancy?
22. What is the sonographic appearance of a dichorionic and diamniotic pregnancy in the first trimester?

REFERENCES

1. Bateman BG and others: Vaginal sonography findings and HCG dynamics of early intrauterine and tubal pregnancies, *Obstet Gynecol* 75:421, 1990.

2. Bohm-Velez M, Mendelson EB: Transvaginal sonography: applications, equipment and technique. In Nyberg DA and others, editors: *Transvaginal ultrasound,* St Louis, 1992, Mosby.

3. Bowerman RA: Sonography of fetal midgut herniation: normal size criteria and correlation with crown-rump length, *J Ultrasound Med* 5:251, 1993.

4. Bromley B and others: Small sac size in the first trimester: a predictor of poor fetal outcome, *Radiology* 178:375, 1991.

5. Callen P: *Ultrasonography in obstetrics and gynecology,* Philadelphia, 1994, WB Saunders.

6. Cullen MT: Comparison of transvaginal and abdominal ultrasound, *J Ultrasound Med* 8:565, 1990.

7. Cyr DR and others: Bowel migration in the normal fetus: US detection, *Radiology* 1986:161, 1986.

8. Cyr DR and others: Fetal rhombencephalon: normal ultrasound findings, *Radiology* 166:691, 1988.

9. Dubose TJ, Cunyus JA, Johnson LF: Embryonic heart rate and age, *J Diag Med Sonogr* 6:151, 1990.

10. Ectopic pregnancy–United States, 1987, *Morb Mortal Wkly Rep* 103:401, 1990.

11. Frates MC, Benson CB, Doubilet PM: Pregnancy outcome after first trimester sonogram demonstrating fetal cardiac activity, *J Ultrasound Med* 12:383, 1993.

12. Gamberdella FR, Marrs RP: Heterotopic pregnancy associated with assisted reproductive technology, *Am J Obstet Gynecol* 160:1520, 1989.

13. Hadlock FP and others: Fetal crown-rump length: reevaluation of relation to menstrual age (5-18 weeks) with high resolution real time US, *Radiology* 182:501, 1992.

14. Hertzberg BS and others: Normal sonographic appearance of the fetal neck late in the first trimester: the pseudomembrane, *Radiology* 171:427, 1989.

15. Hertzberg BS, Mahony BS, Bowie JD: First trimester fetal cardiac activity: sonographic documentation of a progressive early rise in heart rate, *J Ultrasound Med* 7:573, 1988.

16. Kurjak A, Zalud I: Doppler and color flow imaging. In Nyberg DA and others, editors: *Transvaginal ultrasound,* St Louis, 1992, Mosby.

17. Laboda LA, Estroff JA, Benaceraff BR: First trimester bradycardia: a sign of impending fetal loss, *J Ultrasound Med* 8:561, 1989.

18. Leibman AJ, Kruse B, McSweeney MB: Transvaginal sonography: comparison with transabdominal sonography in the diagnosis of pelvic masses, *Am J Roentgenol* 151:89, 1988.

19. Lemire RJ and others: *Normal and abnormal development of the human nervous system,* Hagerstown, Md, 1975, Harper & Row.

20. Levi CS: Sonographic evaluation of multiple gestation pregnancy. In Fleischer AC, editor: *Principles and practices of ultrasonography,* East Norwalk, Conn, 1991, Appleton & Lange.

21. Levi CS, Lyons EA, Dashefsky SM: The first trimester. In Rumack CM, Wilson SR and Charboneau JW, editors: *Diagnostic ultrasound,* St Louis, 1992, Mosby.

22. Lindsay DJ and others: Yolk sac diameter and shape at endovaginal ultrasound: predictors of pregnancy outcome in the first trimester, *Radiology* 183:115, 1992.

23. Mendelson EB and others: Gynecologic imaging: comparison of transabdominal and transvaginal sonography, *Radiology* 166:321, 1988.

24. Moore KL: *The developing human: clinically oriented embryology,* ed 4, Philadelphia, 1988, WB Saunders.

25. Moore KL: The placenta and fetal membranes. In Moore KL, editor: *The developing human: clinically oriented embryology,* Philadelphia, 1988, WB Saunders.

26. Neiman HL: Transvaginal ultrasound embryology, *Semin Ultrasound CT MR* 11:22, 1990.

27. Neiman HL: Sonoembryology. In Nyberg DA and others, editors: *Transvaginal ultrasound,* Philadelphia, 1992, Mosby.

28. Nyberg DA, Hill LM: Normal early intrauterine pregnancy: sonographic development and hCG correlation. In Nyberg DA and others, editors: *Transvaginal ultrasound,* St Louis, 1992, Mosby.

29. Nyberg DA, Laing FC, Filly RA: Threatened abortion: sonographic distinction of normal and abnormal gestation sacs, *Radiology* 158:397, 1986.

30. Nyberg DA and others: Early gestation: correlation of HCG levels and sonographic identification, *Am J Roentgenol* 144:951, 1985.

31. Nyberg DA and others: Value of the yolk sac in evaluating early pregnancies, *J Ultrasound Med* 7:129, 1988.

32. Peisner DB, Timor-Tritsch IE: The discriminatory zone of beta-hCG for vaginal probes, *J Clin Ultrasound* 18:280, 1990.

33. Rempen A: Diagnosis of viability in early pregnancy with vaginal sonography, *J Ultrasound Med* 9:711, 1990.

34. Rizk B and others: Heterotopic pregnancies after in vitro fertilization and embryo transfer, *Am J Obstet Gynecol* 164:161, 1991.

35. Robinson HP: "Gestational sac" volumes as a journal by sonar in the first trimester of pregnancy, *Br J Obstet Gynecol* 82:100, 1975.

36. Robinson HP: The diagnosis of early pregnancy failure by sonar, *Br J Obstet Gynecol* 82:849, 1975.

37. Sadler TW: *Langman's medical embryology,* ed 5, Baltimore, 1985, Williams & Wilkins.

38. Schats R and others: Embryonic heart activity: appearance and development in early human pregnancy, *Br J Obstet Gynecol* 97:989, 1990.

39. Shenker L and others: Embryonic heart rates before the seventh week of pregnancy, *J Reprod Med* 31:333, 1986.

40. Timor-Tritsch IE, Farine D, Rosen MG: A close look at early embryonic development with high-frequency transvaginal transducer, *Am J Obstet Gynecol* 159:676, 1988.

41. Townsend R: Membrane thickness in ultrasound prediction of chorionicity of twins, *J Ultrasound Med* 7:327, 1988.

Sonography of the Abnormal First-Trimester Pregnancy

Sandra L. Hagen-Ansert

OBJECTIVES

- Describe the cranial abnormalities seen in the first trimester
- Distinguish among normal bowel herniation, gastroschisis, and omphalocele
- Discuss the sonographic findings with cystic hygroma
- Name the types of umbilical cord masses that may be seen with ultrasound
- Differentiate between a hemorrhagic corpus luteum cyst and a dermoid
- Discuss the difference between a fibroid and uterine contraction on sonography
- Describe the clinical and sonographic findings in ectopic pregnancy
- List the other types of abnormal pregnancies
- Discuss the normal range for fetal cardiac rhythm
- Distinguish between an incomplete abortion and blighted ovum
- Describe the sonographic findings in molar pregnancy

DIAGNOSIS OF EMBRYONIC ABNORMALITIES IN THE FIRST TRIMESTER

CRANIAL ANOMALIES
ABDOMINAL WALL DEFECTS
CYSTIC HYGROMA
FIRST-TRIMESTER UMBILICAL CORD CYSTS
PLACENTAL HEMATOMAS

FIRST-TRIMESTER PELVIC MASSES

OVARIAN
UTERINE

ECTOPIC PREGNANCY

SONOGRAPHIC FINDINGS IN ECTOPIC PREGNANCY
ADNEXAL MASS WITH ECTOPIC PREGNANCY

HETEROTOPIC PREGNANCY
INTERSTITIAL PREGNANCY
CERVICAL PREGNANCY
OVARIAN PREGNANCY

ABNORMAL PREGNANCY: ULTRASOUND FINDINGS

EMBRYONIC BRADYCARDIA
EMBRYONIC OLIGOHYDRAMNIOS AND GROWTH RESTRICTION
COMPLETE ABORTION
INCOMPLETE ABORTION
ANEMBRYONIC PREGNANCY (BLIGHTED OVUM)
GESTATIONAL TROPHOBLASTIC DISEASE IN THE FIRST TRIMESTER

REVIEW QUESTIONS

KEY TERMS

anembryonic pregnancy (blighted ovum) - ovum without an embryo

bowel herniation - during the first trimester the bowel normally herniates outside the abdominal cavity between 8 and 12 weeks

complete abortion - complete removal of all products of conception, including the placenta

corpus luteum cyst - may persist until the 20th to 24th week of pregnancy

cystic hygroma - fluid-filled structure (often with septations), initially surrounding the neck, may extend upward to the head or laterally to the body

ectopic pregnancy - pregnancy outside the uterus

gastroschisis - congenital fissure that remains open in the wall of the abdomen just to the right of the umbilical cord; bowel and other organs may protrude outside the abdomen from this opening

gestational trophoblastic disease - condition in which trophoblastic tissue overtakes the pregnancy and propagates throughout the uterine cavity

heterotopic pregnancy - simultaneous intrauterine and extrauterine pregnancy

incomplete abortion - retained products of conception

interstitial pregnancy - pregnancy occurring in the cornu of the uterus

omphalocele - congenital hernia of the umbilicus that is covered with a membrane; the cord may be seen in the middle of the mass

pseudogestational sac - decidual reaction that occurs within the uterus in a patient with an ectopic pregnancy

Turner's syndrome - congenital endocrine disorder caused by failure of the ovaries to respond to pituitary hormone stimulation; cystic hygroma often seen

DIAGNOSIS OF EMBRYONIC ABNORMALITIES IN THE FIRST TRIMESTER

Normal embryologic processes that are sonographically visible in the first-trimester embryo have been described. These normal processes should not be mistaken for anomalies, and the sonographer should be aware of the pathology that can be diagnosed in the first trimester.

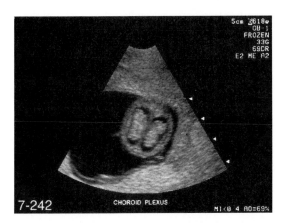

Figure 27-1 Transvaginal axial scan of the choroid plexus in a first-trimester fetus.

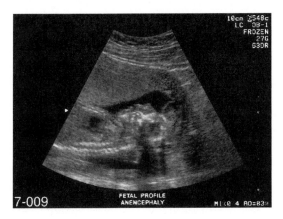

Figure 27-2 Fetal profile of an anencephalic fetus in the second trimester. The fetus is lying in a vertex position with the spine down. The face is pointing toward the anterior placenta; the skull is absent from the fetal forehead to the top of the cranium.

CRANIAL ANOMALIES

Although the embryonic head can be sonographically identified by 7 weeks, the cerebral hemisphere continues to evolve through the second trimester. The dominant structure seen within the embryonic cranium within the first trimester is that of the choroid plexus, which fills the lateral ventricles that in turn fill the cranial vault (Figure 27-1). Thus the diagnosis of hydrocephalus in the first trimester is impossible. However, anomalies of cranial organization, such as holoprosencephaly, have been described in the first trimester.[53] The previously described rhombencephalon-hindbrain is a cystic structure within the posterior aspect of the embryonic cranium that should not be confused with abnormality.[18] A diagnosis of hydranencephaly, which is brain necrosis from occlusion of the internal carotid arteries, has been reported during the first trimester, which sonographically demonstrated loss of all intracranial anatomy.[51] In the first trimester, anencephaly should be diagnosed with caution. Reports have shown normal amounts of brain matter seen in the first trimester embryo with anencephaly, unlike classic sonographic appearances in the second and third trimesters (Figure 27-2). Ossification of the cranial vault is not complete in the first trimester; the resulting false cranial border definition may give rise to a false-negative diagnosis.[6,30]

Extreme caution is advised if an embryonic cranial abnormality is suspected. Because traditional cranial anatomy can be visualized after 12 to 14 weeks of gestation, repeat the sonogram at this time to either confirm or rule out abnormality.

ABDOMINAL WALL DEFECTS

Although the diagnosis of omphalocele, gastroschisis, and limb-body-wall complex has been reported in the first trimester, such diagnoses should be made with care.[16,33,39,45,85]

Abdominal wall defects must be distinguished from normal physiologic midgut herniation.[17] As stated previously, normal **bowel herniation** sonographically appears as an echogenic mass at the base of the umbilical cord between 8 and 12 weeks. Because liver is never herniated into the base of the umbilical cord, normally, any evidence of liver outside the anterior abdominal wall should be considered abnormal (Figure 27-3). Although the diagnosis of **gastroschisis** in the first trimester may be more difficult, reports have shown bowel to be separate and eviscerated from the umbilical cord and its attachment to the fetus.[33] The bowel-only **omphaloceles** that have been reported to be highly associated with chromosomal abnormalities cannot be differentiated from normal physiologic bowel migration and should be diagnosed after 12 to 14 weeks.[32,59]

CYSTIC HYGROMA

Cystic hygroma is one of the most common abnormalities seen sonographically in the first trimester (Figure 27-4).[6,12,15] Cystic hygromas, especially those seen in the first trimester, are highly associated with chromosomal

abnormalities.[40,47,48] Several authors recently reported that in fetuses detected with cystic hygroma in the second and third trimesters, **Turner's syndrome** is the most common karyotype abnormality.[40,47,48] In fetuses with cystic hygroma in the first trimester, however, trisomies 21, 18, and 13 were most prevalent. If the hygroma resolves by 18 weeks, most fetuses were chromosomally normal, whereas all persistent hygromas were karyotypically abnormal. If cystic hygroma or nuchal thickening is seen in the first trimester, genetic counseling and further sonographic monitoring are required.[40]

Cystic hygroma visualized in the first trimester may vary in size, but all appear on the posterior aspect of the fetal neck and upper thorax. Soft-tissue thickening may also be present and should be considered as nuchal thickening. Although cystic hygroma and nuchal thickening may be concordant, differentiation may be difficult. A potential diagnostic pitfall for the sonographer is misinterpreting the hypoechoic or sonolucent embryonic skin surface in the region of the posterior neck. This has been described as the pseudomembrane sign and should not be confused with cystic hygroma, encephalocele, cervical meningomyelocele, teratoma, or hemangioma.[34] Caution should also be observed in differentiating the pseudomembrane from the normal amniotic membrane on which the embryo is lying (Figure 27-5).[34]

FIRST-TRIMESTER UMBILICAL CORD CYSTS

Sonographic identification of first-trimester umbilical cord cysts has been reported.[68] One study found a 0.4% incidence of umbilical cord cysts between 8 and 12 weeks of gestation.[75] Cyst size varied with a range of 2.0 to 7.5 mm, and embryos whose cysts resolved by the second trimester progressed to normal delivery. Differential diagnostic considerations of umbilical cord cysts include: (1) amniotic inclusion cysts, (2) omphalomesenteric duct cysts, (3) allantoic cysts, (4) vascular anomalies, (5) neoplasms, and (6) Wharton's jelly abnormalities. Umbilical cord cysts that persist through the second trimester or are associated with other abnormalities warrant further investigation and genetic evaluation (Figure 27-6).[24,38]

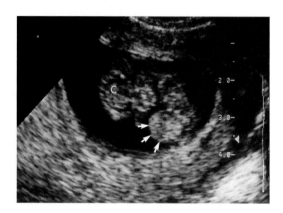

Figure 27-3 Sonogram of a 9-week gestation demonstrating herniated liver contents into the base of the umbilical cord *(arrows)*, consistent with first trimester omphalocele. This was confirmed at 14 weeks' gestation. *C,* Embryonic cranium.

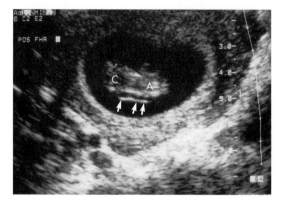

Figure 27-5 A 9-week embryo demonstrating the "hammocking" effect of the embryo lying on top of amniotic membrane *(arrows)*. This may give a false impression of cystic hygroma/nuchal thickening. *A,* Embryonic abdomen *C,* embryonic cranium.

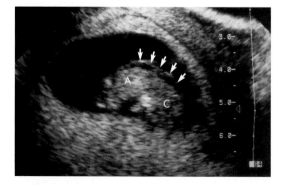

Figure 27-4 A 9-week embryo demonstrating sonolucent cystic hygroma with nuchal thickening *(arrows)*. Genetic analysis demonstrated trisomy 18. *A,* Embryonic abdomen; *C,* embryonic cranium.

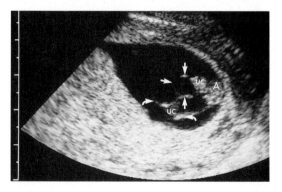

Figure 27-6 An 8.5-week gestation demonstrating umbilical cord cyst *(arrows)*. This cyst resolved by 14 weeks' gestation and went on to normal delivery. *A,* Embryonic abdomen; *UC,* umbilical cord; *curved arrows,* amniotic membrane.

PLACENTAL HEMATOMAS

The embryonic placenta, or frondosum, may become detached, resulting in the formation of a hematoma, which typically causes vaginal bleeding (Figure 27-7). Most of these hemorrhages are contiguous with a placental edge, which is consistent with the second- or third-trimester placental marginal abruption.[58] Although no risk factors have been associated with first-trimester placental separation, it has been reported to have a 50% or greater fetal loss rate.[54] Although the prognosis seems to depend on hematoma size, no specific volumes have been correlated in the first trimester with fetal outcomes. Improved outcomes do seem to be consistent with smaller hematomas (Figure 27-8).[54]

FIRST-TRIMESTER PELVIC MASSES

OVARIAN

The **corpus luteum cyst** is by far the most common ovarian mass seen in the first trimester of pregnancy. The cor-

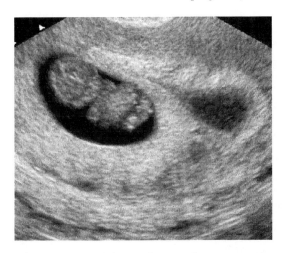

Figure 27-7 Transvaginal scan of a 10-week pregnancy; the gestational sac and embryo are clearly visible. The placenta is anterior; the prominent hypoechoic area visible between the gestational sac and the placenta represents a subchorionic hemorrhage.

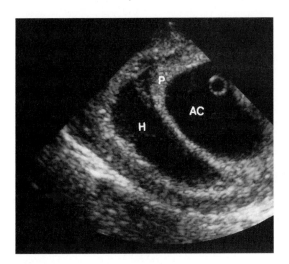

Figure 27-8 An 8-week gestation demonstrating subchorionic hematoma *(H)*. This embryo went on to normal delivery. *AC,* Amniotic cavity; *P,* edge of placenta.

pus luteum cyst is necessary to preserve the embryo because it secretes progesterone. The corpus luteum cyst typically measures less than 5 cm in diameter and does not contain septations.[25] Occasionally, corpus luteum cysts are large, reaching sizes of more than 10 cm, with internal septations and echogenic debris, which are thought to be secondary to internal hemorrhage (Figure 27-9).[25,64] Because of high metabolic activity, color-flow imaging may demonstrate a ring of increased vascularity surrounding the corpus luteum, giving low-resistance (high-diastolic) waveforms on pulsed Doppler imaging. Such findings are similar to decidual flows characterized in ectopic pregnancies but are intraovarian in location.

A hemorrhagic corpus luteum cyst cannot be differentiated from other pathologic cysts such as ovarian cancer or dermoid (Figure 27-10). As the pregnancy progresses, corpus luteum cysts regress and are typically not seen beyond 16 to 18 weeks of gestation. If ovarian cystic masses persist beyond 18 weeks of gestation or increase in size, surgical removal is often required because benign and malignant processes cannot be distinguished using sonography. A high incidence of torsion of ovarian masses during the second and third trimesters has been reported.[77] All persistent ovarian masses in pregnancy should be followed closely.[25,64]

UTERINE

Uterine leiomyomas or fibroids are common throughout pregnancy. If fibroids coexist with a first-trimester pregnancy, the fibroid should be identified in relation to the placenta. Fibroids may increase in size throughout the first trimester and early second trimester because of estrogen stimulation. A rapid increase in fibroid size may lead to necrosis of the leiomyoma, giving rise to significant maternal symptoms that may require myomectomy.[9] Rapidly growing fibroids may compress the gestational sac, causing spontaneous abortion (Figure 27-11).

Sonographically, fibroids may be hypoechoic, echogenic, or isoechoic in relation to myometrium. They typically cause deformity or displacement of the uterus, endometrium, or both. Fibroids are high-acoustic attenuators, which give rise to poor acoustic transmission (Figure 27-12). It may be difficult to differentiate fibroid from focal uterine contraction, although preliminary data sug-

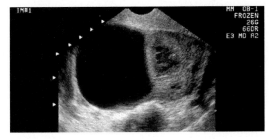

Figure 27-9 Transvaginal scan of the adnexal area in a patient in her first trimester shows a large corpus luteum cyst with anechoic and internal septations with debris.

gest that color Doppler imaging shows a more hypovascular appearance with uterine contractions than with fibroids.[76] Fibroids may also be differentiated from focal myometrial contractions by observing the focal lesion over time (typically 20 to 30 minutes); the myometrial contraction should disappear, whereas a fibroid would still be present.[53]

ECTOPIC PREGNANCY

Ectopic pregnancy is one of the most crucial diagnoses made in any modality of ultrasound. Approximately 10% of maternal deaths are related to ectopic pregnancy.[22] In a typical ultrasound practice, ectopic pregnancy is not an uncommon finding, with a reported incidence varying from 1 in 64 to 1 in 241 pregnancies.[78] The incidence of ectopic pregnancy has increased in recent years. Associated risk factors include previous pelvic infections, use of intrauterine contraceptive devices (IUCD), fallopian tube

surgeries, infertility treatments, and a history of ectopic pregnancies.[1]

Clinical findings may vary and are nonspecific. Pelvic pain has been reported in 97% of patients, although pain may be consistent with other pathologic processes, such as appendicitis or pelvic inflammatory disease. Other clinical findings associated with ectopic pregnancy are vaginal bleeding and a palpable adnexal mass. These clinical findings are found in 75% and 50% of patients, respectively.[83]

Pathologically, ectopic pregnancy is diagnosed by the invasion of trophoblastic tissue within the fallopian tube mucosa.[79] This causes the bleeding often associated with ectopic pregnancy, which may cause hematosalpinx, hemoperitoneum, or both.[7]

Ectopic pregnancy occurs within the fallopian tube in approximately 95% of cases. Other sites, such as the ovary, broad ligament, peritoneum, and cervix, account for the remaining cases (Figure 27-13).[3]

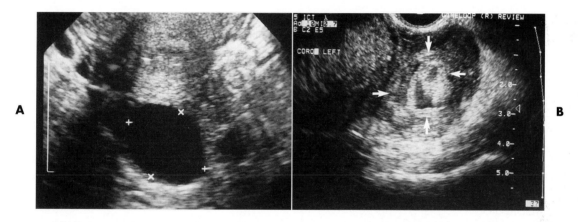

Figure 27-10 A, Sonogram demonstrating a typical corpus luteum cyst *(calipers)* within the right ovary in an 8-week gestation. Sonographic characteristics of this cyst are simple, which is typical. **B,** Sonographic example of hemorrhagic corpus luteum cyst *(arrows).* This may be difficult to differentiate from hematosalpinx, distal tubal ectopic pregnancy, ovarian ectopic pregnancy, or other ovarian neoplasms.

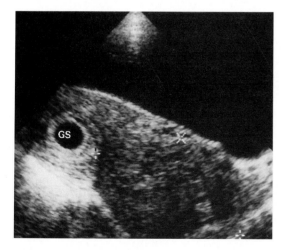

Figure 27-11 Sagittal sonogram demonstrating an 8-cm fibroid/leiomyoma *(calipers)* coexisting with a 6-week gestational sac *(GS)*. This fibroid continued to grow compressing this young gestation, causing demise.

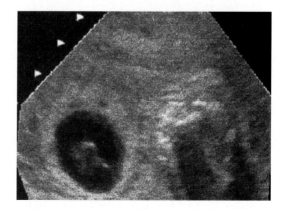

Figure 27-12 Transvaginal three-dimensional scan of an early pregnancy that shows the gestational sac on the left of the image with the echogenic fibroid *(with shadowing)* to the right.

Correlating clinical tests with sonographic findings in ectopic pregnancy is imperative for diagnosis. Specific assays for human chorionic gonadotropin (hCG) allow the sonographer/sonologist to have expectations of sonographic findings, or lack thereof. The beta subunit of human chorionic gonadotropin (beta-hCG) is quantified from maternal blood by two preparations, the First International Reference Preparation (1st IRP) or the Second International Standard (2IS). It is crucial that the sonographer understand which hCG assay a particular institution or laboratory is using. Quantification of hCG is directly correlated with gestational age throughout the first trimester. Generally, the 1st IRP has hCG quantities double those of the 2IS.

Given the complexities of hCG testing, it is vital that the sonographer have a good understanding of the discriminatory level of hCG and sonographic findings. Simply put, the discriminatory level of hCG in pregnancy should be thought of as a minimum level of hCG in normal intrauterine or ectopic pregnancy.[56] Using transvaginal techniques, the hCG discriminatory level in detecting an intrauterine pregnancy has been shown to be 800 to 1000 IU/L based on the 2IS and 1000 to 2000 IU/L based on the first IRP.[52,62]

If discriminatory levels of beta-hCG are met or surpassed and no intrauterine gestational sac is seen, an ectopic pregnancy should be suspected. Caution should be taken if beta-hCG levels are below discriminatory levels. Ectopic pregnancy may or may not exist, given that ectopic gestations do not produce hCG at normal levels (hCG levels double every other day) and 90% of ectopic gestations are not viable, and so may not reflect typical correlation between gestational age and hCG levels. Also, early intrauterine pregnancy may have an intrauterine appearance similar to ectopic pregnancy. Thus, in nonemergent cases, serial beta-hCG levels are preferred because trending of these levels would demonstrate a continuing pregnancy if hCGs rise normally or slowly or plateau, whereas falling hCG levels may indicate missed or incomplete abortion.

ULTRASOUND FINDINGS IN ECTOPIC PREGNANCY

The sonographic appearances of ectopic pregnancy have been well documented with both transabdominal and transvaginal techniques (Figure 27-14).[20,23,67] The most important finding when scanning for ectopic pregnancy is identification of a normal intrauterine gestation (Table 27-1). Again, the expectation of visualizing a normal intrauterine gestation is directly correlated to beta-HCG levels. Although the visualization of an intrauterine gestational sac that includes embryonic heart motion firmly makes the diagnosis of intrauterine pregnancy, earlier gestations (5 to 6 weeks) may normally not demonstrate these findings. As many as 20% of patients with ectopic pregnancy demonstrate an intrauterine saclike structure known as the **pseudogestational sac.**[36,55]

Although difficult, differentiating between normal early gestation and pseudogestational sac often is possible (Figure

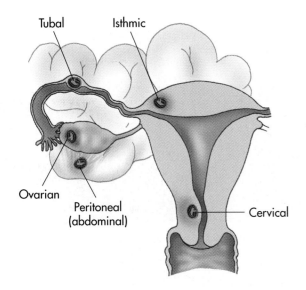

Figure 27-13 Schematic demonstrating sites of ectopic pregnancy.

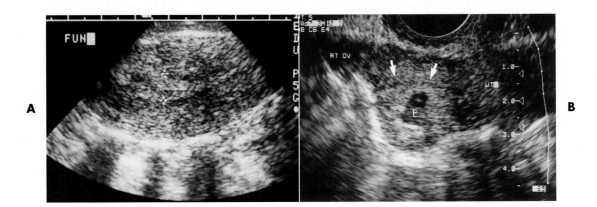

Figure 27-14 **A,** Sagittal sonogram demonstrating an empty uterus with normal endometrial canal *(calipers)*. **B,** Coronal sonogram demonstrating uterus *(UT)*; and right ovary *(RT OV)*, with an echogenic concentric ring with embryo seen centrally with fetal heart motion. Consistent with ectopic pregnancy. *Arrows,* Decidua/trophoblastic villi; *E,* embryo.

27-15). The following guidelines may be helpful: (1) pseudogestational sacs do not contain either a living embryo or yolk sac; (2) pseudogestational sacs are centrally located within the endometrial cavity, unlike the burrowed gestational sac, which is eccentrically placed; (3) homogeneous level echoes are commonly observed in pseudogestational sacs, unlike normal gestational sacs. These findings are most commonly observed using transvaginal techniques.

Color Doppler imaging and spectral analysis may also be helpful in distinguishing normal from pseudogesta-

TABLE 27-1 ABNORMAL ULTRASOUND FINDINGS

Ultrasound Findings	Differential Diagnosis
Empty uterus*	Normal intrauterine pregnancy (3 to 5 weeks) Recent spontaneous abortion

Ultrasound Findings	Differential Diagnosis
Ectopic pregnancy	Intrauterine debris Incomplete spontaneous abortion Intrauterine blood

Ultrasound Findings	Differential Diagnosis
Molar pregnancy	Sac, no embryo Viable intrauterine pregnancy (5 to 6.5 weeks)

Ultrasound Findings	Differential Diagnosis
Nonviable intrauterine pregnancy	Pseudogestational sac of ectopic pregnancy Embryo, no cardiac motion Nonliving intrauterine pregnancy Embryo, cardiac motion Living intrauterine pregnancy

From Nyberg DA, Laing FC: In Nyberg DA and others, editors: *Transvaginal ultrasound,* St Louis, 1992, Mosby.
*Cardiac motion may occasionally be absent in embryos measuring 4 mm or less.
For larger embryos, a potential pitfall is blood clot.

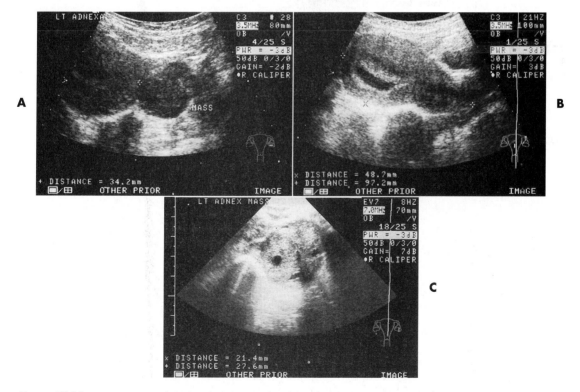

Figure 27-15 A young female in her first trimester presented in the emergency room with elevated human chorionic gonadotropin levels, bleeding, and pelvic pain. **A,** The transabdominal scan clearly shows a mass in the left adnexal area separate from the uterus. **B,** The longitudinal scan of the uterus shows the pseudogestational sac in the fundus of the uterus. **C,** A transvaginal scan showed a gestational sac within the left adnexal area.

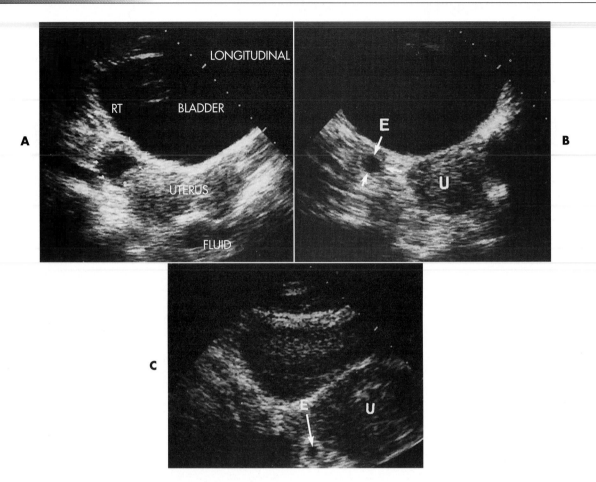

Figure 27-16   A, Longitudinal scan depicting an empty uterus, fluid in the cul-de-sac, and "rindlike" cystic mass anterior to the uterus *(arrows)* representing an ectopic gestational sac. *RT,* Right. **B** and **C,** Transverse representations of ectopic gestational sacs *(E).* In **C** the ectopic sac is in close proximity to the uterine wall. *U,* Uterus.

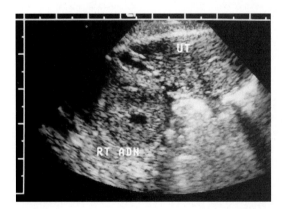

Figure 27-17   Coronal section demonstrating empty uterus *(UT),* and a right adnexal *(RT ADN)* mass with an echogenic ring and sonolucent center consistent with gestational sac. This is consistent with ectopic pregnancy with extrauterine sac.

tional sac with the demonstration of peritrophoblastic flow associated with intrauterine pregnancy. Typically, peritrophoblastic flow demonstrates a low-resistance (high-diastolic) pattern with fairly high peak velocities (approximately 20 cm per second). The decidual cast of the endometrium, as seen in pseudogestational sac, typically demonstrates a high-resistance pattern (low-diastolic component) with low peak velocities.[11,24]

The adnexa should always be sonographically examined when evaluating for ectopic pregnancy. The identification of a live embryo within the adnexa is the most specific for ectopic gestation. Unfortunately, this occurs only 17% to 28% of the time.[11,41] It is important to note that only 10% of live ectopic pregnancies are identified using transabdominal sonography (Figure 27-16).[13]

The identification of an extrauterine sac within the adnexa is one of the most frequent findings of ectopic pregnancy. It has been reported that more than 71% of patients with ectopic pregnancy demonstrate an extrauterine sac or ring, although this study did include living extrauterine ectopic fetuses.[26] The extrauterine gestational sac has sonographic appearances and characteristics similar to the intrauterine gestational sac. Extrauterine gestational sacs often demonstrate a thickened echogenic ring, separate from the ovary, which represents trophoblastic tissue or chorionic villi; there is a possibility that the embryo or yolk sac will be seen (Figure 27-17).

Color-flow imaging and Doppler waveforms may also help diagnose extrauterine gestational sacs. One study reported color flow detection in and around suspicious ex-

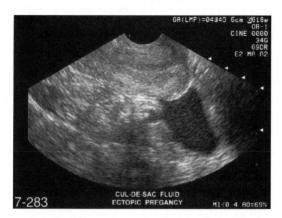

Figure 27-18   Transvaginal scan of the lower uterine segment shows the hypoechoic fluid collection in the cul-de-sac secondary to a ruptured ectopic pregnancy.

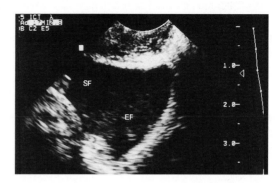

Figure 27-19   Transvaginal sonogram demonstrating echogenic free intraperitoneal fluid in an ectopic gestation. *EF,* Echogenic fluid; *SF,* simple fluid.

trauterine lesions in 95 of 106 ectopic gestations with Doppler waveforms of less than 0.40 resistivity, using the resistive index.[42,43] The positive predictive value of this technique was 96.8%, with sensitivity and specificity of 89.3% and 96.3%, respectively. Other studies must be performed to correlate this criteria.

ADNEXAL MASS WITH ECTOPIC PREGNANCY

A risk of ectopic pregnancy has been reported to be greater than 90% when intrauterine gestation is absent and there is a corresponding adnexal mass.[49] Complex adnexal masses, aside from extrauterine gestational sacs, often represent hematoma within the peritoneal cavity, which is usually contained within the fallopian tube or broad ligament (hematosalpinx).[70] In early-gestational ectopic pregnancy, hematoma may be the only sonographic sign of ectopic pregnancy. It should be distinguished, however, from ovarian cyst, such as the corpus luteum, which is typically hypoechoic, although a hemorrhagic corpus luteum cyst may mimic an extrauterine gestational sac or a distal hematosalpinx.

Often, ovarian processes such as corpus luteum cysts and endometriomas can be differentiated based on their location within the ovary, and one can often visualize surrounding ovarian tissue, although this does not rule out the rare ovarian ectopic gestation.

It has been reported that approximately 80% of patients with ectopic pregnancy demonstrate at least 25 ml of blood within the peritoneum, caused by blood escaping from the distal tube (fimbria). Sonographically detected free intraperitoneal fluid is also a common finding in ectopic pregnancy.[2,26] Approximately 60% of women with ectopic pregnancy demonstrate intraperitoneal fluid, using transvaginal techniques (Figure 27-18). These studies have correlated an increased risk of ectopic pregnancy with moderate to large quantities of free intraperitoneal fluid and an associated adnexal mass.[49,82]

The presence of echogenic free fluid has been shown to be very specific for hemoperitoneum and to be highly correlated with ectopic pregnancy. A 92% risk of ectopic pregnancy with echogenic free fluid has been reported, with

15% of cases demonstrating echogenic free fluid to be the only sonographic finding (Figure 27-19).[60] Another study has shown that the combination of an adnexal mass and free pelvic fluid was the best sonographic correlation in the diagnosis of ectopic pregnancy.[71]

Although intrauterine and adnexal findings are crucial in diagnosing ectopic pregnancy, it is clear that the previously described sonographic findings are not routine. One report states 52.5% of cases with ectopic pregnancy could not accurately demonstrate an adnexal mass or masses.[61] Of that 52.5%, over half (25.5%) were overshadowed by coexisting findings, such as bowel segments that were echogenic or had isoechoic acoustic properties, that did not allow sonographic demarcation of tissue from surrounding ovary or adnexa. Another study demonstrated that in 74% of ectopic pregnancies a confident diagnosis was made of an intrauterine pregnancy using transvaginal techniques and that 26.3% of ectopic pregnancies had a normal transvaginal sonogram at initial presentation.[71] The definition of normal transvaginal sonogram in this study was no adnexal masses or pelvic fluid identified and no evidence of intrauterine gestation.

These findings reiterate the need for meticulous scanning when looking for evidence of ectopic pregnancy, and for an understanding of the limitations of all ultrasound techniques.

HETEROTOPIC PREGNANCY

Fortunately, simultaneous intrauterine and extrauterine pregnancy are uncommon, with recent studies suggesting prevalence rates of 1 in every 6000 to 8000 pregnancies, including those in patients undergoing an infertility workup.[28] This emphasizes that the sonographic observer should be aware that ovulation induction and in vitro fertilization with embryo transfer not only lead to higher risk of **heterotopic pregnancy** but also to an overall increase in ectopic pregnancies, including bilateral ectopic pregnancies.[69]

INTERSTITIAL PREGNANCY

Interstitial pregnancy, or cornual pregnancy, is potentially the most life threatening of all ectopic gestations. This is because of the location of the ectopic pregnancy, which lies in the segment of the fallopian tube that enters the uterus. This site involves the parauterine and myometrial vasculature, creating life-threatening hemorrhage when rupture occurs.[31] Interstitial pregnancies have been reported to occur in approximately 2% of all ectopic pregnancies. Sonographic identification of an interstitial ectopic pregnancy is difficult, but it has been described as an eccentrically placed gestational sac within the uterus that has an incomplete myometrial mantel surrounding the sac (Figure 27-20).[32,74]

CERVICAL PREGNANCY

Cervical pregnancy has a reported incidence of 1 in 16,000 pregnancies.[37] Sonographic demonstration of a gestational sac within the cervix suggests a cervical pregnancy, although a spontaneous abortion may have a similar appearance.

OVARIAN PREGNANCY

An ovarian pregnancy is also very rare, accounting for less than 3% of all ectopic pregnancies.[66] The sonographic diagnosis of ovarian pregnancy may be difficult; reported cases have demonstrated complex adnexal masses that involve or contain ovary. Thus, distinguishing ovarian pregnancy from hemorrhagic ovarian cyst or from other ovarian processes may be difficult.

ABNORMAL PREGNANCY: ULTRASOUND FINDINGS

Sonographic differentiation of normal and abnormal appearances of the first-trimester pregnancy may be subtle.[63] Distinguishing living from nonliving gestations is crucial, but recent studies have shown that demonstration of a living embryo does not necessarily mean a normal outcome.[27,68] Recent data prospectively looked at 556 pregnancies between 6 and 13 weeks of gestation and identified embryonic heart motion. Overall, the pregnancy loss rate after identification of an intrauterine pregnancy with positive cardiac motion was 8.8%. If sonographic abnormalities were detected (subchorionic hematoma being the most frequent), the loss rate was 15.2%, compared with 8.8% when sonogram findings were normal. It is of interest that the loss rate after a normal sonogram was similar in symptomatic patients (10.6%) and asymptomatic patients (9.1%).[27]

Obviously, identifying an intrauterine pregnancy with or without cardiac activity is the first conclusive sonographic sign of normality or abnormality. With transvaginal sonography, a living embryo should be detected by 46 menstrual days.[35,72,73] Other sonographic appearances allow the ultrasound clinician to differentiate normal and abnormal findings within the gestational sac period. To conclusively demonstrate normal or abnormal findings, more than one sonogram may be needed. These are discussed throughout this chapter and are outlined in Table 27-1.

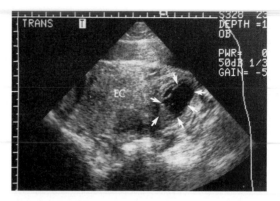

Figure 27-20 Sonogram of an 8.5-week gestation demonstrating the cystic rhombencephalon within the fetal cranium *(arrows)*. Note yolk sac between calipers. *EC,* Endometrial cavity.

EMBRYONIC BRADYCARDIA

The variations in embryonic cardiac rate during the first trimester range between 90 and 170 beats per minute. Embryonic cardiac rates of less than 90 beats per minute at any gestational age within the first trimester have been shown to be a poor prognostic finding. In fact, no reported embryo survived beyond the second trimester with this finding.[21,35,46,72]

EMBRYONIC OLIGOHYDRAMNIOS AND GROWTH RESTRICTION

Studies have indicated that growth delay and oligohydramnios within the first trimester have poor outcomes. If the gestational sac is 4 mm less than the crown-rump length, embryonic oligohydramnios may be suspected. Universal demise was reported in embryos with this characteristic.[4,14]

Embryonic growth restriction can be determined only by relative sonographic dating either by reliable menstrual history or by growth delay of the embryo or gestational sac in relation to serial sonograms. Chromosome abnormalities, such as triploidy, have been associated with embryonic growth restriction and embryonic oligohydramnios.[4]

COMPLETE ABORTION

Characteristics for the sonographic diagnosis of **complete abortion** are of an empty uterus with no adnexal masses or free fluid and positive hCG levels. Serial hCG levels demonstrate rapid decline. Caution should be taken when a positive pregnancy test and an empty uterus are seen, given the possibility that an early normal intrauterine pregnancy between 3 and 5 weeks of gestation may be present. Consequently, serial hCG levels should always be obtained.

INCOMPLETE ABORTION

Incomplete abortion may show several sonographic findings, ranging from an intact gestational sac with a nonliving embryo to a collapsed gestational sac that is grossly misshapen (Figure 27-21).[64] Often, women who are clinically undergoing abortion or who have had elective termination require follow-up sonography to determine if re-

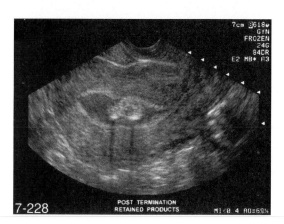

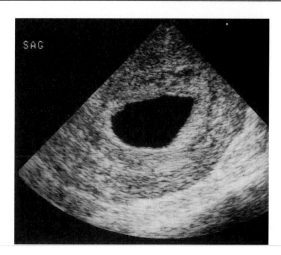

Figure 27-21 Transvaginal scan of a patient who presented with fever, pain, and bleeding secondary to an abortion two days previously. The endometrial cavity is distended, with retained products of conception casting small shadows into the myometrial cavity.

Figure 27-23 Transvaginal sonogram in a sagittal plane demonstrating a large empty gestational sac that does not contain yolk sac, amnion, or embryo. This is consistent with anembryonic pregnancy.

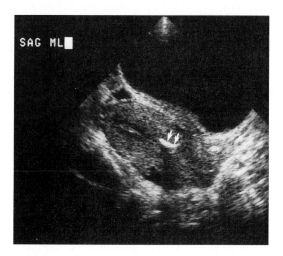

Figure 27-22 Transabdominal sagittal sonogram demonstrates an echogenic focus causing acoustic shadowing *(arrows)*. This patient had a positive pregnancy test and was experiencing vaginal bleeding. The echogenic source most likely represents retained products, possibly skeletal structures.

tained products of conception are present. Sonography of retained products may be subtle; a thickened endometrium greater than 5 mm may be the only sonographic evidence of such a diagnosis. Obvious embryonic parts, which may or may not cause acoustic shadowing, are obvious evidence of retained products of conception (Figure 27-22).[44]

ANEMBRYONIC PREGNANCY (BLIGHTED OVUM)

By definition, **anembryonic pregnancy,** or **blighted ovum,** is a gestational sac in which the embryo fails to develop. The typical sonographic appearance of anembryonic pregnancy is of a large, empty gestational sac that does not demonstrate yolk sac, amnion, or embryo. The sac size typically is clearly abnormally large (greater than 18 mm mean sac diameter); no intragestational sac

anatomy is seen (Figure 27-23). Box 27-1 outlines several sonographic intrauterine findings associated with abnormal pregnancies.

GESTATIONAL TROPHOBLASTIC DISEASE IN THE FIRST TRIMESTER

Gestational trophoblastic disease is a proliferative disease of the trophoblast after a pregnancy. It represents a spectrum of disease from a relatively benign form, hydatidiform mole, to a more malignant form, invasive mole, or choriocarcinoma. The clinical hallmark of gestational trophoblastic disease is vaginal bleeding in the first or early second trimester. The serum levels of beta-hCG are dramatically elevated, often greater than 100,000 IU/ml. The patient may also experience symptoms of hyperemesis gravidarum or preeclampsia.[50, 81]

In the United States, gestational trophoblastic disease affects approximately 1 out of every 1500 to 2000 pregnancies. The highest reported incidence is in some Asian countries, where it affects more than 1 in 100 pregnancies.[65,84] Associations with women over age 40 and with molar pregnancy have been reported.[30] Genetic studies indicate that a complete hydatidiform mole has a normal diploid karyotype of 46XX, which is usually entirely derived from the father and has proven malignant biologic potential. A partial mole, in contrast, is karotypically abnormal, triploidy being the most prevalent abnormality.[80]

Ultrasound Findings. The sonographic appearance of molar pregnancy varies with gestational age. The characteristic "snowstorm" appearance of hydatidiform mole, which includes a moderately echogenic soft tissue mass filling the uterine cavity and studded with small cystic spaces representing hydropic chorionic villi, may only be specific for a second-trimester mole (Figure 27-24).[50] Sonographic identification of the disease in the first trimester has been considered difficult. The appearance of first-

BOX 27-1 SONOGRAPHIC FINDINGS OF GESTATIONAL SACS ASSOCIATED WITH ABNORMAL INTRAUTERINE PREGNANCIES

EMBRYO
Absence of cardiac motion in embryos 5 mm or larger
Absence of cardiac motion after 6.5 menstrual weeks

YOLK SAC AND AMNION
Large yolk sac or amnion without a visible embryo
Calcified yolk sac

LARGE GESTATIONAL SAC
>18 mm lacking a living embryo
>8 mm lacking a visible yolk sac

SHAPE
Irregular or bizarre

POSITION
Low

TROPHOBLASTIC REACTION
Irregular
Absent double decidual sac finding
Thin trophoblastic reaction <2 mm
Intratrophoblastic venous flow

GROWTH
Gestational sac growth of <0. 6 mm/day
Absent embryonic growth

hCG CORRELATION
Discrepancy in sac size with HCG levels

From Nyberg DA, Laing FC: In Nyberg DA and others, editors: *Transvaginal ultrasound,* St Louis, 1992, Mosby.

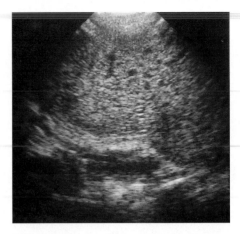

Figure 27-24 Longitudinal scan of the pregnant uterus in a patient who presented larger than appropriate for dates and with bleeding. The uterus is filled with tiny grapelike clusters of tissues that represent a hydatidiform mole.

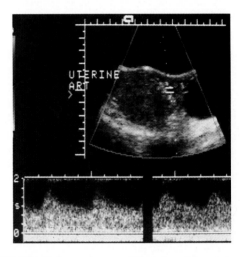

Figure 27-25 Color and spectral Doppler of the molar pregnancy shows high-velocity flow throughout the abnormal tissue.

trimester molar pregnancy may simulate a missed abortion, incomplete abortion, blighted ovum, or hydropic degeneration of the placenta associated with missed abortion (Figure 27-25).[9,50] It may also be seen as a small echogenic mass filling the uterine cavity without the characteristic vesicles.[9] The vesicles or cystic spaces may be too small to be seen by ultrasound in the first trimester.

The primary treatment of molar pregnancy is uterine curettage followed by serial measurements of serum hCG levels.[29] The serum hCG level falls toward normality within 10 to 12 weeks after evacuation.[30] The reported incidence of residual disease after curettage is approximately 20%. The use of ultrasound for direct visualization of the uterine content to ensure complete evacuation during the curettage procedure has been shown to substantially reduce the incidence of residual gestational trophoblastic disease.[19]

ACKNOWLEDGMENT

The author acknowledges the work of Dale Cyr on this chapter in the fourth edition of this book.

REVIEW QUESTIONS

1. Name the most likely cranial abnormalities that can be diagnosed with ultrasound in the first trimester.
2. How does the insertion of the umbilical cord differ in abdominal wall defects?
3. Where does the cystic hygroma first appear?
4. What is the most common ovarian mass seen in the first trimester of pregnancy?
5. Describe the sonographic technique for differentiating a fibroid from a uterine contraction.
6. What clinical findings are important to know in a patient with ectopic pregnancy?
7. Discuss the sonographic appearance of an ectopic pregnancy.
8. Describe the other complications of pregnancy that occur in the first trimester.
9. What is the normal cardiac heart rate in the first trimester?
10. How can the sonographer distinguish a complete versus incomplete abortion?

11. What are the clinical signs and sonographic findings in gestational trophoblastic disease?

REFERENCES

1. Atrash HK, Franks A: Causes of the increase in ectopic pregnancy, *Am J Obstet Gynecol* 162:1130, 1990.

2. Bateman BG and others: Vaginal sonography findings and HCG dynamics of early intrauterine and tubal pregnancies, *Obstet Gynecol* 75:421, 1990.

3. Bayless RB: Nontubal ectopic pregnancy, *Clin Obstet Gynecol* 30:191, 1987.

4. Bromley B and others: Small sac size in the first trimester: a predictor of poor fetal outcome, *Radiology* 178:375, 1991.

5. Bronshtein M and others: First-trimester and early second-trimester diagnosis of nuchal cystic hygroma by transvaginal sonography: diverse prognosis of the septated from the non-septated lesion, *Am J Obstet Gynecol* 161:78, 1989.

6. Bronshtein M and others: Detection of fetal chromosomal anomalies by transvaginal sonography at 12 to 16 weeks of gestation, Presented to the first World Congress of the International Society of Ultrasound in Obstetrics and Gynecology, London, January 6-10, 1991.

7. Budowick M and others: The histopathology of the developing tubal ectopic pregnancy, *Fertil Steril* 34:169, 1980.

8. Buschi AJ and others: Hydropic degeneration of the placenta simulating hydatidiform mole, *J Clin Ultrasound* 7:60, 1979.

9. Buttram VC Jr, Reiter RC: Uterine leiomyomata: etiology, symptomatology, and management, *Fertil Steril* 36:433, 1981.

10. Callen, P: *Ultrasonography in obstetrics and gynecology,* ed 3, Philadelphia, 1994, WB Saunders.

11. Cartier MS and others: Diagnostic efficacy of endovaginal color flow Doppler in an ectopic pregnancy screening program. Presented to the Seventy-sixth Annual Assembly of the Radiologic Society of North America, Chicago, Nov 1990, *Radiology* 177(suppl):117, 1990.

12. Chervenak FA and others: Fetal cystic hygroma: cause and natural history, *N Engl J Med* 309:822, 1983.

13. Coleman BG and others: Ectopic embryo detection using real-time sonography, *J Clin Ultrasound* 13:545, 1985.

14. Crade M: First trimester growth retardation, *J Ultrasound Med* 8:56, 1989 (letter).

15. Cullen MT: Comparison of transvaginal and abdominal ultrasound, *J Ultrasound Med* 8:565, 1990.

16. Curtis JA, Watson L: Sonographic diagnosis of omphalocele in the first trimester of fetal gestation, *J Ultrasound Med* 7:97, 1988.

17. Cyr DR and others: Bowel migration in the normal fetus: US detection, Radiology 1986:161, 1986.

18. Cyr DR and others: Fetal rhombencephalon: normal ultrasound findings, *Radiology* 166:691, 1988.

19. Cyr DR and others: Sonography as an aid in molar pregnancy evaluation. Presented to the 35th Annual Convention of the American Institute of Ultrasound in Medicine, Atlanta, 1991, vol 10, pp s44, American Institute of Ultrasound in Medicine, Baltimore.

20. Dashefsky SM and others: Suspected ectopic pregnancy: endovaginal and transvesical US, *Radiology* 169:181, 1988.

21. Dubose TJ, Cunyus JA, Johnson LF: Embryonic heart rate and age, *J Diag Med Sonogr* 6:151, 1990.

22. Ectopic pregnancy-United States, 1987, MMWR 39:401, 1990.

23. Filly RA: Ectopic pregnancy: the role of sonography, *Radiology* 162:661, 1987.

24. Fink IJ, Filly RA: Omphalocele associated with umbilical cord allantoic cyst: sonographic evaluation in utero, *Radiology* 149:473, 1983.

25. Fleischer AC: Sonographic evaluation of pelvic masses and maternal disorders. In James AE Jr, editor: *The principles and practices of ultrasonography and obstetrics and gynecology,* Norwalk, Conn, 1985, Appleton-Century-Crofts.

26. Fleischer AC and others: Ectopic pregnancy: features at transvaginal sonography, *Radiology* 174:375, 1990.

27. Frates MC, Benson CB, Doubilet PM: Pregnancy outcome after first trimester sonogram demonstrating fetal cardiac activity, *J Ultrasound Med* 12:383, 1993.

28. Gamberdella FR, Marrs RP: Heterotopic pregnancy associated with assisted reproductive technology, *Am J Obstet Gynecol* 160:1520, 1989.

29. Goldstein DP, Berkowitz RJ, Cohen SM: The current management of molar pregnancy, *Curr Probl Obstet Gynecol* 3:1, 1979.

30. Goldstein RB, Filly RA: Prenatal diagnosis of anencephaly: spectrum of sonographic appearances and distinction from the amniotic band syndrome, *Am J Roentgenol* 151:547, 1988.

31. Graham M, Cooperberg PL: Ultrasound diagnosis of interstitial pregnancy: findings and pitfalls, *J Clin Ultrasound* 7:433, 1979.

32. Gray DL, Martin CM, Crane JP: Differential diagnosis of first trimester ventral wall defect, *J Ultrasound Med* 8:255, 1989.

33. Guzman ER: Early prenatal diagnosis of gastroschisis with transvaginal ultrasonography, *Am J Obstet Gynecol* 162:1253, 1990.

34. Hertzberg BS and others: Normal sonographic appearance of the fetal neck late in the first trimester: the pseudomembrane, *Radiology* 171:427, 1989.

35. Hertzberg BS, Mahony BS, Bowie JD: First trimester fetal cardiac activity: sonographic documentation of a progressive early rise in heart rate, *J Ultrasound Med* 7:573, 1988.

36. Hill LM, Kislak S, Martin JG: Transvaginal sonographic detection of the pseudogestational sac associated with ectopic pregnancy, *Obstet Gynecol* 75:986, 1990.

37. Hofmann HM and others: Cervical pregnancy: case reports and current concepts in diagnosis and treatment, *Arch Gynecol Obstet* 241:63, 1987.

38. Jauniaux E and others: Umbilical cord pseudocyst in trisomy 18, *Prenat Diagn* 8:557, 1988.

39. Jauniaux E and others: Early sonographic diagnosis of body stalk anomaly, *Prenat Diagn* 10:127, 1990.

40. Johnson MP: First trimester simple hygroma, *Am J Obstet Gynecol* 168:156, 1993.

41. Kivikoski AI, Martin CM, Smeltzer JS: Transabdominal and transvaginal ultrasonography in the diagnosis of ectopic pregnancy: a comparative study, *Am J Obstet Gynecol* 163:123, 1990.

42. Kurjak A, Zalud I: Doppler and color flow imaging. In Nyberg DA, Hill LM, Bohm-Velez M, Mendelson EB, editors: *Transvaginal ultrasound,* St. Louis, 1992, Mosby.

43. Kurjak A, Zalud I, Schulman H: Ectopic pregnancy: transvaginal color Doppler of trophoblastic flow in questionable adnexa, *J Ultrasound Med* 10:685, 1991.

44. Kurtz A and others: Detection of retained products of conception following spontaneous abortion of first trimester, *J Ultrasound Med* 10:387, 1991.

45. Kushnir O and others: Early transvaginal sonographic diagnosis of gastroschisis, *J Clin Ultrasound* 18:194, 1990.

46. Laboda LA, Estroff JA, Benaceraff BR: First trimester bradycardia: a sign of impending fetal loss, *J Ultrasound Med* 8:561, 1989.

47. Langer JC and others: Cervical cystic hygroma in the fetus: clinical spectrum and outcome, *J Pediatr Surg* 25:58, 1990.

48. Macken MB, Grantmyre EB, Vincer MJ: Regression of nuchal cystic hygroma in utero, *J Ultrasound Med* 8:101, 1989.

49. Mahony BS and others: Sonographic evaluation of ectopic pregnancy, *J Ultrasound Med* 4:221, 1985.

50. Munyer TP and others: Further observations on the sonographic spectrum of gestational trophoblastic disease, *J Clin Ultrasound* 9:349, 1981.

51. Neiman HL: Transvaginal ultrasound embryology, *Semin Ultrasound CT MR* 11:22, 1990.

52. Nelson LH, King M: Early diagnosis of holoprosencephaly, *J Ultrasound Med* 11:57, 1992.

53. Nyberg DA, Hill LM: Normal early intrauterine pregnancy: sonographic development and hCG correlation. In Nyberg DA and others, editors: *Transvaginal ultrasound,* St Louis, 1992, Mosby.

54. Nyberg DA, Laing FC, Filly RA: Threatened abortion: sonographic distinction of normal and abnormal gestation sacs, *Radiology* 158:397, 1986.

55. Nyberg DA and others: Ultrasonographic differentiation of the gestational sac of early intrauterine pregnancy from the pseudogestational sac of ectopic pregnancy, *Radiology* 146:755, 1983.

56. Nyberg DA and others: Early gestation: correlation of HCG levels and sonographic identification, *Am J Roentgenol* 144:951, 1985.

57. Nyberg DA and others: Endovaginal sonographic evaluation of ectopic pregnancy: a prospective study, *Am J Roentgenol* 149:1181, 1987.

58. Nyberg DA and others: Sonographic spectrum of placental abruption, *Am J Roentgenol* 148:161, 1987.

59. Nyberg DA and others: Chromosomal abnormalities in fetuses with omphalocele: significance of omphalocele contents, *J Ultrasound Med* 8:299, 1989.

60. Nyberg DA and others: Extrauterine findings of ectopic pregnancy at transvaginal US: importance of echogenic fluid, *Radiology* 178:823, 1991.

61. Parvey HR, Maklad W: Pitfalls in the transvaginal sonographic diagnosis of ectopic pregnancy, *J Ultrasound Med* 3:139, 1993.

62. Peisner DB, Timor-Tritsch IE: The discriminatory zone of beta-hCG for vaginal probes, *J Clin Ultrasound* 18:280, 1990.

63. Pennell RG and others: Complicated first trimester pregnancies: evaluation with endovaginal vs. transabdominal technique, *Radiology* 165:79, 1987.

64. Pennes DR, Bowerman RA, Silver TM: Echogenic adnexal masses associated with first-trimester pregnancy: sonographic appearance and clinical significance, *J Clin Ultrasound* 13:391, 1985.

65. Poen HJT, Djojopranoto M: The possible etiologic factors of hydatidiform mole and choriocarcinoma, *Am J Obstet Gynecol* 92:510, 1965.

66. Raziel A and others: Ovarian pregnancy: a report of 20 cases in one institution, *Am J Obstet Gynecol* 163:1182, 1990.

67. Rempen A: Sonographic first trimester diagnosis of umbilical cord cyst, *J Clin Ultrasound* 17:53, 1989.

68. Rempen A: Diagnosis of viability in early pregnancy with vaginal sonography, *J Ultrasound Med* 9:711, 1990.

69. Rizk B and others: Heterotopic pregnancies after in vitro fertilization and embryo transfer, *Am J Obstet Gynecol* 164:161, 1991.

70. Romero R and others: The value of adnexal sonographic findings in the diagnosis of ectopic pregnancy, *Am J Obstet Gynecol* 158:52, 1988.

71. Russell SA, Filly RA, Damato N: Sonographic diagnosis of ectopic pregnancy with endovaginal probes: what really has changed? *J Ultrasound Med* 3:145, 1993.

72. Schats R and others: Embryonic heart activity: appearance and development in early human pregnancy, *Br J Obstet Gynecol* 97:989, 1990.

73. Shenker L and others: Embryonic heart rates before the seventh week of pregnancy, *J Reprod Med* 31:333, 1986.

74. Sherer DM and others: Transvaginal sonographic diagnosis of an unruptured interstitial pregnancy, *J Clin Ultrasound* 18:582, 1990.

75. Skibo LK, Lyons EA, Levi CS: First trimester umbilical cord cyst, *Radiology* 182:719, 1992.

76. Smith K: Color flow imaging of leiomyomas and focal myometrial contractions during pregnancy, *J Diagn Med Sonogr,* 1993.

77. Sommerville M and others: Ovarian neoplasms and the risk of ovarian torsion, *Am J Obstet Gynecol* 164:577, 1991.

78. Stabile I, Grudzinskas JG: Ectopic pregnancy: a review of incidence, etiology, and diagnostic aspects, *Obstet Gynecol Surv* 45:335, 1990.

79. Stock RJ: Histopathologic changes in tubal pregnancy, *J Reprod Med* 30:923, 1985.

80. Szulman AE, Surti U: The syndromes of hydatidiform mole. I. Cytogenetic and morphologic correlations, *Am J Obstet Gynecol* 131:665, 1978.

81. Szulman AE, Surti U: The syndromes of hydatidiform mole. II. Morphologic evolution of the complete and partial mole, *Am J Obstet Gynecol* 132:20, 1978.

82. Thorsen MK and others: Diagnosis of ectopic pregnancy: endovaginal vs. transabdominal sonography, *Am J Roentgenol* 155:307, 1990.

83. Weckstein LN: Clinical diagnosis of ectopic pregnancy, *Clin Obstet Gynecol* 30:236, 1987.

84. Wei P, Ouyang P: Trophoblastic disease in Taiwan, *Am J Obstet Gynecol* 85:844, 1963.

85. Wilson RD, McGillivray BC: Omphalocele: early prenatal diagnosis by ultrasound, *J Clin Ultrasound* 12:A-2, 1984.

BIBLIOGRAPHY

Bronson RA, VandeVegte GL: An unusual first trimester sonographic finding associated with development of hydatidiform mole: the hyperechoic ovoid mass, *Am J Roentgenol* 160:137, 1993.

Crane JP: Sonographic evaluation of multiple pregnancy, *Semin Ultrasound CT MR* 5:144, 1984.

England MA: *Color atlas of life before birth: normal fetal development,* Chicago, 1983, Mosby.

Sauerbrei EE, Pham DH: Placental abruption and subchorionic hemorrhage in the first half of pregnancy: ultrasound appearance and clinical outcome, *Radiology* 160:109, 1986.

Townsend R: Membrane thickness in ultrasound prediction of chorionicity of twins, *J Ultrasound Med* 7:327, 1988.

CHAPTER 28

Ultrasound of the Second and Third Trimesters

Sandra L. Hagen-Ansert

REVIEW QUESTIONS

KEY TERMS

apex - the ventricles of the heart come to a point called the *apex;* normally the apex is directed toward the left hip

breech - indicates the fetal head is toward the fundus of the uterus

ductus venosus - structure that carries oxygenated blood from the umbilical vein to the inferior vena cava

frontal bossing - slight indentation of the frontal bones of the skull; also known as "lemon head"

gravidity - total number of pregnancies

human chorionic gonadotropin (hCG) - hormone within the maternal urine and serum; hCG is elevated during pregnancy

menstrual age - gestational age of the fetus is determined from the last menstrual period (LMP)

micrognathia - abnormally small chin

midline echo complex (the falx) - widest transverse diameter of the skull; proper level to measure the biparietal diameter

normal situs - indicates normal position of the abdominal organs (liver on right, stomach on left, heart apex to the left)

parity - number of live births

transverse lie - indicates fetus is lying transversely (horizontal) across the abdomen

trimester - pregnancy is divided into three 13-week segments called *trimesters*

vertex - indicates that the fetus is positioned head down in the uterus

---

The second and third **trimesters** are the ideal time to image detailed fetal anatomy with ultrasound. To perform a complete evaluation of the fetus, the sonographer should follow a specific protocol/guideline as recommended by the national organizations who have an interest in obstetric ultrasound procedures.

The guidelines for obstetric scanning as outlined by the American College of Radiology (ACR), the American

Institute of Ultrasound in Medicine (AIUM), and the American College of Obstetricians and Gynecologists (ACOG) are described in Chapter 25. This chapter focuses on the specific fetal anatomy the sonographer needs to understand in order to develop a systematic scanning protocol.

PROTOCOL/GUIDELINES FOR AN OBSTETRIC ULTRASOUND EXAMINATION

The protocol/guidelines for the second- and third-trimesters ultrasound examination include a biometric and anatomic survey of the fetus. The guidelines suggest the following[24]:

1. Observation of fetal viability by visualization of cardiovascular pulsations.
2. Demonstration of presentation (fetal lie).
3. Demonstration of the number of fetuses. In multiple gestations, individual studies should be performed on each fetus, growth comparison studies between fetuses performed, placental number determined, and amniotic sacs assessed.
4. Estimation of the quantity of amniotic fluid. Abnormal fluid amounts should be described.
5. Localization of the placenta. Placenta previa should be excluded by examination of the cervical area.
6. Assessment of fetal age. At least two dating parameters should be evaluated. Fetal growth studies include a serial growth analysis when multiple examinations are performed.
7. Biometric parameters that may be used include the following:
   • Biparietal diameter
   • Head circumference
   • Femur length
   • Abdominal circumference
   • Head circumference to abdominal circumference ratio (used in cases in which head to abdomen disproportion is suspected or unusual head or body contours are observed)
8. Evaluation of uterus, adnexae, and cervix to exclude masses that may complicate obstetric management.
9. Anatomic survey of fetal anatomy to exclude major congenital malformations. Comprehensive studies may be necessary when a fetal anomaly is suspected.
10. Basic ultrasound examinations to evaluate the anatomic areas listed below. More detailed studies may be performed. Documentation of required anatomy should be completed.
    • Cerebral ventricles (exclusion of ventriculomegaly)
    • Spine (exclusion of large spinal defects)
    • Stomach (exclusion of gastrointestinal obstruction)
    • Heart (four-chamber and outflow views)
    • Kidneys and urinary bladder (exclusion of severe renal disease)
    • Fetal insertion of umbilical cord (exclusion of an anterior abdominal wall defect)
    • Renal regions (exclusion of severe renal malformations)

The sonographer should establish a systematic scanning protocol encompassing all criteria of the guidelines. An organized approach to scanning ensures completeness and reduces the risk of missing a birth defect.

OBSTETRIC PARAMETERS

The length of the average human pregnancy is 40 weeks (280 days), beginning from the first day of the last menstrual period (LMP).[36] Ovulatory age is approximately 266 days (38 weeks); ovulation generally occurs on the fourteenth day of the menstrual cycle.[36] When the LMP is unknown or when the patient has irregular menstrual cycles, the estimated date of confinement (EDC), or due date, is derived by other clinical parameters (uterine size, Doptone [auscultation of fetal heart tones], ultrasound, ovulation indicators).

TRIMESTERS

Pregnancy is divided into trimesters, or thirds (Box 28-1). The first trimester covers the first week of pregnancy through the twelfth week, the second trimester continues from the thirteenth week through the twenty-sixth week, and the third trimester commences with the twenty-seventh week and concludes at the forty-second week of pregnancy. A pregnancy extending beyond the forty-second week is considered a postterm or postdate gestation.[36]

NÄGELE'S RULE

The EDC may be calculated using Nägele's rule (Box 28-2). According to this method, the EDC is derived by subtracting 3 months from the LMP and adding 7 days. For example, an LMP of 10/17 would result in an EDC of 7/24 (10/17 − 3 months = 7/17 + 7 days = 7/24).[36] Commercial date wheels simplify this method to determine the due date and to assign fetal age at the time of the ultrasound study.

In clinical practice the gestational age of the fetus or fetal age is determined from the LMP. This is also referred to as the **menstrual age.** Ovulatory age is not used in practice because of inconsistent ovulatory patterns found among women.

Pregnancy can be clinically detected approximately 6 to 8 days after ovulation. **Human chorionic gonadotropin (hCG)** is the hormone present within the maternal urine and serum predictive of pregnancy.

BOX 28-1 TRIMESTERS

• First trimester = 0 to 12 weeks of gestation
• Second trimester = 13 to 26 weeks of gestation
• Third trimester = 27 to 42 weeks of gestation
• Postterm pregnancy = >42 weeks of gestation

BOX 28-2 NÄGELE'S RULE

Nägele's Rule: EDC = LMP − 3 months + 7 days
Menstrual Age = Date of pregnancy from last menstrual period (LMP)

GRAVIDITY AND PARITY

The sonographer should understand the clinical labeling of pregnancy. Pregnancy history includes **gravidity** (G) (number of pregnancies, including the present one) and parity (P). **Parity** is described using a numeric system describing all pregnancy outcomes. The numeric sequence, P0000, is commonly used. Numbers are assigned to follow the parity symbol, P. The numbers represent, in order, full-term pregnancies, premature births, abortions, and living children. For instance, a G4P2103 describes a patient undergoing her fourth pregnancy. She has had two full-term pregnancies, one premature birth, no abortions, and three living children.

NORMAL FETOPLACENTAL ANATOMY OF THE SECOND AND THIRD TRIMESTERS

Recognizing normal fetal anatomy is critical to the performance of obstetric ultrasound studies. Once normal anatomic structures are identified, the investigator is prepared to detect malformations in fetal development. The task of identifying standard anatomic planes and organs poses a considerable challenge for the sonographer. Image resolution continually improves; therefore more detailed anatomy must be recognized as more sophisticated equipment becomes available. The sonographer must continuously update his or her knowledge of sonographic techniques and fetal anatomy. This section describes basic fetal anatomy imaged in the second and third trimesters.

One of the most important technical considerations in developing scanning expertise is to become organized and systematic in assessing the fetus, placenta, and amniotic fluid (Box 28-3).

The sonographer should initially determine the position of the fetus in relationship to the position of the mother (Figure 28-1). For example, with the probe held in a sagittal orientation on the maternal abdomen, the fetal plane or position may be sagittal, coronal, or transverse, depending on fetal position (spine up or down, on its side, or in a **transverse lie**) (Figure 28-2).

In determining fetal position and in surveying the uterine contents the transducer is systematically directed toward the uterine fundus, maintaining a midline path. By moving the probe from side to side, fetal position, cardiac activity, the number of fetuses, the presence of uterine and placental masses, and any obvious fetal anomalies may be recognized and the amniotic fluid assessed.

BOX **SCANNING TECHNIQUES**
28-3
• Survey uterus
• Observe cardiac activity
• Determine position and number of the fetus and placenta
• Assess amniotic fluid
• Look for uterine or placental masses and fetal anomalies

It is important to remember to view cardiac activity at the beginning of each study to ensure both patient and scanner that the fetus is alive. If a fetal demise or an obvious anomaly is initially recognized, the sonographer is better prepared to perform the study and involve the physician immediately.

After fetal position is understood, the sonographer determines the direction and orientation necessary to find fetoplacental anatomy and to obtain measurements. Assessment of the fetus may begin by progressively studying anatomy and measuring the fetus from the cranial to caudal poles. The placenta, amniotic fluid, uterus, and adnexae are then examined.

FETAL PRESENTATION

Vertex. A simple method to determine fetal presentation consists of a midline scan at the symphysis pubis, which is directed upward toward the fundus. Immediately cephalad to the symphysis the maternal bladder is visualized. This allows the investigator to determine which fetal part is presenting and to check the relationship between the cervix and placenta. The fetal head is visualized at this level when the fetus is in a **vertex** or cephalic presentation. Proceeding fundally, if the fetal body is noted to follow the head, a vertex lie is confirmed (Figure 28-3). The fetal body may lie in an oblique axis to the right or left of the maternal midline. If the body is not initially recognized in the midline, the sonographer should direct the transducer from side to side to search for the abdomen. Identification of the vertebral column entering the cranium further delineates the fetal lie. Fetuses generally assume a longitudinal, transverse, or oblique lie within the uterus (Figure 28-4).

Breech. When the lower extremities or lower body are found to be in the lower uterine segment and the head is visualized in the uterine fundus, a **breech** presentation should be suspected (Figure 28-5). In fetuses near term, determination of the specific type of breech lie provides important clinical information for the obstetrician to plan the safest route of delivery. Some fetuses in a breech position (e.g., those in a frank breech position with the thighs flexed at the hips and the lower legs extended in front of the body and up in front of the head) (Figure 28-6) may be safely turned, or verted, allowing vaginal delivery, whereas fetuses in other breech lies (e.g., complete breech when both the hips and lower extremities are found in the lower pelvis) need to be delivered by cesarean section. A footling breech is found when the hips are extended and one (single footling) or both feet (double footling) are the presenting parts closest to the cervix.

Transverse. When a transverse cross-section of the fetal head or body is noted in the sagittal plane, a transverse lie should be considered (Figure 28-7). By rotating the transducer perpendicularly, the long axis of the fetus should be observed.

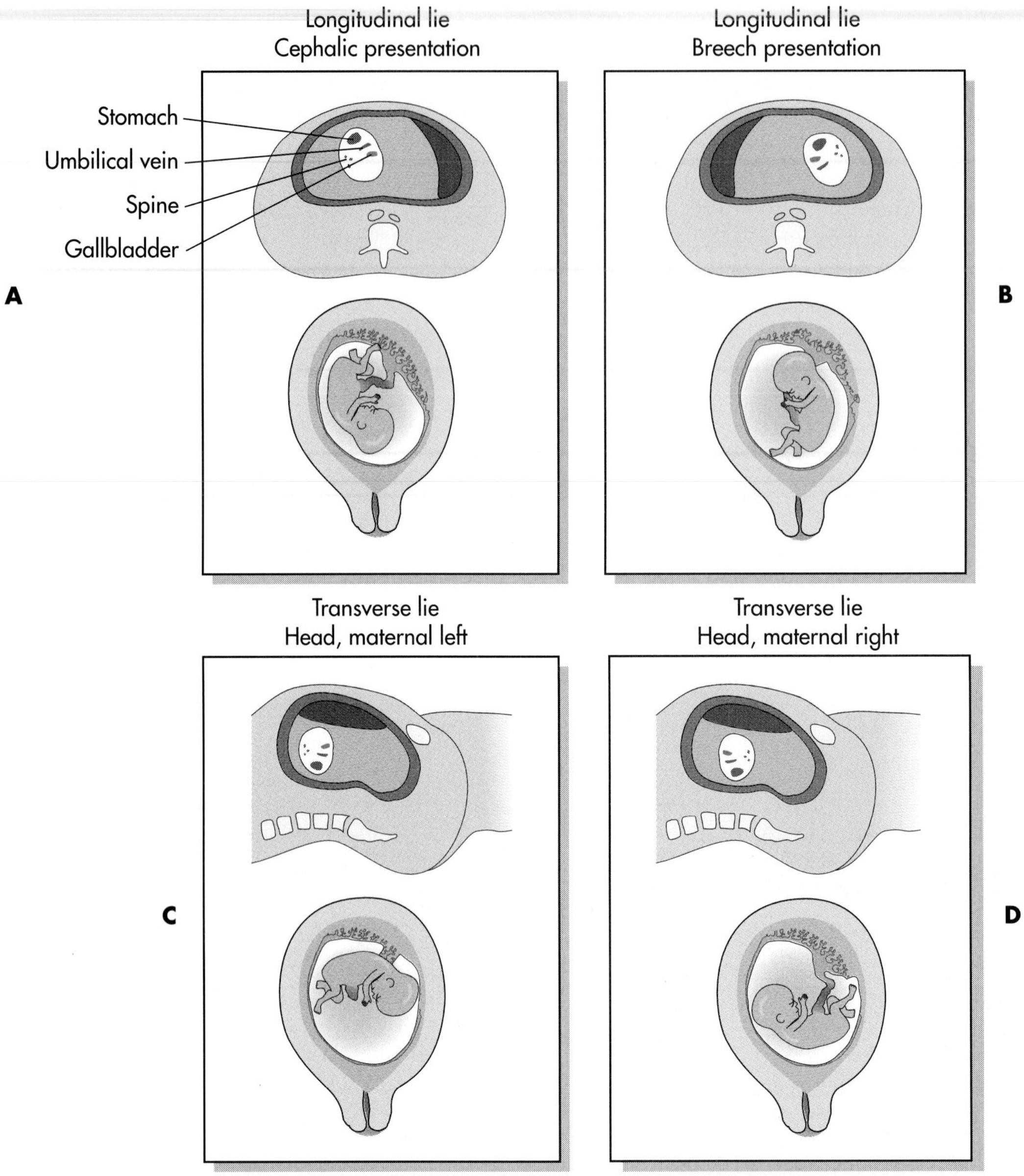

Figure 28-1 Knowledge of the plane of section across the maternal abdomen (longitudinal or transverse), as well as the position of the fetal spine and left-side (stomach) and right-side (gallbladder) structures, can be used to determine fetal lie and presenting part. **A,** This transverse scan of the gravid uterus demonstrates the fetal spine on the maternal right with the fetus lying with its right side down (stomach anterior, gallbladder posterior). Because these images are viewed looking up from the patient's feet, the fetus must be in longitudinal lie and cephalic presentation. **B,** When the gravid uterus is scanned transversely and the fetal spine is on the maternal left with the right side down, the fetus is in a longitudinal lie and breech presentation. **C,** When a longitudinal plane of section demonstrates the fetal body to be transected transversely and the fetal spine is nearest the uterine fundus with the fetal left side down, the fetus is in a transverse lie with the fetal head on the maternal left. **D,** When a longitudinal plane of section demonstrates the fetal body to be transected transversely and the fetal spine is nearest the lower uterine segment with the fetal left side down, the fetus is in a transverse lie with the fetal head on the maternal right. Although real-time scanning of the gravid uterus quickly allows the observer to determine fetal lie and presenting part, this maneuver of identifying specific right- and left-side structures within the fetal body forces one to determine fetal position accurately and identify normal and pathologic fetal anatomy.

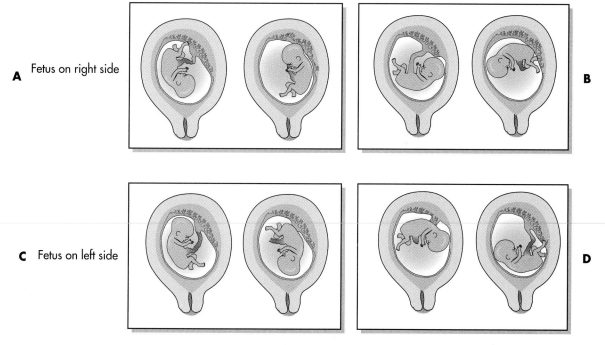

Figure 28-2   Various fetal positions and the method used to differentiate the left side from the right side. **A-B,** Fetus lying on right side. **C-D,** Fetus lying on left side.

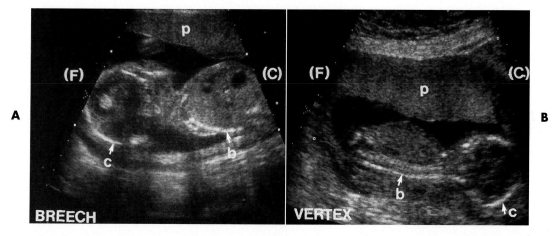

Figure 28-3   A, A breech presentation. The body *(b)* is closest in proximity to the direction of the cervix *(C)* (right of image), and the cranium *(c)* is directed toward the uterine fundus *(F). p,* Placenta. **B,** A vertex presentation. The cranium *(c)* is closest in proximity to the direction of the cervix *(C)* (to the right of image) and the body *(b)* is directed toward the uterine fundus, *(F). p,* Placenta.

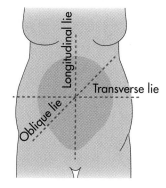

Figure 28-4   These vectors demonstrate the three major possible axes that a fetus may occupy. A fetal lie does not necessarily indicate whether the vertex or the breech is closest to the cervix.

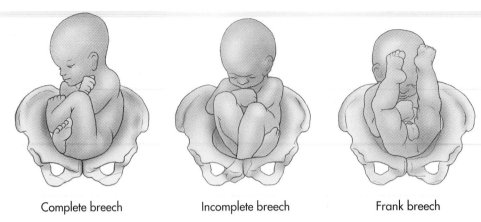

Complete breech   Incomplete breech   Frank breech

Figure 28-5   Three possible breech presentations. The complete breech demonstrates flexion of the hips and knees. The incomplete breech demonstrates intermediate deflexion of one hip and knee (single or double footling). The frank breech shows flexion of the hips and extension of both knees.

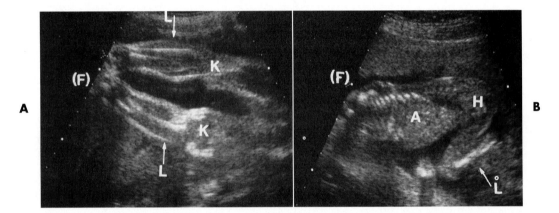

Figure 28-6   **A,** A fetus in a frank breech presentation with both legs extended upward toward the uterine fundus *(F). K,* Knee; *L,* lower leg. **B,** Complete breech presentation with one leg flexed at the hips, with the lower leg *(L)* and foot positioned under the hips *(H).* The other leg was in a similar position. *A,* Abdomen; *(F),* fundus.

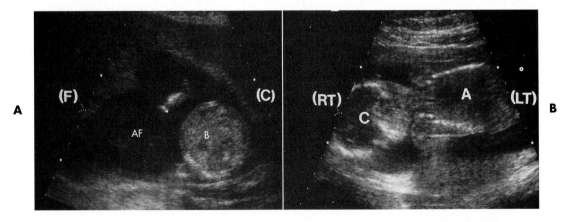

Figure 28-7   **A,** A scan obtained in an 18-week fetus using a sagittal scanning plane reveals the fetal body in a transverse position rather than a sagittal or coronal orientation (compare with Figure 28-3). *AF,* Amniotic fluid; *B,* body; *(C)* toward cervix; *(F),* fundus. **B,** In the same fetus, by rotating the transducer 90 degrees, the abdomen may be connected to the head to reveal the transverse lie with the head oriented to the maternal right side *(RT)* and the abdomen *(A)* to the maternal left side *(LT).*

Situs. In addition to determining fetal lie, the right and left sides of the fetus should be determined to ensure **normal situs** (positioning) of fetal organs. For example, if the fetus is in a vertex presentation with the fetal spine toward the maternal right side, the right side of the fetus is down and the left side is up.

One should further differentiate the right from left sides by identifying anatomic landmarks. For example, the fetal stomach lies on the fetal left side, the gallbladder on the right side, and the **apex** of the heart toward the fetal left side. The fetal aorta lies slightly to the left of midline, anterior to the spine, and the inferior vena cava is to the right of midline and slightly more anterior to the aorta. Various fetal positions are encountered during obstetric studies; therefore the sonographer should be familiar with basic fetal positions (see Figure 28-2). An atypical fetal presentation should be noted, such as face, brow, or shoulder presentation, because this may complicate delivery. Similarly, hyperextension of the fetal head may alter obstetric management.

The key to effective obstetric scanning stems from the operator's ability to determine fetal position.

NORMAL FETOPLACENTAL LANDMARKS

THE CRANIUM

The sonographer must be adept at recognizing the normal appearances and developmental changes of the fetal brain throughout pregnancy. The scanner must be able to identify neuroanatomy at specific levels where measurements are obtained, such as biparietal diameter or cerebellar diameter, and to screen for malformations in brain development (see Chapter 16, Neonatal Echoencephalography). The sonographer must understand these developmental changes, recognize normal anatomic variations, and develop an ability to detect malformations.

Several important principles must be understood when viewing the fetal brain. First, brain tissue, a solid structure, may appear hypoechoic or cystic because of the low density of the tissue. Brain tissue does not exhibit typical solid appearances because of the small size of the reflective interfaces; echoes are not generated unless the reflectors are large enough to cause reflections. The water content of the fetal brain is high, contributing to the cystic appearances of various brain structures. Second, as the brain develops, structures change their sonographic appearances. For example, the choroid plexuses seem large early in pregnancy, but as the brain grows, these structures appear small in relationship to the entire brain.

By the 12th week of gestation, the cranial bones ossify. By 18 weeks of gestation, the texture characteristics of each brain structure have been determined. From this point on in the pregnancy, the appearance of each brain structure should remain the same.

In general, two types of brain tissues are highly echogenic, the dura (pachymeninx) and the pia arachnoid

(leptomeninx), which covers the inner and outer brain surfaces.[14] The appearance of the brain structures largely depends on the amount of pia arachnoid tissue and cerebrospinal fluid (CSF) making up a specific structure. For example, a subarachnoid space contains a large amount of CSF and will then appear cystic. In contrast, an area that contains both CSF and pia arachnoid has both echo-free and echogenic appearances. Pia arachnoid tissue appears echogenic.[14]

In evaluating the cranium, the long axis of the fetus is determined. The transducer is aligned in a longitudinal or sagittal position over the fetus and then specifically positioned over the fetal head. Rotation of the transducer perpendicular to the sagittal plane generates transverse sections of the brain. Brain anatomy and measurements are assessed in these transverse scanning planes (occipitotransverse position) (Figure 28-8).

The first step in surveying the brain is to check the contour or outline of the skull bones. This is accomplished by sweeping the transducer through the cranium from the highest level (roof) in the brain to the skull base. The cranium appears as a circle at the highest levels and as an oval at the ventricular, peduncular, and basal levels. Check for any irregularities in the contour of the skull bones. Keep in mind that extracranial masses (e.g., cephaloceles) distort the normal configuration of the skull table; therefore exclusion of cranial masses should be routinely attempted.

When the fetal cranium is difficult to view, search deep in the pelvis, because it may be low in the late third trimester of pregnancy, limiting study of brain anatomy and growth. Maternal bladder filling or tilting of the patient into Trendelenburg position (maternal head directed down) may free the head from the pelvis. In some cases, especially when a brain anomaly is suspected, use of a transvaginal probe may define the skull and brain. In all cases, at a minimum, the outline of the cranium should be visible; if it is not, cranial absence (anencephaly) or deformity should be considered.

Optimal studies of the fetal brain may not be possible when the fetal head is in an occipitoposterior position (looking up) or when the head is in an occipitoanterior position (looking down).

The next step in the fetal profile is to assess the development of the brain. Although all fetal brain structures are not visible prenatally, commonly recognized neuroanatomic structures are described.

In a transverse plane, at the most cephalad level within the skull (Figure 28-9), the contour of the skull should be round or oval (depending on exact level) and should have a smooth surface (excluding a cephalocele in which the meninges, brain, or both herniate from the skull). At this level, the interhemispheric fissure (IHF), or falx cerebri, is observed as a membrane separating the brain into two equal hemispheres. The IHF is an important landmark to visualize because its presence implies that separation of the cerebrum has occurred (this excludes the severe anomaly alobar holoprosencephaly, in which there is only a single

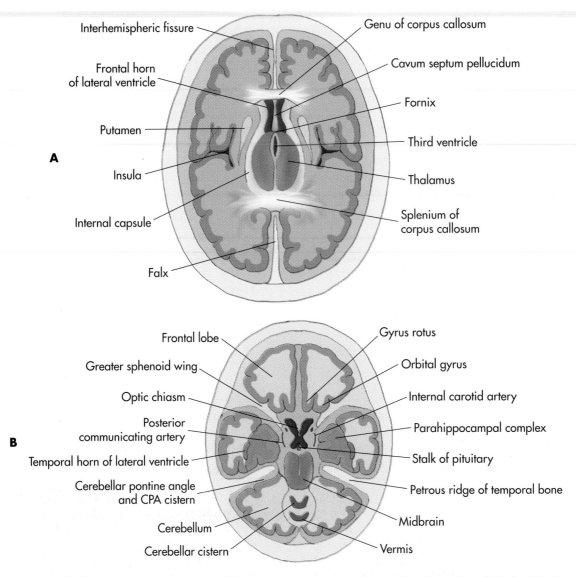

Figure 28-8 **A,** Transverse view of the fetal intracranial anatomy taken at the midsection of the fetal head. **B,** Transverse view inferior to **A** taken at the level of the cerebellum and vermis.

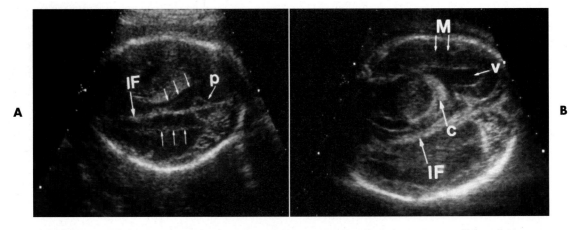

Figure 28-9 **A,** Transverse cross-section revealing white-matter tracts *(arrows)* coursing parallel to the interhemispheric fissure *(IF)* at 26 weeks of gestation. *p,* Peduncles. **B,** The choroid plexus *(C)* is located in the proximal or near hemisphere within the ventricular cavity *(v)*. Note the homogeneous appearance of the brain tissue. *M,* Mantle.

ventricle and an absent IHF). Lateral and running parallel to the IHF, two linear echoes representing deep venous structures (white-matter tracts) are viewed (see Figure 28-9). It is important to recognize that the white-matter tracts are positioned above the level of the lateral ventricles.

The fetal ventricular system consists of two paired lateral ventricles, a midline third ventricle, and a fourth ventricle. CSF travels from the lateral ventricles to the third ventricle through the foramen of Monroe and then to the fourth ventricle from the aqueduct of Sylvius (within the third ventricle) and into the cerebral and spinal subarachnoid spaces from the interventricular foramina and foramina of Luschka. CSF then enters the venous system (e.g., cranial venous sinuses).[32]

CSF, which coats the brain and spinal cord, is manufactured by the choroid plexuses, which are located within the roofs of each ventricle except the frontal ventricular horns. The fetal ventricles are important to assess because ventriculomegaly or hydrocephalus (dilated ventricular system) represents one of the most common neural tube defects. Ventriculomegaly is commonly observed in fetuses with central nervous system disorders and may be the first clue that such a problem exists.[8]

The lateral ventricles are viewed at a level just below the white-matter tracts (Figure 28-10). The lumen of the ventricles may be recognized by the bright reflection of their borders and the presence of the large choroid plexuses that normally fill the cavity of the ventricles early in gestation. The lateral borders of the ventricular chambers (LVB) are represented as echogenic lines coursing parallel to the IHF. The LVB is more easily imaged in the distal hemisphere, as opposed to the proximal or nearest ventricle, because of reverberation artifacts in the near field. The ventricular cavity is represented sonographically as an echo-free space, filled with choroid plexus and housed between the medial ventricular border and LVB (Figure 28-11).

As a general rule in early pregnancy (approximately 12 to 22 weeks), the LVB appears to be large in relation to the developing cranial hemispheres. Later in pregnancy, the LVB assumes a more medial position (Figure 28-12).

The glomus, or body, of the choroid plexus marks the site at which the size of the ventricle may be assessed. The

glomus should fill the entire ventricle. If the glomus appears to float or dangle within the cavity, measurements of ventricular size are recommended to exclude abnormally enlarged or dilated ventricles (ventriculomegaly). Atrial diameter measurements are clinically practical because the size of the ventricular atria remains the same throughout gestation.[5]

When measuring the size of the ventricle, locate the glomus and measure directly across the posterior portion, measuring perpendicular to the long axis of the ventricle rather than the falx, while placing the calipers at the junction of the ventricular wall and lumen or cavity of the ventricle (see Figure 28-10). The normal ventricle measures 6.5 mm. Any ventricle measuring greater than 10 mm is considered outside of normal error ranges and is therefore abnormal, warranting further consultation and prenatal testing.

The texture of the choroid plexus should be assessed to exclude the formation of cysts. It is thought that CSF may become trapped during development within the neuroepithelial folds and result in the formation of a choroid plexus cyst. This commonly represents a normal variation in fetal development, but these cysts are known to be associated with chromosomal problems, such as trisomy 21 (Down syndrome), trisomy 13, and trisomy 18.

Moving the transducer in a more caudal direction identifies the echogenic **midline echo complex.** This is the widest transverse diameter of the skull and is therefore the proper level at which to measure the biparietal diameter and to assess the development of the midline brain structures (see Figure 28-11). Along the midline echo, the paired thalamus lies on either side and resembles a heart with the apex projected toward the fetal occiput. This orientation aids in deciding in which direction the face is positioned.

Between the thalamic structures lies the cavity of the third ventricle (see Figure 28-12). In the same scanning plane the box-shaped cavum septum pellucidi (CSP) is observed in front of the thalamus. The CSP is the space between the leaves of the septum pellucidum. By viewing the CSP an anomaly known as complete agenesis of the corpus callosum may be excluded because the presence of the CSP signifies normal development of the frontal midline.[8]

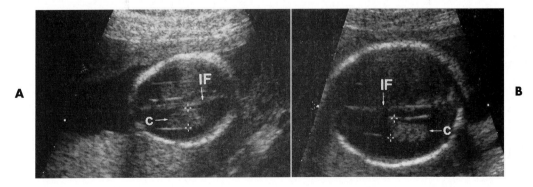

Figure 28-10   A, Transverse view demonstrating ventricular atrial diameter of 6 mm *(calipers)* at 16 weeks of gestation representing a normal-size ventricle. *C,* Choroid plexus; *IF,* interhemispheric fissure. **B,** In a 19-week gestation the atrial diameter of 6 mm corresponds to a normal-size ventricle.

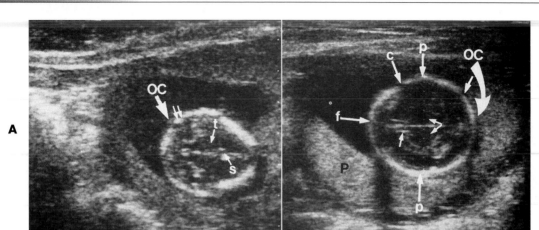

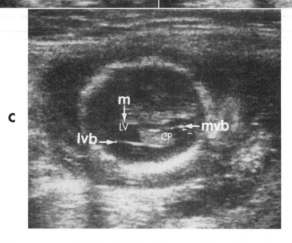

Figure. 28-11 **A,** Cranial anatomy at the level of the thalamus *(t)* in a 14-week gestation. Note the contour of the bony calvarium *(double arrows)*. *OC,* Occiput; *s,* cavum septum pellucidum. **B,** Cranial anatomy at the same level in an 18-week gestation. *Curved arrow,* Thalamus; *single arrow,* cavum septum pellucidum; *c,* coronal suture; *f,* frontal bone; *OC,* occiput; *P,* placenta; *p,* parietal bones. **C,** Cerebral ventricles at 19 weeks of gestation. The midline echo from the interhemispheric fissure *(m)* is noted. The medial ventricular border *(mvb)* and lateral ventricular border *(lvb)* are identified. The ventricular cavity *(LV)* and echogenic choroid plexus *(CP)* are demonstrated.

The frontal horns of the ventricles may be seen as two diverging echo-free structures within the frontal lobes of the brain and are prominent in the presence of ventricular dilation. The corpus callosum is ill-defined sonographically and represented as the band of tissue between the frontal ventricular horns.[14]

The ambient cisterns are pulsatile structures vascularized by the posterior cerebral artery bordering the thalamus posteriorly. When scanning laterally in the brain, brain tissue from the temporal lobe of the brain is visible along with evidence of the insula (i.e., Sylvian cistern complex). The insula appears to pulsate because of blood circulation through the middle cerebral artery, which courses through the insula (see Figure 28-12). The subarachnoid spaces may be seen projecting from the inner skull table.

The sonographer should be careful when studying anatomy in the proximal (near) cranial hemisphere because reverberation artifacts often preclude evaluation of the brain. Interpretation of the normalcy of the brain should, in general, be based on the anatomy seen in the distal hemisphere, because most brain anomalies represent symmetric processes. In most cases, the defect is present bilaterally, even though the anatomy may not be adequately discerned.[4] The sonographer may be able to achieve better visualization by angling cephalad or by scanning transvaginally.

As the transducer is moved caudally, the heart-shaped cerebral peduncles are imaged (Figure 28-13). Although similar to the thalamus in shape, they are smaller. Pulsations from the basilar artery are observed between the lobes of the peduncles at the interpeduncular cistern. The circle of Willis may be seen anterior to the midbrain and appears as a triangular region that is highly pulsatile as a result of the midline-positioned anterior cerebral artery and lateral convergence of the middle cerebral arteries. The suprasellar cistern may be recognized in the center of the circle of Willis.

The cerebellum is located in back of the cerebral peduncles within the posterior fossa. The cerebellar hemispheres are joined together by the cerebellar vermis (Fig-

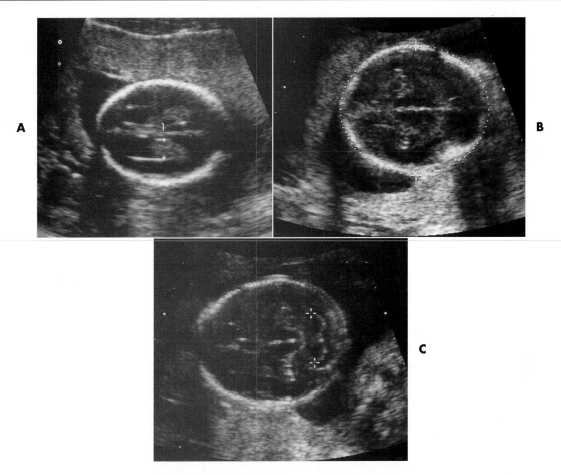

Figure 28-12 A, Transverse view at the level of the ventricles. The width of the lateral ventricle is measured from medial to lateral edges *(1)*. **B,** Transverse view slightly inferior to the level of the ventricles, near the thalamus (hypoechoic "heart" structure in the center of the skull). This is the level at which the biparietal diameter and head circumference are measured. **C,** Transverse view inferior to the level of **B;** the cerebellum is demarcated by the calipers.

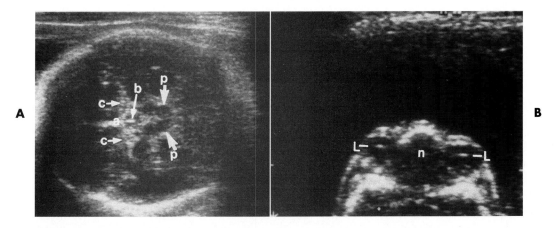

Figure 28-13 A, Circle of Willis *(c)* identified anterior to the cerebral peduncles *(p)*. Arterial pulsations may be observed from the basilar artery *(b)* and anterior cerebral artery *(a)* in real-time imaging. The middle cerebral artery pulsations may be seen at the lateral margins of the circle of Willis. **B,** The lenses *(L)* of the eyes are noted when the fetus is looking upward (occipitoposterior position). The nasal cavities are identified *(n)*.

ure 28-14). It is important to recognize the usual configuration of the cerebellum, because distortion may represent findings suggestive of an open spina bifida (the "banana sign,"or Arnold-Chiari malformation in which the cerebellum may be small or displaced downward into the foramen magnum). Measurements of cerebellar width allow assessment of fetal age and permit necessary follow-up in fetuses with spinal defects and other anomalies of the cerebellum.

The cisterna magna (a posterior fossa cistern filled with CSF) lies directly behind the cerebellum (Figure 28-15). This area should be evaluated routinely when in the cerebellar plane, because a normal-appearing cisterna magna may exclude almost all open spinal defects. The cisterna magna is almost always effaced (thinned out) or obliterated in fetuses with the Arnold-Chiari malformation (cranial changes associated with spina bifida).[29] Therefore, in patients at low risk of spinal defect, confirmation of a normal posterior fossa suggests the absence of spina bifida. Because evaluation of the fetal spine remains challenging in excluding small spinal defects, cranial findings associated with this disorder may be more helpful in screening for these lesions.

Conversely, enlargement of the cisterna magna may indicate a space-occupying cyst, such as a Dandy-Walker malformation or other abnormalities of the posterior fossa.

The normal cisterna magna measures 3 to 11 mm, with an average size of 5 to 6 mm. Measurements of cisterna magna size are obtained by measuring from the vermis to the inner skull table of the occipital bone.[25] Within the cisterna magna space, linear echoes, which are paired, may be observed posteriorly. These echogenic structures represent dural folds that attach the falx cerebelli (see Figure 28-14).[33]

When scanning inferior to or below the cerebellar plane, the orbits may be visualized. It is important to note that both fetal orbits (and eyes) are present and that the spacing between both orbits appears normal. Measurements of orbital width have been reported to aid in gestational age assignment and in detecting abnormalities of spacing between the orbits (Table 28-1).[18,28] There are con-

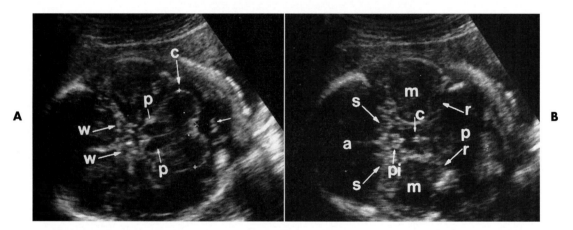

Figure 28-14 **A,** Anatomic depiction at the cerebellar level in a 25-week fetus showing the cerebral peduncles *(p)* positioned anteriorly to the cerebellum *(c)*. The circle of Willis *(w)* is outlined. The dural folds that connect the bottom of the falx cerebelli are seen within the cisterna magna *(arrow)*. **B,** In the same fetus, at a level slightly below the cerebellar level, the anterior *(a)*, middle *(m)*, and posterior fossae are shown. Note the sphenoid bones *(s)*, and petrous ridges *(r)*. *C,* Suprasellar cistern; *pi,* piarachnoid tissue in the basilar cistern.

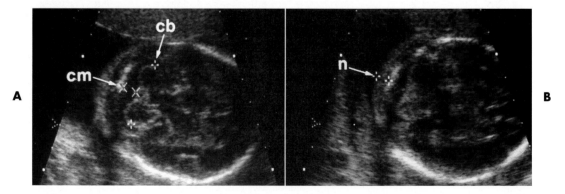

Figure 28-15 **A,** Depiction of a normal cerebellum *(cb)* and cisterna magna *(cm)* in a 24-week fetus. The cerebellum measures 26 mm and the cisterna magna measures 5 mm in diameter. **B,** In the same fetus, at the same level, the skin behind the neck is measured. A normal nuchal skin fold *(n)* of 5 mm is shown. This measurement is unreliable after 20 weeks of gestation.

ditions in which eyes may be missing (anophthalmia), fused or closely spaced (hypotelorism), or abnormally widened (hypertelorism).

The fetal orbits are observed and measured in two planes when the fetal head is in an occipitotransverse position (fetal cranium on the side): (1) a coronal scan posterior to the glabelloalveolar line (Figure 28-16) and (2) a transverse scan at a level below the biparietal diameter (along the orbitomeatal line) (Figure 28-17). In these views the individual orbital rings, nasal structures, and maxillary processes can be identified. When the fetus is in an occipitoposterior position (fetal orbits directed up), orbital distances can also be determined. In this view the orbital rings, lens, and nasal structures may be demonstrated (Figure 28-18). Measurements of the inner orbital distance (IOD) should be made from the medial border of the or-

bit to the opposite medial border, and the outer orbital (or binocular) distance (OOD) is measured from the lateral border of one orbit to the opposite lateral wall (see Figures 28-16 to 28-18).[28] Nomograms for orbital distance spacing have been published.[18,28]

At the base of the skull the anterior, middle, and posterior cranial fossae are observed (see Figure 28-14). The sphenoid bones create a V-shaped appearance as they separate the anterior fossa from the middle fossa, with the petrous bones further dividing the fossa posteriorly. At the junction of the sphenoid wings and petrous bones lies the sella turcica (site of the pituitary gland).[15]

THE FACE

The architecture and morphology of the fetal face are easily appreciated by the 17th to 22nd weeks of gestation. By

TABLE 28-1	PREDICTED BIPARIETAL DIAMETER (BPD) AND WEEKS OF GESTATION FROM THE INNER AND OUTER ORBITAL DISTANCES						
BPD (cm)	Ges (wks)	IOD (cm)	OOD (cm)	BPD (cm)	Ges (wks)	IOD (cm)	OOD (cm)
1.9	11.6	0.5	1.3	5.8	24.3	1.6	4.1
2.0	11.6	0.5	1.4	5.9	24.3	1.6	4.2
2.1	12.1	0.6	1.5	6.0	24.7	1.6	4.3
2.2	12.6	0.6	1.6	6.1	25.2	1.6	4.3
2.3	12.6	0.6	1.7	6.2	25.2	1.6	4.4
2.4	13.1	0.7	1.7	6.3	25.7	1.7	4.4
2.5	13.6	0.7	1.8	6.4	26.2	1.7	4.5
2.6	13.6	0.7	1.9	6.5	26.2	1.7	4.5
2.7	14.1	0.8	2.0	6.6	26.7	1.7	4.6
2.8	14.6	0.8	2.1	6.7	27.2	1.7	4.6
2.9	14.6	0.8	2.1	6.8	27.6	1.7	4.7
3.0	15.0	0.9	2.2	6.9	28.1	1.7	4.7
3.1	15.5	0.9	2.3	7.0	28.6	1.8	4.8
3.2	15.5	0.9	2.4	7.1	29.1	1.8	4.8
3.3	16.0	1.0	2.5	7.3	29.6	1.8	4.9
3.4	16.5	1.0	2.5	7.4	30.0	1.8	5.0
3.5	16.5	1.0	2.6	7.5	30.6	1.8	5.0
3.6	17.0	1.0	2.7	7.6	31.0	1.8	5.1
3.7	17.5	1.1	2.7	7.7	31.5	1.8	5.1
3.8	17.9	1.1	2.8	7.8	32.0	1.8	5.2
4.0	18.4	1.2	3.0	7.9	32.5	1.9	5.2
4.2	18.9	1.2	3.1	8.0	33.0	1.9	5.3
4.3	19.4	1.2	3.2	8.2	33.5	1.9	5.4
4.4	19.4	1.3	3.2	8.3	34.0	1.9	5.4
4.5	19.9	1.3	3.3	8.4	34.4	1.9	5.4
4.6	20.4	1.3	3.4	8.5	35.0	1.9	5.5
4.7	20.4	1.3	3.4	8.6	35.4	1.9	5.5
4.8	20.9	1.4	3.5	8.8	35.9	1.9	5.6
4.9	21.3	1.4	3.6	8.9	36.4	1.9	5.6
5.0	21.3	1.4	3.6	9.0	36.9	1.9	5.7
5.1	21.8	1.4	3.7	9.1	37.3	1.9	5.7
5.2	22.3	1.4	3.8	9.2	37.8	1.9	5.8
5.3	22.3	1.5	3.8	9.3	38.3	1.9	5.8
5.4	22.8	1.5	3.9	9.4	38.8	1.9	5.8
5.5	23.3	1.5	4.0	9.6	39.3	1.9	5.9
5.6	23.3	1.5	4.0	9.7	39.8	1.9	5.9
5.7	23.8	1.5	4.1				

Modified from Mayden KL and others: *Am J Obstet Gynecol* 144:289, 1982.

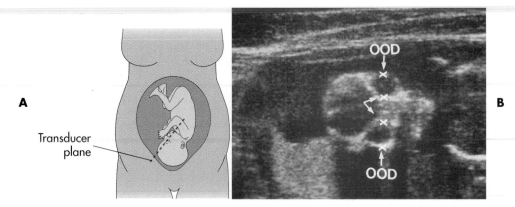

Figure 28-16   A, Frontal view demonstrating a fetus in a vertex presentation with the fetal cranium in an occipitotransverse position. The transducer is placed along the coronal plane (approximately 2 cm posterior to the glabella-alveolar line). **B,** Sonogram demonstrating the orbits in the coronal view. The outer orbital diameter *(OOD)* and inner orbital diameter IOD *(angled arrows)* are viewed. The IOD is measured from the medial border of the orbit to the opposite medial border *(angled arrows).* The *OOD* is measured from the outermost lateral border of the orbit to the opposite lateral border.

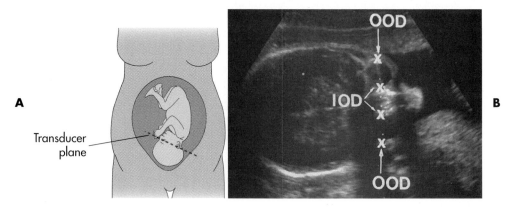

Figure 28-17   A, Frontal view demonstrating the orbits in an occipitotransverse position. The transducer is placed along the orbitomeatal line (approximately 2 to 3 cm below the level of the biparietal diameter). **B,** Sonogram demonstrating the orbits in the occipitotransverse position. *OOD,* Outer orbital diameter; *IOD,* inner orbital diameter.

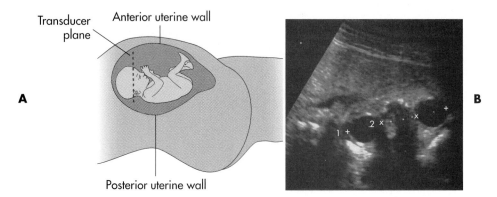

Figure 28-18   A, Side view demonstrating the fetus in an occipitoposterior position. The transducer is placed in a plane that transects the occiput, orbits, and nasal processes. **B,** Sonogram of the orbits in an occipitoposterior position.

understanding the normal appearance of the developing face, the sonographer may recognize when it is deformed. Viewing facial behaviors produces an enlightening scanning session, because fetal yawning, swallowing, and eye movements may be observed. These behaviors may provide insightful clues to fetal well-being.

The fetal face may be recognized even in the first trimester of pregnancy. Facial morphology becomes more apparent in the second trimester, but visualization relies heavily on ideal fetal positioning, adequate amounts of amniotic fluid, and excellent visualization. The incorporation of three-dimensional ultrasound imaging has brought increased understanding to determining facial detail.

Anatomic Landmarks of the Facial Profile. Views of the fetal forehead and facial profile are achieved by imaging the facial profile (Figure 28-19). In this view the contour of the frontal bone, the nose, the upper and lower lips, and the chin may be assessed. Profile views of the face are useful in determining the relationship of the nose to the lips, in excluding forehead malformations (e.g., anterior cephaloceles, cleft lip and palate, **frontal bossing** [as seen in some forms of skeletal dysplasias]), and in assessing the formation of the chin (to exclude an abnormally small chin **[micrognathia]).**

Anatomic Landmarks of the Coronal Facial View. By placing the transducer in a coronal scanning plane, sectioning through the face reveals both orbital rings, the parietal bones, ethmoid bones, nasal septum, zygomatic bone, maxillae, and mandible (Figure 28-20). Scans obtained in an anterior plane over the orbits demonstrate the eyelids and, when directed posterior to this plane, the orbital lens. The eyeglobes, hyaloid artery, and vitreous matter have been sonographically identified.[2]

The oral cavity and tongue are frequently outlined during fetal swallowing (see Figure 28-19). Tangential views of the face help differentiate the nostrils, nares, nasal septum, maxillae, and mandible (Figure 28-21). This view is helpful in the diagnosis of craniofacial anomalies, such as cleft lip. It is important to recognize facial landmarks because bony shadowing and normal tissues may simulate defects.

The fetal ears may be defined in the second trimester as lateral protuberances emerging from the parietal bones. Later in pregnancy the components of the external ear, helix, lobule, and antitragus may be seen (Figure 28-22).[14] The semicircular canals and internal auditory meatus have been sonographically recognized.[14,22]

Fetal hair is often observed along the periphery of the skull and must not be included in the biparietal diameter measurement (Figure 28-23).

THE VERTEBRAL COLUMN

The anatomy of the vertebral column should be assessed in all fetuses referred for obstetric evaluation. A gross anatomic survey of the spine should be attempted to exclude major spinal malformations (e.g., meningomyelocele). The fetal spine is studied in coronal, transverse, and sagittal scanning planes.

Coronal In a coronal section the spine appears as two curvilinear lines extending from the cervical spine to the sacrum. The normal fetal spine tapersnear the sacrum and widens near the base of the skull (Figures 28-24 to 28-26). This double line appearance of the spine is referred to as the "railway sign" and is generated by echoes from the posterior and anterior laminae and spinal cord.[16]

When the scanning plane cross-sects both laminae and equal amounts of tissue are noted on either side of the spinal echoes, the transverse processes and vertebral bodies are delineated.[16] This is the coronal plane in which to screen for spinal defects.[16]

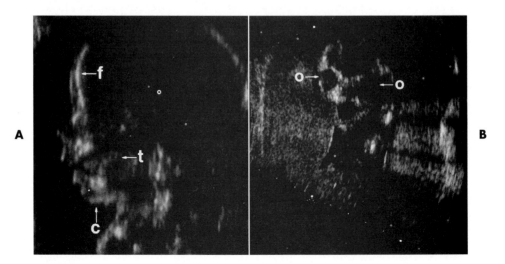

Figure 28-19 A, Sagittal view in a 23-week fetus, showing the contour of the face in profile. Note the smooth surface of the frontal bone *(f),* the appearance of the nose and upper and lower lips; tongue *(t),* and chin *(c).* **B,** Coronal facial view in an 18-week fetus, revealing a wide-open mouth. Note the nasal bones between the orbits *(o).*

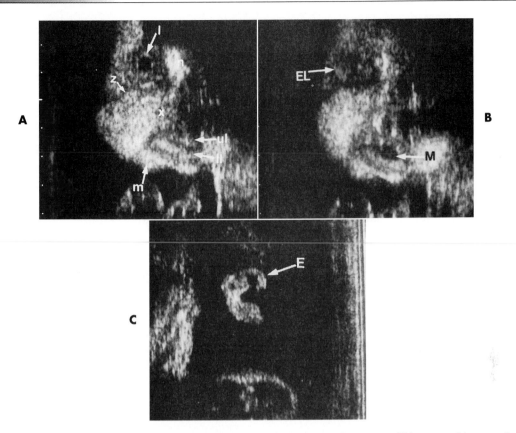

Figure 28-20   **A,** Coronal view showing facial features. *l,* Lens; *ll,* lower lip; *m,* mandible; *n,* nasal bones; *ul,* upper lip; *x,* maxilla; *z,* zygomatic bone. **B,** In the same fetus the eyelids *(EL)* and mouth *(M)* are shown. **C,** In the same fetus the ear *(E)* is shown.

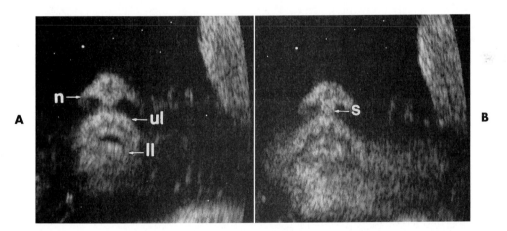

Figure 28-21   **A,** Axial view through the upper *(ul)* and lower lip *(ll)* in a fetus with an open mouth. Note the nares *(n)* and nasal septum. This is the view used to check for a cleft of the upper lip. **B,** In the same fetus, same anatomy viewed with a closed mouth. *s,* Nasal septum.

Transverse. In a transverse plane the spinal column appears as a closed circle, indicating closure of the neural tube. The circle of echoes represents the center of the vertebral body and the posterior elements (laminae or pedicles) (Figure 28-27).[12] These elements should be identified in the normal fetus, whereas the pedicles appear splayed in a V-, C-, or U-shaped configuration and the posterior ossification echo (vertebral arch) is absent in a fetus with a spinal defect.

Sagittal. When evaluating the spine in the sagittal plane, it is imperative for the sonographer to align the transducer in a perpendicular axis to the spinal elements. Incorrect angles may falsely indicate an abnormality. The spinal muscles and posterior skin border are viewed posterior to the circular ring of the ossification centers (see Figure 28-27). It is important to note the integrity of the skin surface because this membrane is absent in fetuses with open spina bifida. Inspection of the spine is often impossible when the fetus is lying with the

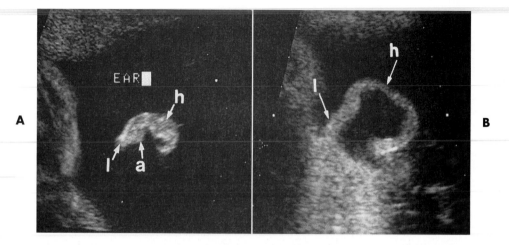

Figure 28-22 A, The external ear observed in a 26-week fetus showing the helix *(h),* lobule *(l),* and antitragus *(a).* At 36 weeks of gestation, the lobule *(l)* and helix *(h)* are observed.

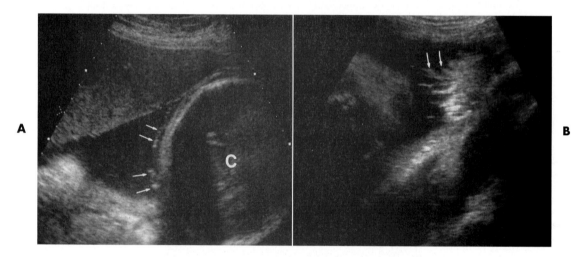

Figure 28-23 A, Fetal hair *(arrows)* observed as a series of dots around the periphery of the fetal cranium in a 39-week fetus. *C,* Cranium. **B,** Long hair *(arrows)* observed in a 34-week fetus.

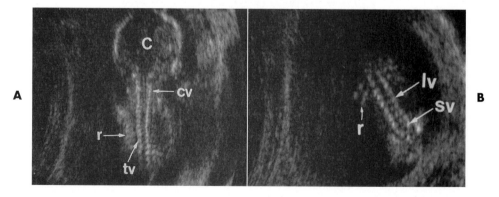

Figure 28-24 A, Coronal view of the fetal spine in a 15-week fetus outlining the cervical vertebrae, *(cv)* and cranium *(C).* The thoracic vertebrae *(tv)* are visualized distally. The rib *(r)* aids in localizing the thorax. **B,** In the same fetus a coronal plane outlines the lumbar *(lv)* and sacral vertebrae *(sv). r,* Rib.

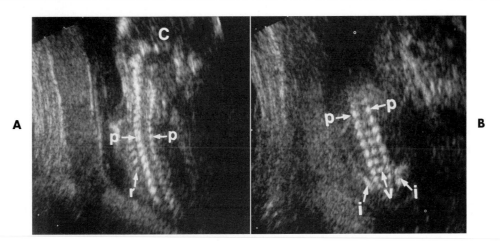

Figure 28-25   **A,** Coronal view of the spine in a 19-week fetus, demonstrating the parallel nature of the posterior elements, or laminae *(p),* of the cervical and thoracic vertebrae. *C,* Cranium; *r,* rib. **B,** In the same fetus the lumbosacral vertebrae are observed in the coronal plane. The posterior elements *(p),* or laminae, and vertebral body *(v)* are noted. In fetuses with spina bifida, widening across the posterior elements may be found (see Chapter 32). *i,* Iliac crest.

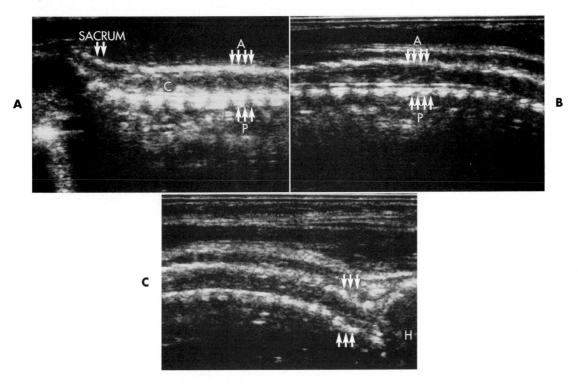

Figure 28-26   Longitudinal sections of the lumbosacral **(A),** thoracic **(B),** and cervical **(C)** spine in a 37-week fetus displaying the anterior *(A)* and posterior *(P)* elements, or laminae. Note the tapering of the spine at the sacrum **(A)** and the widening at the entrance into the base of the skull **(C, H** [head]). Between the posterior elements lies the spinal canal **(A, C)** and cord (may be seen as a linear echo within the spinal canal).

spine down. Optimal viewing of the spine occurs when the fetus is lying on its side in a transverse direction. Often the sonographer will need to ask the mother to turn to either side in an effort to encourage the fetus to change positions so a better scanning window may be obtained.

THE THORAX

Although the fetus is unable to breathe air in utero, the lungs are important landmarks to visualize within the tho-

racic cavity. The lungs serve as lateral borders for the heart and are therefore helpful in assessing the relationship and position of the heart in the chest. Fetal breathing movements are also observed at this level. Like all fetal organs, the lungs are subject to abnormal development. Lung size, texture, and location should be assessed routinely to exclude a lung mass.

The fluid-filled fetal lungs are observed as solid, homogeneous masses of tissue bordered medially by the heart,

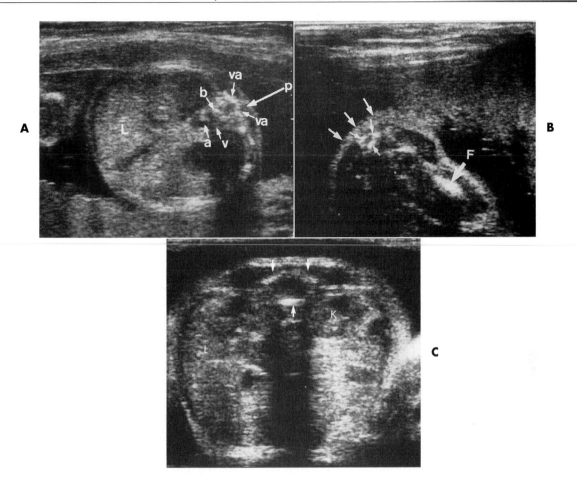

Figure 28-27   A, Transverse scans of the vertebral column showing the echogenic ring produced by the vertebral body and posterior elements, or laminae. Thoracic vertebrae with typical landmarks. *L,* Liver; *a,* aorta; *b,* body; *p,* posterior vertebral muscles; *v,* vena cava; *va,* vertebral arch or posterior elements. **B,** Sacral vertebra outlined *(small arrows).* Note the intact posterior skin wall in this normal fetus *(large arrows). F,* Femur. **C,** Transverse view through the spine at kidney level *(K)* demonstrating the closed-circle appearance *(arrows)* of the spine created by the intact vertebral arch. *L,* Liver.

inferiorly by the diaphragm, and laterally by the rib cage (Figure 28-28). The heart occupies a midline position within the chest; its displacement warrants further study to exclude a possible mass of the lung that may alter the position of the heart.

In sagittal views, lung tissue is present superior to the diaphragm and lateral to the heart (see Figure 28-28). Investigators have attempted to define textural variations of the lung in comparison to the liver.[1] Fetal lung tissue appears more dense than the liver as pregnancy progresses.

The ribs, scapulae, and clavicles are bony landmarks of the chest cavity. Because these structures are composed of bone, acoustic shadowing occurs posteriorly. Portions of the rib cage may be identified when sections are obtained through the posterior aspects of the spine and rib cage (Figure 28-29). Oblique sectioning of the ribs reveals the total length of the ribs, as well as floating ribs. On sagittal planes the echogenic rib interspersed with the intercostal space creates the typical "washboard" appearance of the rib cage (see Figure 28-29). Sound waves strike the rib and are reflected upward, leaving the characteristic void

of echoes posterior to the bony element, whereas sound waves pass through the intercostal space.

On a transverse cross-section through the chest and upper abdomen, the curvature of the rib may be appreciated below the skin. It is important to differentiate the rib from the skin wall, especially when measuring the abdominal circumference. The entire rib cage is impractical to routinely examine, but study of the ribs is warranted in fetuses at risk for congenital rib anomalies (e.g., rib fractures found in osteogenesis imperfecta).

The clavicles are observed in coronal sections through the upper thorax (Figure 28-30). The clavicular length may aid in determining gestational age.[37] In this same view the spinal elements, esophagus, and carotid arteries maybe seen. The clavicles may also be demonstrated as echogenic dots superior to the ribs. Measurements of the clavicles may be useful in predicting congenital clavicular anomalies.

The scapula may be recognized on sagittal sections as a dense linear echo adjacent to the rib shadows, whereas on transverse sections it is viewed medial to the humeral head

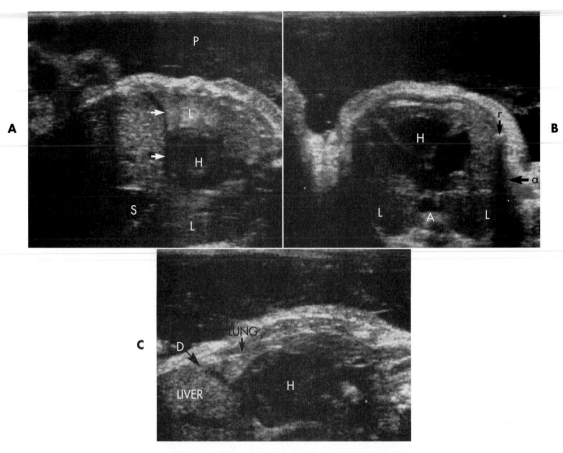

Figure 28-28 **A,** Sagittal scan showing the homogeneous lungs positioned lateral to the heart *(H),* and superior to the diaphragm *(arrows).* Note the normal placement of the stomach *(s)* inferior to the diaphragm. *L,* Lungs; *P,* placenta. **B,** In same fetus a transverse section demonstrates the position of the lungs *(L)* in relationship to the heart *(H).* Note the apex of the heart to the left side of the chest. The base of the heart is in the midline and anterior to the aorta *(A).* Displacement or shifting of the heart should alert the scanner to search for a mass of the lungs, heart, or diaphragm. Note the rib *(r)* and resultant acoustic shadow *(a).* **C,** In the late third trimester of pregnancy the lung tissue can be observed and compared with the liver texture. *D,* Diaphragm; *H,* heart.

(see Figure 28-30). Oblique views demonstrate the entire length of the scapula. The sternum may be seen in axial sections as a bony sequence of echoes beneath the anterior chest wall.

THE HEART

Most major anomalies of the fetal heart are excluded when cardiac anatomy appears normal in the four-chamber view of the heart. The four-chamber assessment is commonly undertaken during a basic fetal scan. The four cardiac chambers and related valves and structures may be observed when the fetus is on its side or in the spine-down position (Figure 28-31). The fetal heart is positioned transversely in the chest. The scanner should assess the following in the four-chamber view:

- Cardiac position, proper situs, and axis. The apex of the heart should point to the fetal left side.
- Presence of the right ventricle (the ventricle found when a line is drawn from the spine to the anterior chest wall) and left ventricle.

- Equal-size ventricles. By the end of pregnancy, the right ventricle may be larger than the left ventricle.[34]
- Presence of equal-size right and left atria, with the foramen ovale opening toward the left atrium as blood is shunted from the right atrium, bypassing the lungs.
- An interventricular septum that appears uninterrupted. The septum appears wider toward the ventricles and thin as it courses cephalad within the heart.
- Normal placement of the tricuspid and mitral valves. The tricuspid valve inserts lower, or closer to the apex, than the mitral valve. Both valves should open during diastole and close during systole.
- Normal rhythm and rate (120 to 160 beats per minute).

In fetuses at high risk for a cardiac anomaly, targeted fetal echocardiography is recommended to evaluate the outflow tracts (aorta and pulmonary artery relationships) (Figure 28-32), pulmonic valve and veins, and other complex cardiac relationships beyond the scope of a basic scan. (For further discussion of normal cardiac anatomy, physiology, and targeted echocardiography see Chapter 40.)

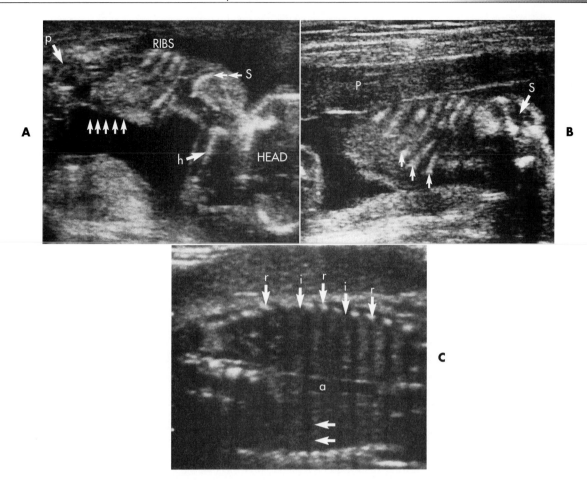

Figure 28-29 A, Sagittal view showing the rib cage, scapula *(S)*, anterior abdominal wall *(arrows)*, and humerus *(h)* in a fetus in a back-up position. *p,* Pelvis. **B,** Tangential view depicting the length of the ribs *(arrows)*. *P,* Placenta; *S,* shoulder. **C,** Sagittal view of the rib cage. Note that the sound waves are unable to pass through the bony rib, resulting in a shadow of echoes *(arrows)* posterior to the ribs *(r)*. Sound passes through the intercostal space *(i)*. *a,* Aorta.

THE DIAPHRAGM AND THORACIC VESSELS

The diaphragm is the muscle that separates the thorax and abdomen and is commonly viewed in the longitudinal plane. The diaphragm lies inferior to the heart and lungs and superior to the liver, stomach, and spleen (Figure 28-33).

The diaphragm may be more obvious on the right side because of the strong liver interface, but attempts to observe an intact left diaphragm are encouraged because diaphragmatic defects occur on both sides of the diaphragm. The stomach should be viewed inferior to the diaphragm, which generally excludes a left-side diaphragmatic hernia.

Vascular structures may be observed within the thoracic cavity and neck. Vessels emanating from the heart are visible within the fetal neck. The carotid arteries (lateral to the esophagus) and the jugular veins (lateral to the carotid arteries) are frequently noted when the fetal neck is extended (Figure 28-34).

The trachea may be identified as a midline structure in both sagittal and transverse planes. The esophagus and oropharynx help determine the location of the carotid arteries and are outlined when amniotic fluid is swallowed by the fetus (Figure 28-35).

The aorta, inferior vena cava, and superior vena cava are routinely observed. The aorta is recognized on sagittal planes as it exits the left ventricle and forms the aortic arch (see Figure 28-33). The vessels branching cephalad into the brain may be observed in the cooperative fetus as they arise from the superior wall of the aortic arch. The innominate artery, left common carotid artery, and left subclavian artery may be identified (Figure 28-36).[20]

As the vessels course posteriorly, the thoracic aorta and descending aorta are observed coursing into the bifurcation of the common iliac arteries (Figure 28-37). The sonographer should recognize the characteristic arterial pulsations from the aorta and its branches. Further divisions of the aorta may be observed as the sonographer views the common iliac vessels, internal iliac vessels, and umbilical arteries (diverging laterally around the bladder) (see Figure 28-40). The external iliac arteries are observed as they en-

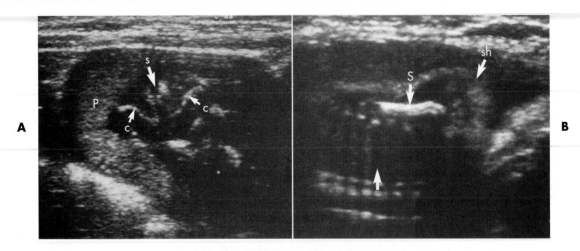

Figure 28-30 **A,** Coronal section of upper thoracic cavity showing the clavicles *(c)* and spine *(s)*. *P,* Placenta. **B,** Sagittal section demonstrating the scapula *(s)* in relationship to the shoulder *(sh)* and ribs *(arrow)*.

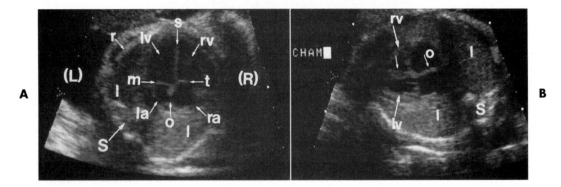

Figure 28-31 **A,** The four-chambered heart view is demonstrated in a 31-week fetus with the spine in the 7-o'clock position. The fetal right side is down and the left side is up. Structures observed are the right *(rv)* and left *(lv)* ventricles; the interventricular septum *(s)*, dividing the two ventricular chambers; and the left *(la)* and right *(ra)* atria. The foramen ovale *(o)*, which allows blood to shunt from the right to left atrium, permits the majority of blood to bypass the lungs. The flap of the foramen ovale is positioned within the left atrium. The atrioventricular valves (mitral and tricuspid) are viewed in systole (closed position). The tricuspid valve allows blood to move from the right atrium to the right ventricle *(rv)*, and the mitral valve *(m)* regulates blood flow from the left atrium to the left ventricle *(lv)*. Note the normal central position of the heart bordered by the lungs *(l)*. The apex of the heart is pointed to the fetal left side *(L)*. When a line is drawn from the spine *(S)* to the anterior chest wall the right ventricle is found. *R,* Fetal right side; *r,* rib. **B,** In a 30-week fetus the heart is observed in the 5-o'clock position. The fetal left side is down. The lungs *(l)* are viewed bordering the heart laterally. The muscularity of the interventricular septum *(arrow)* is observed along with the foramen ovale *(o)*, separating the atrial chambers. *lv,* Left ventricle; *rv,* right ventricle; *S,* spine.

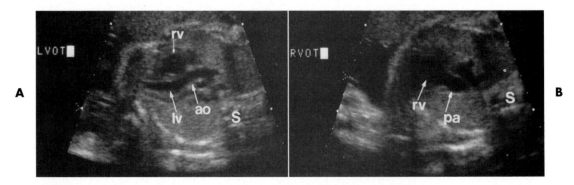

Figure 28-32 **A,** The left ventricular outflow tract *(LVOT)* is observed as the aorta *(ao)* exits the left ventricle *(lv)*. *rv,* Right ventricle; *S,* spine. **B,** The right ventricular outflow tract *(RVOT)* is observed as the pulmonary artery *(pa)* exits the right ventricle. The *LVOT* and *RVOT* should course perpendicularly to each other. *S,* Spine.

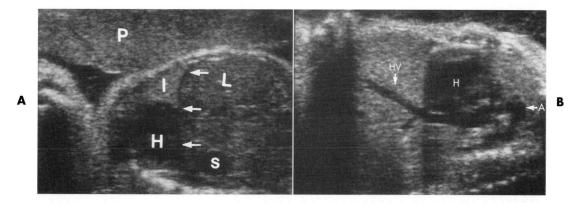

Figure 28-33 A, Sagittal scan showing the diaphragm *(arrows)* separating the thoracic and abdominal cavities. *H,* Heart; *L,* liver; *l,* lung; *P,* placenta; *s,* stomach;. **B,** Sagittal view showing a hepatic vessel *(HV)* coursing through the liver before joining the inferior vena cava as it passes through the diaphragm and empties into the right atrium. Note the aortic arch, *(A)* exiting the heart *(H)* superiorly.

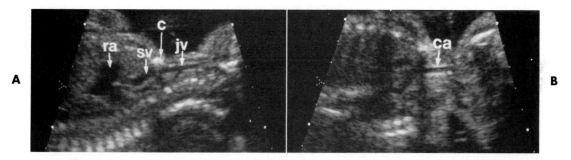

Figure 28-34 A, The jugular vein *(jv)* is observed laterally as it empties into the superior vena cava *(sv)* with drainage into the right atrium *(ra)* in a 25-week fetus. *c,* Clavicle. This sagittal position is helpful in looking for neck masses such as a goiter (enlarged thyroid gland). **B,** A carotid artery *(ca)* is observed in a more medial location coursing cephalad into the brain.

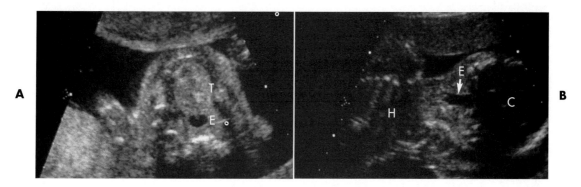

Figure 28-35 A, Cross-section through the tongue *(T)* and esophagus *(E)* or oropharynx in a 24-week fetus. Recent swallowing of amniotic fluid by the fetus allows visualization of these structures. **B,** Fluid-filled esophagus *(E)* or oropharynx seen in a longitudinal view. The bolus of swallowed amniotic fluid will travel to the stomach. *C,* Cranium; *H,* heart.

ter the femoral arteries.[20] The aorta is observed in a transverse plane to the left of the spine.

The inferior vena cava is identified coursing to the right and parallel with the aorta.[20] Transversely, the inferior vena cava is seen anterior and to the right of the spine. It is important to note that the inferior vena cava appears anterior to the aorta within the chest as the vena cava enters anteriorly at the junction of the right atrium.[20]

The hepatic veins may be imaged in sagittal planes or in cephalad-directed transverse planes. The right, left, and middle hepatic vessels are often delineated and followed as they drain into the inferior vena cava (see Figure 28-38).[20]

Differentiation of a hepatic and portal vessel may be possible by evaluating the thickness of the vessel wall. In general, the walls of the portal vessels are more echogenic than those of hepatic vessels.

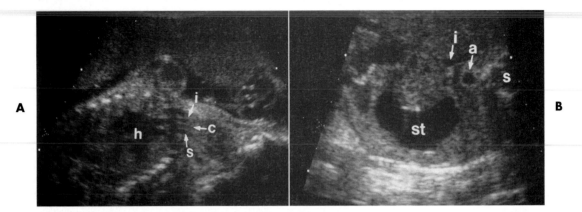

Figure 28-36 **A,** The aortic arch branches are shown in a 35-week fetus with an extended neck. *c,* Left common carotid artery; *h,* heart; *i,* innominate artery; *s,* left subclavian artery. **B,** Aorta *(a)* visualized to the left of the spine *(s)* in a transverse cross-section. *i,* Inferior vena cava; *st,* stomach.

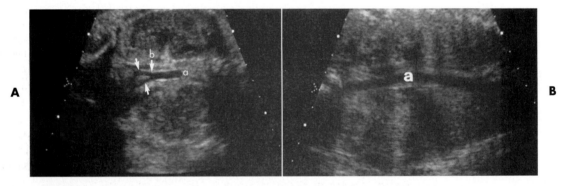

Figure 28-37 **A,** The bifurcation *(b)* of the aorta *(a)* into the common iliac arteries *(small arrows)* is viewed in a 32-week fetus. **B,** In the same fetus a sagittal plane shows the abdominal portion of the aorta *(a).*

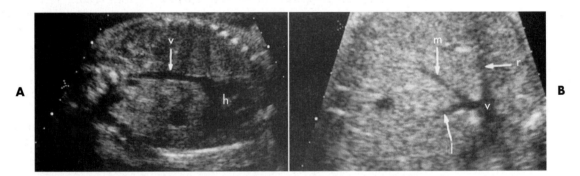

Figure 28-38 **A,** Sagittal view of the inferior vena cava *(v)* entering the right atrium of the heart *(h).* **B,** The left *(l),* middle *(m),* and right *(r)* hepatic veins are shown emptying into the inferior vena cava *(v).*

Divisions of the inferior vena cava (i.e., renal veins, hepatic veins, and iliac veins) may be observed. The superior vena cava may be outlined entering the right atrium from above the heart. By following the superior vena cava into the neck, the jugular veins may be observed.

THE UPPER QUADRANT AND FETAL CIRCULATION
The fetal hepatobiliary system includes the liver, portal venous system, hepatic veins and arteries, gallbladder, and bile ducts. The circulation and purification of fetal blood between the placenta and hepatobiliary system is unique to intrauterine life. The lungs do not purify the blood with oxygen because this occurs within the placenta. The liver serves the important function of shunting oxygen-rich blood from the placenta to the heart, brain, and body organs (Figure 28-39).

Oxygenated blood from the placenta flows through the umbilical vein, within the umbilical cord, to the fetal umbilicus, where it enters the abdomen (Figure 28-40). Deoxygenated blood exits the fetus through the umbilical ar-

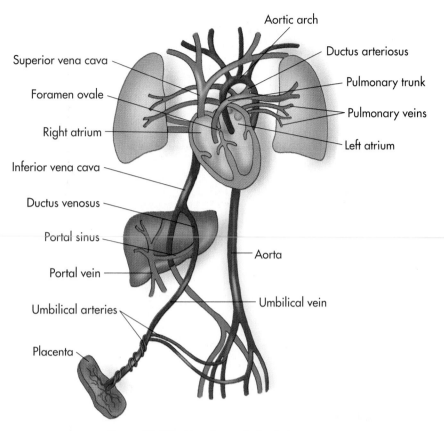

Figure 28-39 Fetoplacental circulation.

teries from the iliac arteries, returning blood to the placenta for purification.

From the umbilicus, the umbilical vein courses cephalad along the falciform ligament to the liver, where it connects with the left portal vein (Figure 28-41). The left portal vein courses posteriorly to meet the right anterior and right posterior portal veins (Figure 28-42). This blood then filters into the liver sinusoids, returning to the inferior vena cava by drainage into the hepatic veins.

A special vascular connection, the **ductus venosus,** carries oxygen-rich blood from the umbilical vein directly to the inferior vena cava, which empties directly into the right atrium. This blood bypasses the liver. Inferior vena cava blood flows from the right atrium through the left atrium by way of the foramen ovale. This blood bypasses the lungs. Less oxygenated blood from the superior vena cava and a small portion of blood from the inferior vena cava empty into the right atrium and into the right ventricle. Both ventricles pump blood into systemic circulation at the same time. Blood ejected from the left ventricle flows to the ascending aorta and to the fetal brain. From the right ventricle, the blood courses from the pulmonary artery into the ductus arteriosus and through the descending aorta to provide oxygenated blood to the abdominal organs. Only 5% to 10% of the blood actually circulates to the lungs.[11]

The liver is a large organ filling most of the upper abdomen. The left lobe of the liver is larger than the right lobe because of the large quantity of oxygenated blood flowing through the left lobe. The liver appears pebble-gray and is discerned by its corresponding portal and hepatic vessels. The liver borders may be seen by viewing the diaphragm at the cephalad margin and the small bowel distally in the sagittal plane (Figure 28-43). The fetal liver is the main storage site for glucose and is very sensitive to disturbances in growth; therefore this is the site at which abdominal measurements reflect liver size. It is important to check for any collections of fluid around the liver margins, because this indicates ascites (fluid retention resulting from anemia, heart failure, or congenital anomalies). Masses of the liver are uncommon but may be detected.

The fetal gallbladder appears as a cone-shaped or teardrop–shaped cystic structure located in the right upper abdomen just below the left portal vein (see Figure 28-42). The gallbladder should not be misinterpreted as the left portal vein. The left portal vein is a midline vessel that appears more tubular and can be traced back to the umbilical insertion.

The fetal pancreas may be seen posterior to the stomach and anterior to the splenic vein when the fetus is lying with the spine down.[16,23]

The spleen may be observed by scanning transversely and posteriorly to the left of the stomach (Figure 28-44). Recognition of the spleen is helpful when assessing the

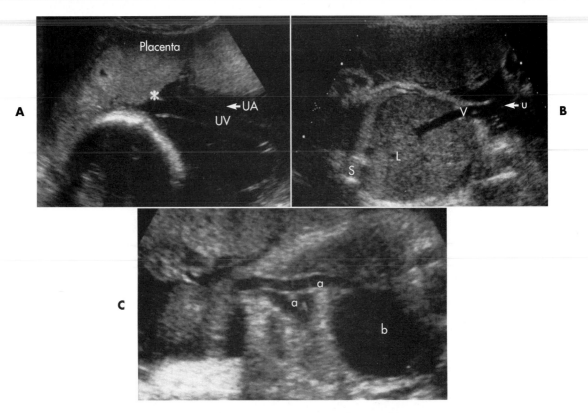

Figure 28-40 **A,** Oxygenated blood leaving the placenta travels through the umbilical vein *(UV)* to the fetal umbilicus. *UA,* Umbilical artery; *asterisk,* placental cord insertion. **B,** The umbilical vein *(v)* after entering at the umbilicus *(u)* courses cephalad and into the liver *(L). s,* Spine. **C,** The umbilical arteries *(a)* enter the umbilicus and course laterally around the bladder *(b)* to meet the common iliac arteries.

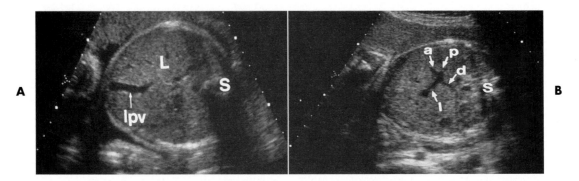

Figure 28-41 **A,** Transverse section of the liver in a 31-week fetus outlining the course of the left portal vein *(lpv)* at its entrance into the liver *(L)* from the fetal umbilical cord insertion. The left portal vein ascends upward and into the liver tissue. *S,* Spine. **B,** The left portal vein *(l)* is shown to bifurcate into the portal sinus, right anterior *(a)* and right posterior *(p)* portal veins. The ductus venosus *(d)* is observed before its drainage into the inferior vena cava. *S,* Spine.

sensitized pregnancy (anti-D) to check for enlargement resulting from increased blood production (hematopoiesis) or to screen for anomalies of the spleen, such as absence of duplication defects.[35]

THE GASTROINTESTINAL SYSTEM

The fetal gastrointestinal tract comprises the esophagus, stomach, and small and large intestines (colon). The esophagus may be recognized after fetal ingestion of am-

niotic fluid, which may be traced during swallowing into the oral cavity, through the hypopharynx, and as it travels downward toward the stomach (see Figure 2-35).

The stomach becomes apparent as early as the 11th week of gestation as swallowed amniotic fluid fills the stomach cavity.[30] The full stomach should be seen in all fetuses beyond the 16th week of gestation. Some conditions prohibit normal filling of the stomach, such as diminished amounts of amniotic fluid (fetuses with rupture of the

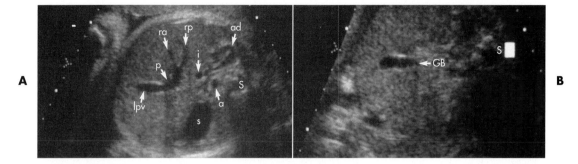

Figure 28-42   A, Transverse section of the liver and related structures in 32-week fetus showing the left portal vein *(lpv)* coursing into the portal sinus *(p).* The blood then moves into the right anterior *(ra)* and right posterior *(rp)* portal veins and ductus venosus (see Figure 28-41, *B*). The right adrenal gland *(ad),* fluid-filled stomach *(s),* aorta *(a),* and inferior vena cava, *(i)* are shown. **B,** The gallbladder *(GB)* is viewed in the right upper quadrant of the abdomen in a 32-week fetus. The teardrop shape of the gallbladder should be distinguished from the left portal vein. *S,* Spine.

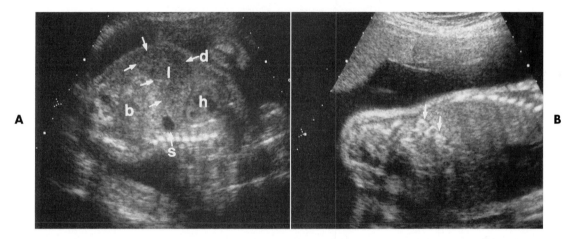

Figure 28-43   A, Liver *(l, arrows)* bordered by the diaphragm *(d)* superiorly and bowel inferiorly in a 29-week fetus. *b,* bowel; *h,* heart; *s,* stomach. **B,** Small bowel *(arrows)* pictured as small fluid-filled rings.

membranes) or blockage that prevents the stomach from filling (esophageal atresia). On occasion, the stomach has emptied into the small bowel before scanning and is not observed. Repeat studies to confirm the presence of the stomach are warranted. Enlargement of the stomach may occur when a fetus ingests a large quantity of amniotic fluid (non–insulin-dependent diabetic pregnancies) or when a congenital anomaly prohibits normal swallowing (duodenal atresia).

Normal bowel may be distinguished prenatally by observing characteristic sonographic patterns for each segment. Beyond 20 weeks of gestation, small bowel may be differentiated from large bowel. Small bowel appears to occupy a central position within the lower abdomen, with a cluster appearance of the bowel loops. Peristalsis and even fluid-filled small bowel loops may be observed (see Figures 28-43 and 28-44).

The large intestine with the ascending, transverse, and descending colon and rectum are identified by their peripheral locations in the lower pelvis (see Figure 28-44). The large bowel typically contains meconium particles and

may measure up to 20 mm in the preterm fetus and even larger near the time of birth or in the postdate fetus.[31]

THE URINARY SYSTEM

The urinary system of the fetus comprises the kidneys, adrenal glands, ureters, and bladder.

The kidneys are located on either side of the spine in the posterior abdomen and are apparent as early as the 15th week of pregnancy.[3] The appearance of the developing kidney changes with advancing gestational age. In the second trimester of pregnancy the kidneys appear as ovoid retroperitoneal structures that lack distinctive borders. The pelvocaliceal center may be difficult to define in early pregnancy, whereas with continued maturation of the kidneys the borders become more defined and the renal pelvis becomes more distinct (Figure 28-45).[3] The renal pelvis appears as an echo-free area in the center of the kidney.

The normal renal pelvis appears to contain a small amount of fluid. This most often represents a normal finding during pregnancy. A renal pelvis that measures greater

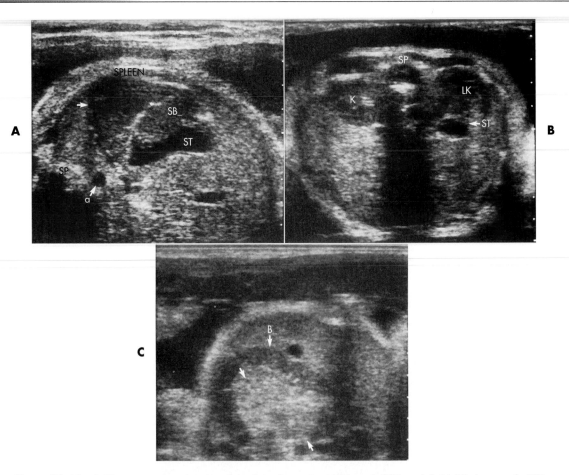

Figure 28-44 **A,** Transverse scan showing the spleen *(arrows)*, small bowel *(SB)*, and fluid-filled stomach *(ST)*. *a,* Aorta; *SP,* spine shadow. **B,** Transverse section showing the right kidney *(K)* and stomach *(ST)* anterior to the left kidney *(LK)* in a fetus in a spine-up position *(SP)*. **C,** Transverse view of the transverse colon *(B)* and small bowel *(arrows)* in a fetus in a spine-down position.

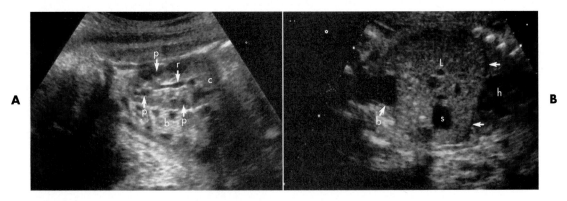

Figure 28-45 **A,** Longitudinal view of the kidney in a 35-week fetus showing the renal cortex *(c)*, pelvis, and pyramids *(p)*. The kidney is marginated by the renal capsule, which is highly visible later in pregnancy because of perirenal fat. *b,* Bowel; *r,* renal pelvis. **B,** Sagittal view of the fluid-filled bladder *(b)* in the pelvis. Note the more cephalic location of the stomach *(s)* in the upper abdomen. *h,* Heart; *L,* liver, Diaphragm *(arrows)*.

than 10 mm beyond 20 weeks of gestation is considered abnormal.[13] It is common to see extra fluid within the renal pelvis in fetuses with extra amounts of amniotic fluid and when the mother has a full bladder. There has been some association of renal pelvis dilation and chromosomal abnormalities.[13]

By the third trimester of pregnancy, internal renal anatomy becomes clear with observation of the renal pyramids (lining up in sequence in anterior and posterior rows), the cortex or medulla, and renal margins (perirenal and sinus fat at this age allows clear visualization) (see Figures 28-44 and 28-45).

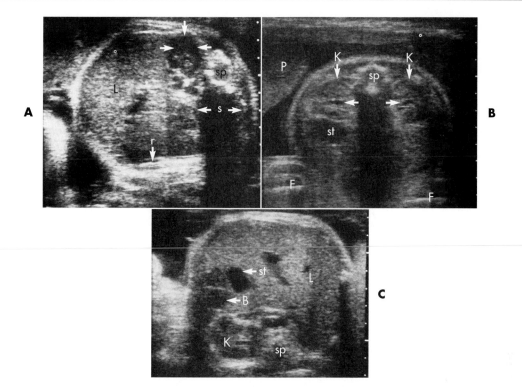

Figure 28-46   A, When the fetus is lying on its side, the upper kidney *(arrows)* is observed adjacent to the spine *(sp)*. The kidney on the bottom is shadowed *(s)* by the spine. *L,* Liver; *r,* rib. **B,** Kidneys *(K)* observed in a spine-up position *(sp)*. Note the renal pelvises *(arrows)*, which are filled with urine—a normal pregnancy finding. The stomach *(st)* is found anterior to the left kidney. Note the spine shadow. *F,* Femurs; *P,* placenta. **C,** When the fetus is lying with the spine *(sp)* down the kidneys are viewed. The left kidney *(K)* is visible posterior to the bowel *(B)* and the stomach *(st)*. The right kidney is located slightly below this level. *L,* Liver.

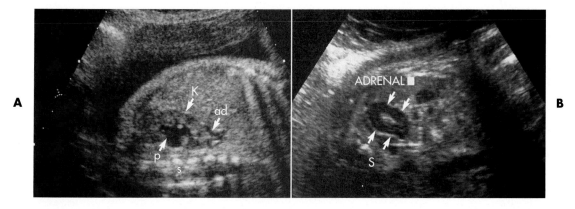

Figure 28-47   A, The adrenal gland *(ad)* is observed in a sagittal view in a 32-week fetus. The adrenal is located above the kidney *(K)* in this spine-down *(s)* position. The texture of the adrenal gland is similar to that of the kidney; often, when a kidney is missing (agenesis), the adrenal is mistaken for the kidney. *p,* Renal pelvis. **B,** The rice-grain appearance of the adrenal gland *(arrows)* is depicted in this transverse plane in a 36-week fetus. Note the dense central interface. *S,* Stomach.

The kidneys appear as elliptic structures when scanning in the longitudinal axis and appear circular in their retroperitoneal locations adjacent to the spine in transverse views. Commonly, in a transverse position the bottom or distal kidney may be shadowed by the acoustic spine. By rotating to the sagittal plane, the distal kidney may be imaged. With the fetus in the spine-up or spine-down position, the kidneys are observed lateral to the spine (see Figure 28-46).

The length, width, thickness, and volume of the kidney have been determined for different gestational ages.[17] This information is useful when a renal malformation is suspected.

The fetal adrenal glands are most frequently observed in a transverse plane just above the kidneys. The adrenals are seen as early as the 20th week of pregnancy and by 23 weeks assume a rice-grain appearance (Figure 28-47).[21] The center of the adrenal gland appears as a central echogenic line surrounded by tissue that is less echogenic. The central midline interface widens after the 35th week of gestation.[21] The transverse aorta may be used to locate the left adrenal because of its close proximity to the anterior surface of the gland. Likewise, the inferior vena cava is helpful in isolating the right adrenal. Occasionally the adrenal glands may be identified in sagittal planes, although rib shadowing may interfere with their recognition.

It is important to realize that adrenal glands may normally appear large in utero and should not be confused with the kidneys. Nomograms for normal adrenal size are available.[21]

The normal fetal ureter, at 1 mm, is too small to be recognized. Dilated or obstructed ureters (hydroureter) are readily apparent.

The urinary bladder is visualized in either transverse or sagittal sections through the anterior lower pelvis (see Figures 28-40 and 28-45). The bladder is located in the midline and appears as a round, fluid-filled cavity. The size of the bladder varies, depending on the amount of the urine contained within the bladder cavity. A fetus generally voids at least once an hour, so failure to see the bladder should prompt the investigator to recheck for bladder filling.

The bladder should be visualized in all normal fetuses. The fetal bladder is an important indicator of renal function. When the bladder and amniotic fluid appear normal, one may assume that at least one kidney is functioning. If one fails to identify the urinary bladder in the presence of oligohydramnios (severe lack of amniotic fluid), one should suspect a renal abnormality or premature rupture of the membranes (the bladder may not be full because of decreased ingestion of fluid).

The fetal bladder size may appear increased in pregnancies complicated by polyhydramnios (large quantities of amniotic fluid).

THE GENITALIA

Identification of the male and female genitalia is possible provided the fetal legs are abducted and a sufficient quantity of amniotic fluid is present. Providing information regarding gender identification is clinically important when a fetus is at risk for a gender-linked disorder (e.g., aqueductal stenosis, hemophilia). Information regarding the gender of the fetus may have significant emotional impact; therefore guidelines should be established within each department regarding whether this information should be given. Only those investigators with proven gender detection skills should attempt to provide this information.

When attempting to localize the genitalia, the scanner should follow the long axis of the fetus toward the hips. The bladder is a helpful landmark within the pelvis by which to identify the anteriorly located genital organs. Tangential scanning planes directed between the thighs are useful in defining the genitalia. The gender of the fetus may be appreciated as early as 14 to 16 weeks of gestation, although clear delineation may not be possible until the 20th to 22nd weeks. When the fetus is in a breech lie, gender may be impossible to determine.

The female genitalia may be seen in a transverse plane. The thighs and labia are identified ventral to the bladder, whereas in tangential projections, the entire labial folds, and often the labia minora, are demonstrated (Figure 28-48). In scans of the perineum obtained parallel to the femurs the shape of the genitalia appears rhomboid (Figure 28-49).[16] Keep in mind that the labia may appear edematous and swollen. This normal finding should not be confused with the scrotum.

The scrotum and penis are fairly easy to recognize in either scanning plane (Figure 28-50). The male genitalia may be differentiated as early as the 15th and 16th weeks of pregnancy. The scrotal sac is seen as a mass of soft tissue between the hips with the scrotal septum and testicles. Fluid around the testicles (hydrocele) is a common benign finding during intrauterine life.

THE UPPER AND LOWER EXTREMITIES

The fetal limbs are accessible to both anatomic and biometric surveillance. Bones of the upper and lower appendicular skeleton have been described extensively, and many nomograms detailing normal growth patterns for each limb have been generated.[19]

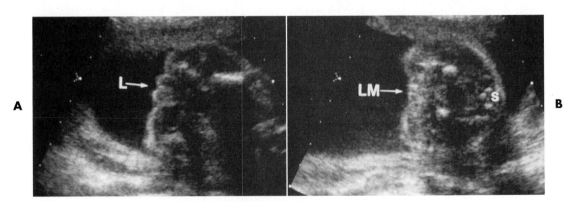

Figure 28-48 **A,** Female genitalia viewed axially in a 23-week fetus, showing the typical appearance of the labia majora *(L).* **B,** In the same fetus the labia minora *(LM)* are represented as linear structures between the labia majora. *s,* Spine.

Fetal long-bone measurements help assess fetal age and growth and allow detection of skeletal dysplasias and various congenital limb malformations. The sonographer must attempt to not only measure fetal limb bones but also survey the anatomic configurations of the individual bones whenever possible for evidence of bowing, fractures, or demineralization, as seen in several common forms of skeletal dysplasias.

The upper extremity consists of the humerus, elbow, radius, ulna, wrist, metacarpals, and phalanges.

Coronally, the hands and fingers may be viewed when opened. When the fingers are viewed in the sagittal plane, individual phalanges, interphalangeal joints, metacarpals, and digits may be observed (Figures 28-51 to 28-54). The hand movement may be studied to assess fetal tone for one component of the biophysical profile. Individual fingers may be assessed and counted. This is more commonly attempted if an anomaly is suspected, as with some chromosome disorders, such as trisomy 18, in which clenching of the hands is common, or when an anomaly is found.

The humerus is found in a sagittal plane by moving the probe laterally away from the ribs and scapula. The long axis of the humerus should be seen lateral to the scapular echo. The cartilaginous humeral head is noted, as well as the cartilage at the elbow (see Figure 28-51). The shaft of the humerus should be seen, along with its characteristic acoustic shadow. Keep in mind that only the first echo interface of the bone is represented. The remainder of the bone is shadowed; therefore the width of the bone is actually larger than what may be appreciated. The muscles and skin may be noted. Epiphyseal ossification centers may be apparent around the 39th week of pregnancy.[26] In transverse planes the humerus appears as a solitary bone surrounded by muscle and skin.

By tracing the humerus to the elbow, the radius and ulna are imaged (see Figures 28-51 and 28-52). In transverse sections, two bones are seen as echogenic dots, whereas in a sagittal plane the long axis of each is identified. The laterally positioned ulna projects deeper into the elbow, which is helpful in differentiating this bone from the medially located radius. When the transducer is moved downward, the wrist and hand are observed.

Adequate amounts of amniotic fluid are essential to evaluate the hands or feet. With oligohydramnios, these areas are generally impossible to localize.

Nomograms have been generated to determine the normal lengths of the humerus, radius, and ulna for age assessment.[19] These values are also beneficial in diagnosing

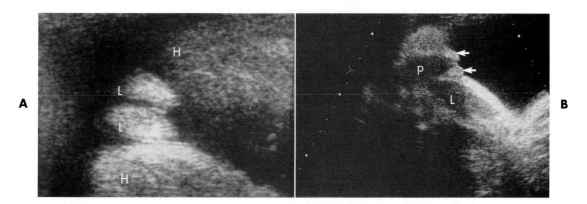

Figure 28-49 **A,** The labia majora *(L)* are imaged in a sagittal plane. *H,* Hips. **B,** The rhomboid-shaped perineum *(p)* is shown in a plane that runs parallel to the femur *(L).* The labia *(arrows)* are observed in a more frontal plane.

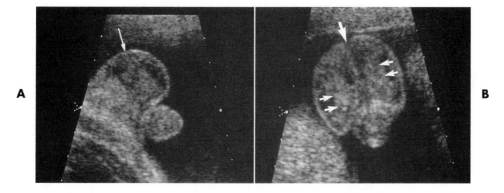

Figure 28-50 **A,** Male genitalia in a 40-week fetus showing the scrotum *(arrow)* and phallus. **B,** Coronal view of the male genitalia outlining descended testicles *(double arrows)* within the scrotum. Note the scrotal septum *(thick arrow)* and phallus.

abnormal developmental growth of the extremities as seen in certain skeletal dysplasias.

Like the upper extremity, the bones of the lower extremity are accessible for dating and for detecting limb anomalies.

The femur is the most widely measured long bone and can be found by moving the transducer along the fetal body down to the fetal bladder. At this junction, the iliac wings are noted. By moving the transducer inferior to the iliac crests, the femoral echo comes into view. With the transducer centered over the femoral echo, one should ro-

tate the probe until the shaft (diaphysis) of the femur is observed. In this view the cartilaginous femoral head, muscles, and occasionally the femoral artery are noted (Figure 28-55).

The distal femoral epiphysis is seen within the cartilage at the knee (see Figure 28-55), and this signifies a gestational age beyond 33 to 35 weeks of gestation.[6] At the tibial end, the proximal tibial epiphyseal center is found after the 35th week of pregnancy (Figure 28-56).[6] Medially, the tibia and laterally positioned fibula (see Figure 28-56) are noted. The tibia is larger than the fibula.

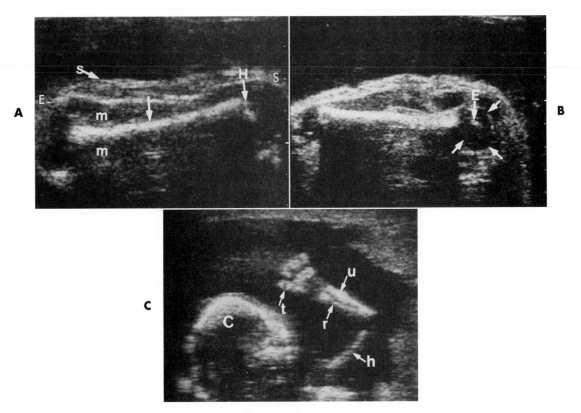

Figure 28-51   **A,** Longitudinal scan of the humeral shaft with the humeral head *(H)* near the shoulder *(s).* Note the muscles *(m)* lateral to the bones and the skin interface *(S). E,* Elbow. **B,** Similar section of a humerus in a 39-week fetus identifying the proximal humeral epiphysis *(E)* within the humeral cartilage *(arrows).* **C,** Sagittal image of the fetal humerus. *c,* Cranium; *h,* hand with thumb, *t,* thumb; *r,* radius; *u,* ulna.

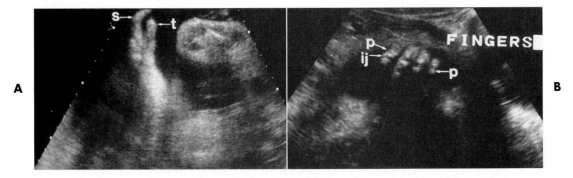

Figure 28-52   **A,** Lateral view of the hand showing the thumb *(t)* and second finger *(s)* in a 36-week fetus. **B,** Curvature of the hand in a 30-week fetus showing the phalanges *(p)* of the second through fifth fingers. The thumb is not imaged in this view because it is located slightly lower. Note the interphalangeal joints *(ij)* between the phalanges.

The ankle, calcaneus, and foot are viewed at the most distal point (Figure 28-57). Individual metatarsals and toes are frequently seen (see Figure 28-57). Like the hands, the fetal feet are prone to malformations, such as extra digits, overlapping, and splaying.

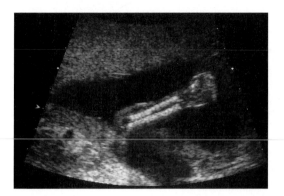

Figure 28-53 Long section of the forearm; the radius is shorter than the ulna (seen along the posterior forearm). The closed fist is shown with the thumb closest to the anterior surface.

THE UMBILICAL CORD

The normal human umbilical cord contains an umbilical vein and two umbilical arteries (Figure 28-58). The umbilical vein transports oxygenated blood from the placenta, whereas the paired umbilical arteries return deoxygenated blood from the fetus to the placenta for purification. The umbilical cord is identified at the cord insertion into the placenta and at the junction of the cord into the fetal umbilicus. The arteries spiral with the larger umbilical vein, which is surrounded by Wharton's jelly (material that supports the cord) (Figure 28-59). Absent cord twists may be associated with a poor pregnancy outcome.[9] The cord is easily imaged in both sagittal and transverse sections. The umbilical vein diameter increases throughout gestation, reaching a maximum diameter of 0.9 cm by 30 weeks of gestation.[27]

Identification of the placental insertion of the cord is important in choosing a site for amniocentesis and in the selection of the appropriate site for cordocentesis. Rarely, the umbilical insertion is atypically located (velamentous insertion).

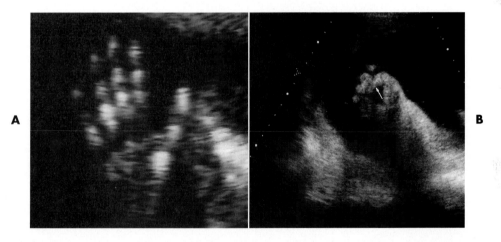

Figure 28-54 **A,** An open hand is shown in a 24-week fetus. **B,** A closed hand is viewed in a 38-week fetus with the thumb crossing in front of the palm of the hand *(arrow)*, with the second through fifth digits identified above the thumb.

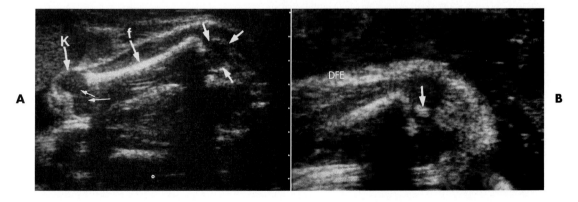

Figure 28-55 **A,** Longitudinal section showing the femoral shaft *(f)*, with the femoral cartilage *(thick arrows)* and epiphyseal cartilage *(thin arrows)* shown at the knee *(K)*. **B,** The distal femoral epiphysis *(arrow)* is clearly shown within the epiphyseal cartilage at the knee in a 42-week fetus. *DFE,* Distal femoral epiphysis.

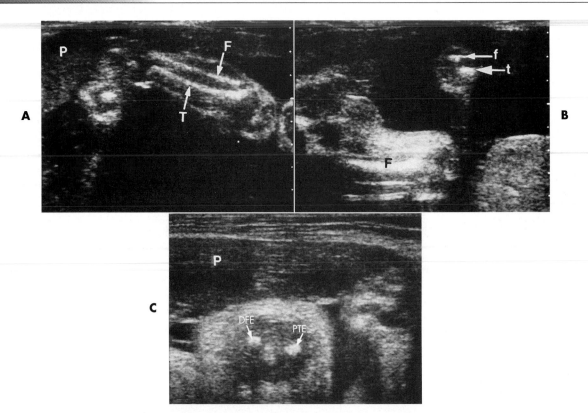

Figure 28-56 **A,** Sagittal view of the medially positioned tibia *(T)* and laterally positioned fibula *(F). P,* Placenta. **B,** In the same fetus a transverse cross-section reveals the two bones. *F,* Fibula; *f,* opposite femur; *t,* tibia. **C,** View of the knee in a 42-week fetus showing both the distal femoral epiphysis (DFE) and proximal tibial epiphysis (PTE). *P,* Placenta.

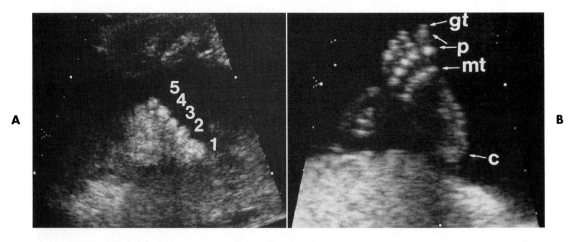

Figure 28-57 **A,** Five toes (*1* to *5*) viewed on end in a 38-week fetus. Note the continuity and shape of each toe. Extra toes, webbing, or clefts are considered abnormal. **B,** Plantar foot view in a 20-week fetus showing five toes and ossified metatarsals *(mt)* and phalanges *(p). c,* Calcaneus; *gt,* great toe.

The insertion of the cord into the fetal umbilicus should be routinely scrutinized in all fetuses because anterior abdominal wall defects are present at this level. Use of color flow imaging may aid in vessel identification (Figure 28-60).

EXTRAFETAL EVALUATION

After the fetus has been studied, evaluation of the placenta, amniotic fluid, and extrauterine areas is recommended. As mentioned previously, the uterus and ovaries should be scrutinized for large masses, such as fibroids or ovarian masses that may alter pregnancy management. This evaluation may be accomplished by surveying the lateral borders of the uterus from the cervix to the fundus along both lateral margins following both sagittal and transverse axes.

The Placenta. The major role of the placenta is to permit the exchange of oxygenated maternal blood (rich in

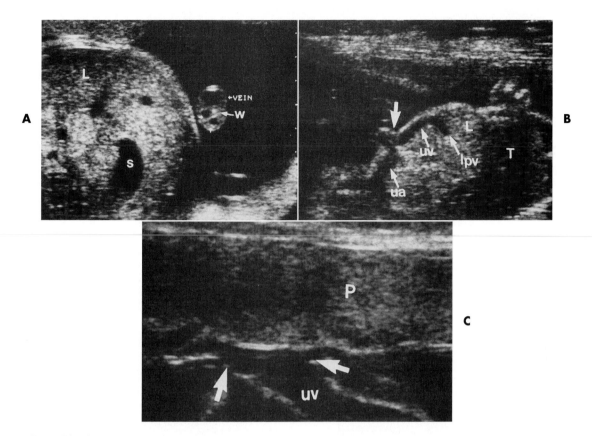

Figure 28-58   A, A three-vessel umbilical cord is shown in a transverse plane represented as paired umbilical arteries *(small arrows)* and a single larger umbilical vein. The vessels are supported by the gelatinous Wharton's jelly *(w)*. A cross-section of the liver *(L)* and stomach *(s)* is in view. **B,** Fetal insertion of the umbilical cord into the umbilicus in a sagittal plane *(arrow)*. The umbilical vein *(uv)* courses superiorly to enter the liver *(L)* and becomes the left portal vein *(lpv)*, whereas the umbilical arteries *(ua)* course posteriorly to join the hypogastric arteries. *T,* Thoracic cavity. **C,** Placental insertion of the umbilical cord showing the umbilical vein *(uv)* at this junction *(arrows)*. *P,* Anterior placenta.

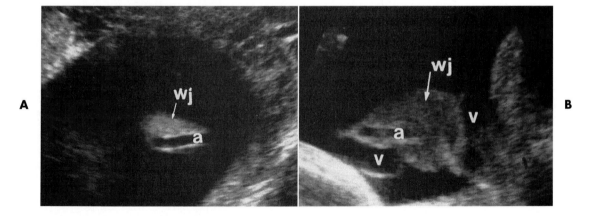

Figure 28-59   A, Wharton's jelly *(wj)* observed in a 30-week fetus. One of the umbilical arteries *(a)* is in view. **B,** Wharton's jelly is present adjacent to one of the umbilical arteries *(a)*, and the single umbilical vein *(v)* is observed in a 35-week fetus. Wharton's jelly is an important structure to recognize in performing cordocentesis procedures when the needle is directed into the cord vessels.

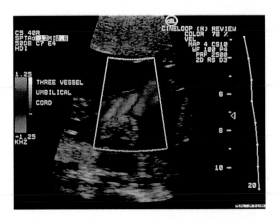

Figure 28-60 Color Doppler image showing the cord insertion into the fetal abdomen.

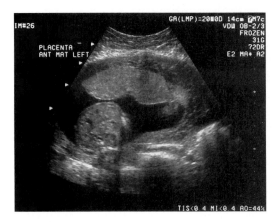

Figure 28-61 The homogeneous placenta is shown along the anterior wall of the uterus. The fetal abdomen is seen in cross-section.

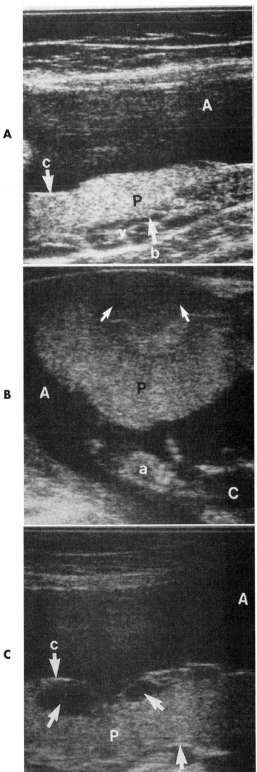

Figure 28-62 A, Posterior placenta (p) at 21 weeks of gestation showing the chorionic plate (c), adjacent to the amniotic cavity (A), and the basal plate (b), closest to the maternal (endometrial) vessels (v). **B,** Anterior placenta (P) at 14 weeks of gestation with evidence of a Braxton-Hicks contraction (arrows). A, Amniotic fluid; C, fetal cranium; a, fetal abdomen. **C,** Posterior placenta (P) at 26 weeks of gestation showing several subchorionic cystic spaces (arrows) that represent blood vessels or fibrin deposits. A, Amniotic fluid; b, basal plate; c, chorionic plate.

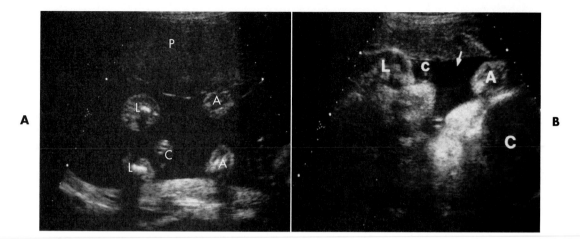

Figure 28-63   A, Amniotic fluid in a 20-week pregnancy outlining the legs *(L)* and arms *(A)*. This is a typical appearance of the abundance of amniotic fluid during this period of pregnancy. *C,* Umbilical cord; *P,* placenta. **B,** Amniotic fluid *(arrow)* in a 35-week pregnancy demonstrating an amniotic fluid pocket *(arrow)* surrounded by fetal parts and the placenta. The amount of amniotic fluid compared with the fetus and placenta is less at this stage of pregnancy. *A,* Arm; *C,* cranium; *c,* umbilical cord; *L,* leg.

oxygen and nutrients) with deoxygenated fetal blood. Maternal vessels coursing posterior to the placenta circulate blood into the placenta, whereas blood from the fetus reaches this point through the umbilical cord.[13]

The substance of the placenta assumes a relatively homogenous pebble-gray appearance during the first part of pregnancy and is easily recognized with its characteristically smooth borders (Figure 28-61). The thickness of the placenta varies with gestational age, with a minimum diameter of 15 mm in fetuses greater than 23 weeks.[16] The size of the placenta rarely exceeds 50 mm in the normal fetus. The sonographer must maintain a perpendicular measurement of the placental width in relation to the myometrial wall when evaluating the width of the placenta.

The position of the placenta is readily apparent on most obstetric ultrasound studies. The placenta may be located within the fundus of the uterus, along the anterior or posterior uterine walls (see Figure 28-62), or laterally, or it may be dangerously implanted over or near the cervix. The sonographer should attempt to carefully define the entire length of the placenta and document both upper and lower margins of this organ.

Occasionally the placenta originates in the fundus and proceeds along the anterior wall (fundal anterior placenta) or along the posterior uterine wall (fundal posterior placenta). When the placenta appears to lie on both anterior or posterior uterine walls, check for a laterally positioned placenta. By moving the transducer laterally one should be able to define the lateral placenta.

The Amniotic Fluid. Amniotic fluid serves several important functions during intrauterine life. It allows the fetus to move freely within the amniotic cavity while maintaining intrauterine temperature and protecting the developing fetus from injury.

Amniotic fluid is produced by the umbilical cord and membranes, lungs, skin, and kidneys.[30] Fetal urination into the amniotic sac accounts for nearly the total volume of amniotic fluid by the second half of pregnancy, so the quantity of fluid is directly related to kidney function.[10] A fetus lacking kidneys or with malformed kidneys produces little or no amniotic fluid. The amount of amniotic fluid is regulated not only by the production of amniotic fluid but also by removal of fluid by swallowing, by fluid exchange within the lungs, and by the membranes and cord. Normal lung development is critically dependent on the exchange of amniotic fluid within the lungs. Inadequate lung development may occur when severe oligohydramnios is present, placing the fetus at high risk for developing small or hypoplastic lungs.

The volume of amniotic fluid increases to the 34th week of gestation and then slowly diminishes.[7] The investigator must be aware of the relative differences in amniotic fluid volume throughout pregnancy. During the second and early third trimesters of pregnancy, amniotic fluid appears to surround the fetus and should be readily apparent (Figure 28-63). From 20 to 30 weeks of gestation, amniotic fluid may appear somewhat generous, although this typically represents a normal amniotic fluid variant. By the end of pregnancy, amniotic fluid is scanty, and isolated fluid pockets may be the only visible areas of fluid. Subjective observation of amniotic fluid volumes throughout pregnancy helps the sonographer determine the norm and extremes of amniotic fluid. The amniotic fluid index aids in estimating the amount of amniotic fluid.

Amniotic fluid generally appears echo-free, although, occasionally, fluid particles (particulate matter) may be seen. Vernix caseosa (fatty material found on fetal skin and in amniotic fluid late in pregnancy) may be seen within the amniotic fluid.

In accordance with the guidelines for obstetric scanning, every obstetric examination should include a thorough evaluation of amniotic fluid volume. When extremes in amniotic fluid volume (hydramnios or oligohydramnios) are found, targeted studies for the exclusion of fetal anomalies are recommended.

ACKNOWLEDGMENT

The author would like to acknowledge the work of Kara L. Mayden Argo on the fourth edition of this book.

REVIEW QUESTIONS

1. What is the purpose of obstetric scanning guidelines as outlined by the ACR, AIUM, and ACOG?
2. Which anatomic and biometric parameters should be included in a basic fetal study?
3. How does a targeted ultrasound study differ from a basic obstetric examination?
4. Why is it important to recognize normal fetal anatomy?
5. Why is determination of fetal presentation clinically important?
6. What is the difference between a cephalic and a breech lie?
7. What is the difference between frank and footling presentation?
8. Why does the fetal cranium appear hypoechoic early in development?
9. Define the following cranial structures: choroid plexus, midline echo complex, ventricular system, cavum septum pellucidi, corpus callosum, circle of Willis, posterior fossa, cerebellar vermis, cisterna magna.
10. Identify the sonographic landmarks of the fetal spine in longitudinal and transverse planes.
11. What is the function of the ductus venosus, foramen ovale, and ductus arteriosus in fetoplacental circulation?
12. Describe how the fetal liver differs from the adult liver.
13. To ensure the presence of a normal genitourinary system when evaluating the fetus during a basic scan, which structures and substances must be observed?
14. At what gestational week should the fetal kidneys be imaged on ultrasound?
15. Describe the protocol utilized by the sonographer to evaluate the upper and lower extremities.
16. Why is the production of amniotic fluid critical to fetal development?

REFERENCES

1. Benson DM and others: Ultrasonic tissue characterization of fetal lung, liver and placenta for the purpose of assessing fetal maturity, *J Ultrasound Med* 2:489, 1983.
2. Birnholz JC: Ultrasonic fetal ophthalmology, *Early Hum Dev* 12:199, 1985.
3. Bowie JD and others: The changing sonographic appearance of fetal kidneys during pregnancy, *J Ultrasound Med* 2:505, 1983.
4. Callen PW, editor: *Ultrasonography obstetrics and gynecology*, ed 2, Philadelphia, 1988, WB Saunders.
5. Cardoza JD, Goldstein RB, Filly RA: Exclusion of fetal ventriculomegaly with a single measurement: the width of the lateral ventricular atrium, *Radiology* 169:711, 1988.
6. Chinn DH and others: Ultrasonic identification of fetal lower extremities epiphyseal ossification centers, *Radiology* 147:815, 1983.
7. Ellis JW: Disorders of the placenta, umbilical cord, and amniotic fluid. In Ellis JW, Beckmann CRB, editors: *A clinical manual of obstetrics*, Norwalk, Conn, 1983, Appleton-Century-Crofts.
8. Filly RA: *The fetal neural axis: a practical approach for identifying anomalous development*, Chicago, 1992, The Society of Radiologists in Ultrasound.
9. Finberg HJ: Avoiding ambiguity in the sonographic determination of the direction of umbilical cord twists, *J Ultrasound Med* 11:185, 1992.
10. Fleischer AC and others, editors: *The principles and practice of ultrasonography in obstetrics and gynecology*, ed 4, Norwalk, Conn, 1991, Appleton & Lange.
11. Gabbe SG, Niebyl JR, Simpson JL, editors: *Obstetrics: normal and problem pregnancies*, New York, 1991, Churchill Livingstone.
12. Gray D, Crane J, Rudolff M: Origin of midtrimester vertebral ossification centers as determined by sonographic waterbath studies of a dissected fetal spine. Paper presented at the annual meeting of the American Institute of Ultrasound in Medicine, Las Vegas, 1986.
13. Grignon A and others: Urinary tract dilatation in utero: classification and clinical applications, *Radiology* 160:645, 1986.
14. Guyton AC: Pregnancy and lactation. In Guyton AC, editor: *Textbook of medical physiology*, Philadelphia, 1981, WB Saunders.
15. Isaacson G, Mintz MC, Crelin ES: Fetal head and neck. In Isaacson G, Mintz MC, Crelin ES, editors: *Atlas of fetal sectional anatomy*, New York, 1986, Springer-Verlag.
16. Jeanty P, Romero R, editors: How does a normal abdomen look? In *Obstetrical Ultrasound*, New York, 1984, McGraw-Hill.
17. Jeanty P, Dramaix-Wilmet MS, Elkasan N: Measurement of the fetal kidney growth on ultrasound, *Radiology* 144:159, 1982.
18. Jeanty P, Dramaix-Wilmet MS, VanGansbeke D: Fetal ocular biometry by ultrasound, *Radiology* 143:513, 1982.
19. Jeanty P, Kirkpatrick C, Dramaix-Wilmet MS: Fetal limb growth, *Radiology* 140:165, 1981.
20. Jeanty P, Romero R, Hobbins JC: Vascular anatomy of the fetus, *J Ultrasound Med* 3:113, 1984.
21. Jeanty P and others: Normal ultrasonic size and characteristics of the fetal adrenal glands, *Prenatal Diagnosis* 4:21, 1984.
22. Jeanty P and others: Facial anatomy of the fetus, *J Ultrasound Med* 5:607, 1986.
23. Johnson ML, Rees GK, Hattan RA: Normal fetal anatomy. In Callen PW, editor: *Ultrasonography in obstetrics and gynecology*, Philadelphia: WB Saunders, 1983.
24. Leopold GR: Obstetrical ultrasound examination guidelines, *J Ultrasound Med* 5:241, 1986 (editorial).
25. Mahony BS and others: The fetal cisterna magna, *Radiology* 153:773, 1984.

26. Mahony BS and others: Epiphyseal ossification centers in the assessment of fetal maturity: sonographic correlation with the amniocentesis lung profile, *Radiology* 159:521, 1986.

27. Mayden KL: The umbilical vein diameter in Rh isoimmunization, *Med Ultrasound* 4:119, 1980.

28. Mayden KL and others: Orbital diameters: a new parameter for prenatal diagnosis and dating, *Am J Obstet Gynecol* 144:289, 1982.

29. Nicolaides KH, Campbell S, Gabbe SG: Ultrasound screening for spina bifida: cranial and cerebellar signs, *Lancet* 2:72, 1986.

30. Nyberg DA, Mahony BS, Pretorius DH, editors: *Diagnostic ultrasound of fetal anomalies: text and atlas,* St Louis, 1990, Mosby.

31. Nyberg DA and others: Fetal bowel: normal sonographic findings, *J Ultrasound Med* 6:3, 1987.

32. O'Rahilly R, Muller F: *Human embryology and teratology,* New York, 1992, Wiley-Liss.

33. Pretorius DH and others: Linear echoes in the fetal cisterna magna, *J Ultrasound Med* 11:125, 1992.

34. Sanders RC: *Clinical sonography: a practical guide,* ed 2, Boston, 1991, Little, Brown.

35. Schmidt W and others: Sonographic measurements of the fetal spleen: clinical implications, *J Ultrasound Med* 4:667, 1985.

36. Work BA: Determination of gestational age and the management of postdatism. In Ellis JW, Beckmann CRB, editors: *A clinical manual of obstetrics,* Norwalk, Conn, 1983, Appleton-Century-Crofts.

37. Yarkoni S and others: Clavicular measurement: a new biometric parameter for fetal evaluation, *J Ultrasound Med* 4:467, 1985.

BIBLIOGRAPHY

Abramovich DR: The volume of amniotic fluid and its regulating factors. In Fairweather D, Eskes T, editors: *Amniotic fluid: research and clinical applications,* ed 2, New York, 1978, Excerpta Medica.

American College of Obstetric and Gynecology: Ultrasound in pregnancy, Tech Bull 116, Washington, DC, May 1988, The College.

Consensus Development Conference: Diagnostic ultrasound imaging in pregnancy,   Pub No 84-667, Washington, DC, US Department of Health and Human Services.

Fiske CE, Filly RA: Ultrasound evaluation of the normal and abnormal fetal neural axis, *Radiol Clin North Am* 20:285, 1982.

Harrison MR, Golbus MS, Filly RA, editors: *The unborn patient, prenatal diagnosis and treatment,* ed 2, Philadelphia, 1990, WB Saunders.

Hoddick WK and others: Minimal fetal renal pyelectasis, *J Ultrasound Med* 4:85, 1985.

CHAPTER *29*

Obstetric Measurements and Gestational Age

Sandra L. Hagen-Ansert

Frank A. Chervenak

OBJECTIVES

- List gestational sac growth and measurements
- Describe how to perform a crown rump measurement
- Calculate the biparietal diameter, head circumference, abdominal circumference, and extremity measurements
- Describe when other measurements should be used to provide additional clinical information

KEY TERMS

abdominal circumference (AC) - measurement at the level of the stomach, left portal vein, and left umbilical vein

anophthalmos - absence of one (cyclops) or both eyes

banana sign - refers to the shape of the cerebellum when a spinal defect is present (cerebellum is pulled downward into the foramen magnum)

biparietal diameter (BPD) - measurement of the fetal head at the level of the thalamus and cavum septum pellucidum

brachycephaly - fetal head is elongated in the transverse diameter and shortened in the anteroposterior diameter

crown-rump length (CRL) - most accurate measurement for determining gestational age; made in the first trimester.

dolichocephaly - fetal head is shortened in the transverse plane and elongated in the anteroposterior plane

femur length (FL) - measurement from the femoral head to the distal end of the femur

gestational sac diameter - used in the first trimester to estimate appropriate gestational age with menstrual dates

growth-adjusted sonar age (GASA) - the method whereby the fetus is categorized into small, average, or large growth percentile

humeral length - measurement from the humeral head to the distal end of the humerus

hypertelorism - condition in which the orbits are spaced far apart

hypotelorism - condition in which the orbits are close together

lemon sign - occurs with spina bifida; frontal bones collapse inward

microphthalmos - small eyes

spina bifida - failure of the vertebrae to close

Reliably assessing gestational age and the growth of the fetus has long posed a challenge to all who care for pregnant women. Clinical parameters, although not without value, lack the necessary consistency to provide for optimal perinatal care. With recent advances in diagnostic imaging, fetal age and growth can now be assessed with high accuracy.

The definition of menstrual age versus fetal age is important to establish in clinical obstetrics. *Fetal age* begins at the time of conception and is also known as *conceptional age.* Conceptional age is restricted to pregnancies in which the actual date of conception is known, as found in patients with in vitro fertilization or artificial insemination. If conceptual age is already known, the menstrual age may be found by adding 14 days to the conceptual age.

Obstetricians date pregnancies in menstrual weeks, which is calculated from the first day of the last normal menstrual period. This method is called *menstrual age or gestational age.*

It is clinically important to know the menstrual age of a patient because this information is used for the following reasons:

- In early pregnancy to schedule invasive procedures (chorionic villus sampling and genetic amniocentesis).
- To interpret maternal serum alpha fetoprotein screening.
- To plan date of delivery.
- For evaluation of fetal growth.

Before the use of ultrasound determination of fetal growth, menstrual age was calculated by three factors: (1) the menstrual history, (2) physical examination of the fundal height of the uterus, and (3) postnatal physical examination of the neonate. This process was not always reliable if the patient could not recall the date of the last period or if other factors such as oligomenorrhea, implantation bleeding, use of oral contraceptives, or irregular menstrual cycle was present.

GESTATIONAL AGE ASSESSMENT: FIRST TRIMESTER

GESTATIONAL SAC DIAMETER
Transvaginal sonography enables visualization and evaluation of intrauterine pregnancies earlier than was previously thought possible. The earliest sonographic finding of an intrauterine pregnancy is thickening of the decidua. Sonographically, this appears as an echogenic, thickening filling of the fundal region of the endometrial cavity occurring at approximately 3 to 4 weeks of gestation (Box 29-1, Figure 29-1).

At approximately 4 weeks of menstrual age, a small hypoechoic area appears in the fundus or midportion of the uterus, known as the *double decidual sac sign.* As the sac embeds further into the uterus it is surrounded by an echogenic rim and is seen within the choriodecidual tissue. This is known as the **chorionic** or **gestational sac.**

At 5 weeks the average internal diameter of the gestational sac, calculated as the mean of the anteroposterior diameter, the transverse diameter, and the longitudinal diameter, can provide an adequate estimation of menstrual age. A gestational sac should be seen within the uterine cavity when the beta human chorionic gonadotropin (beta hCG) is above 500 mIU/mL (second international standard). This becomes especially important when evaluating a pregnancy for ectopic implantation.

The sac grows rapidly in the first 10 weeks, with an average increase of 1 mm per day. According to one report, a gestational sac growing less than 0.7 mm per day is associated with impending early pregnancy loss.[17] Even the most experienced sonographer may incorporate a measuring error; therefore the beta-hCG test in conjunction with a sonographic evaluation are suggested in a sequential time frame.

When the gestational sac exceeds 8 mm in mean internal diameter, a yolk sac should be seen (Figure 29-2). The yolk sac is identified as a small, anechoic circular structure within the gestational sac. It provides early transfer of nutrients from the trophoblast to the embryo. It also aids in the early formation of the primitive gut and vitelline arteries and veins and in the production of the primordial germ cells. Yolk sac size has not been correlated with gestational age determination, but the size, shape, and number of yolk sacs have been well described (Figure 29-3).[10, 17]

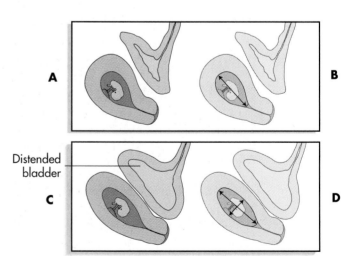

Figure 29-1 Gestational sac measurement. **A,** Longitudinal. **B,** The sac length should be measured from inner to inner borders. **C,** Transverse. **D,** The width of the sac should be measured along the inner to inner borders.

> **BOX 29-1 GESTATIONAL SAC MEASUREMENTS (FIGURE 29-1)**
>
> - A distended urinary bladder has an effect on gestational sac measurement; it changes its shape from round to ovoid or teardrop.
> - If the sac is round, measure one diameter inner to inner.
> - If the sac is ovoid, make two measurements inner to inner: one transverse and the other perpendicular to the length.

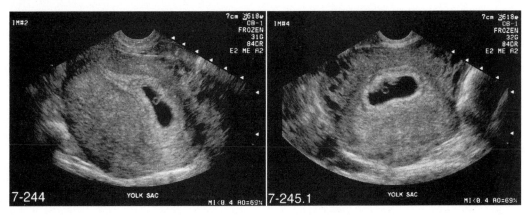

Figure 29-2 Sagittal and coronal images of a yolk sac in a 4-week gestation as seen with transvaginal ultrasound. The small gestational sac is well seen within the endometrial cavity of the uterus.

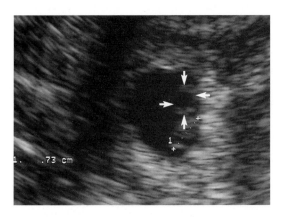

Figure 29-3 Transvaginal ultrasound measuring an early crown-rump length (CRL) *(crosses)*. The yolk sac is noted and outlined *(arrows)*. The CRL is consistent with 6.5 weeks.

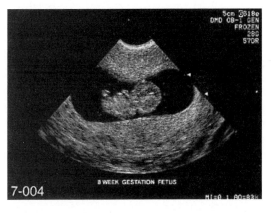

Figure 29-4 Transvaginal image of an 8-week gestation showing a developing embryo.

> **BOX 29-2 TRANSVAGINAL SONOGRAPHIC LANDMARKS FOR EARLY PREGNANCIES**
>
> - 500 mIU/mL beta-hCG = gestational sac seen
> - >8 mm gestational sac = yolk sac seen
> - >16 mm gestational sac = embryo seen
> - < 6-mm yolk sac = normal
> - >8-mm yolk sac = abnormal
> - >7-mm fetal pole = positive cardiac activity

> **BOX 29-3 CROWN-RUMP LENGTH (CRL) (FIGURE 29-5)**
>
> - By transvaginal ultrasound the CRL can be measured from 6 to 12 gestational weeks.
> - Measurements should be made along the long axis of the embryo from the top of the head (crown) to the bottom of the trunk (rump).
> - This is the most accurate fetal age measurement.

Normal yolk sac size should be less than 6 mm; greater than 8 mm has been associated with poor pregnancy outcome (Box 29-2).[10, 17]

When the mean **gestational sac diameter** exceeds 16 mm an embryo with definite cardiac activity should be well visualized with transvaginal scanning. This usually occurs by the 6th menstrual week (Figure 29-4). For the transabdominal scanning approach the maternal urinary bladder must be filled to create an acoustic window. With this technique the sac shape can vary secondary to bladder compression, maternal bowel gas, or myomas and should not be misinterpreted as abnormal.

Assessing gestational age using a single gestational sac diameter or even up to three averaged diameters yields an accuracy of only ±2 to 3 weeks in 90% of cases.[9] Accordingly, gestational sac diameter has not been widely used as an determinant of gestational age.

CROWN-RUMP LENGTH

With transvaginal sonography, embryonic echoes can be identified as early as 38 to 39 days of menstrual age (Box 29-3, Figure 29-5). The **crown-rump length (CRL)** is usually 1 to 2 mm at this stage.[13] The embryo is usually located adjacent to the yolk sac. A CRL is the most accurate

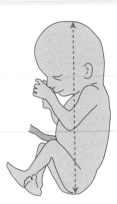

Figure 29-5 The crown-rump length should be measured along the long axis of the embryo from the top of the head to the bottom of the trunk.

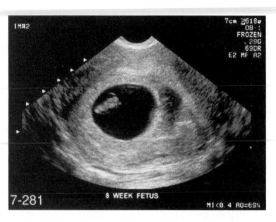

Figure 29-7 Transvaginal image of an 8-week gestation that shows a large gestational sac with a small, undeveloped embryo. No cardiac activity was identified.

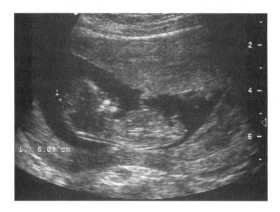

Figure 29-6 Transabdominal ultrasound demonstrating the proper landmarks for an accurate crown-rump length (CRL) measurement. The calipers should be placed at the top of the fetal head and the bottom of the fetal rump, excluding the legs or yolk sac. The CRL is consistent with a gestation of 12 weeks and 3 days.

sonographic technique for establishing gestational age in the first trimester. The reason for this high accuracy is the excellent correlation between fetal length and age in early pregnancy, because pathologic disorders minimally affect the growth of the embryo during this time.[8, 11]

The embryo can be measured easily with real-time dynamic imaging. For transabdominal imaging, the mother's bladder should be full to create an acoustic window. The measurement should be taken from the top of the fetal head to the outer fetal rump, excluding the fetal limbs or yolk sac. The accuracy is ±5 days with a 95% confidence level (Figure 29-6).[20] The average of at least three separate measurements of the CRL should be obtained to determine gestational age.

Cardiac activity should be seen when the CRL exceeds 7 mm, but it is generally accepted to follow patients with small CRL and no fetal heart beat over a few days. In general the CRL should increase at a rate of 8 mm per day.

Occasionally an embryo is seen with no visible cardiac activity and a small CRL for menstrual age. It is advisable to wait a week and rescan to see if the patient spontaneously aborts the products of conception or if she needs medical intervention, such as a dilation and curettage procedure. Infrequently, an appropriate fetal CRL and positive cardiac activity are seen after the week's wait (Figure 29-7). Why this happens is not known, but it has been observed by experienced sonographers.

Absence of an embryo by 7 to 8 weeks of gestation is consistent with a blighted ovum or an anembryonic pregnancy. If a nomogram is not readily available to identify gestational age, a convenient formula is gestational age in weeks = CRL in cm + 6.[8] After the twelfth week a CRL is no longer considered accurate because of flexion and extension of the active fetus; therefore other biometric parameters should be used.

GESTATIONAL AGE ASSESSMENT: SECOND AND THIRD TRIMESTERS

FETAL MEASUREMENTS

In the second trimester the gestational age parameters extend to the biparietal diameter, head circumference, abdominal circumference, and femur length. It is critical for the sonographer to know precisely what landmarks are needed to determine these measurements. Proper gain settings, instrumentation, and fetal lie will all influence the accuracy of gestational age.

Biparietal Diameter. In the second trimester the **biparietal diameter (BPD)** is the most widely accepted means of measuring the fetal head and estimating fetal age. As the pregnancy enters the third trimester, an accurate measurement of fetal age becomes more difficult to obtain because the fetus begins to drop into the pelvic outlet cavity. The reproducibility of the BPD is ±1 mm (±2 standard deviations). When dating a pregnancy between 17

BOX MEASURING THE BIPARIETAL DIAMETER 29-4 (FIGURE 29-8)

- Obtain biparietal diameter (BPD) of the fetal head at the transverse level of the midbrain: falx, cavum septi pellucidi, and thalamic nuclei.
- Make sure the head is symmetric and oval.
- Measure from outer to inner margins of the skull.
- In the third trimester, the BPD is not as accurate in predicting fetal age; may approach ± 3 to 3.5 weeks.

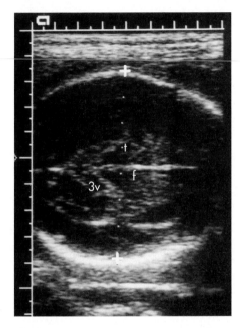

Figure 29-8 The biparietal diameter of the fetal head is made at the transverse level of the midbrain at the level of the falx *(f)*, cavum septi pellucidi, and thalamic nuclei *(t)*. *3v*, Third ventricle.

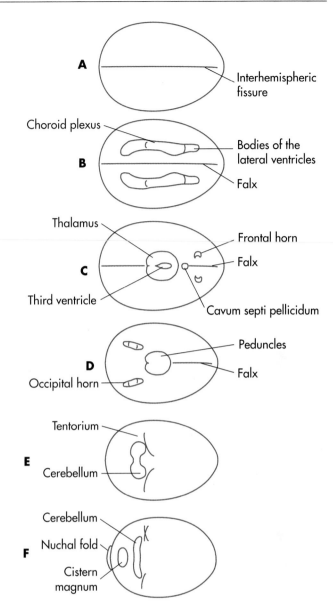

Figure 29-9 Progression of the fetal head anatomy in the transaxial plane from the level of the **A,** interhemispheric fissure; **B,** choroid plexus, falx, and bodies of the lateral ventricles; **C,** falx, thalamus, third ventricle, cavum septi pellucidum, frontal horns; **D,** falx, peduncles, occipital horns; **E,** tentorium, cerebellum; **F,** cerebellum, cistern magnum, nuchal fold.

and 26 weeks of gestation the predictive value is ±11 days in 95% of the population.[20] After 26 weeks the correlation of BPD with gestational age decreases because of the increased biologic variability. The predictive value decreases to +3 weeks in the third trimester. The growth of the fetal skull slows from 3 mm per week in the second trimester to 1.8 mm per week in the third trimester.

When measuring the BPD, it is important to accurately determine the landmarks (Box 29-4, Figures 29-8 and 29-9). The fetal head should be imaged in a transverse axial section, ideally with the fetus in a direct occiput transverse position. The BPD should be measured perpendicular to the fetal skull at the level of the thalamus and the cavum septi pellucidi. Intracranial landmarks should include the falx cerebri anteriorly and posteriorly, the cavum septi pellucidi anteriorly in the midline, and the choroid plexus in the atrium of each lateral ventricle. With real-time ultrasound equipment, one can identify the middle cerebral artery pulsating in the insula (Figure 29-10).

The head shape should be ovoid, not round (brachycephaly), because this can lead to overestimation of gestational age, just as a flattened or compressed head (dolicho-

cephaly) can lead to underestimation of gestational age. The calipers should be placed from the leading edge of the parietal bone to the leading edge of the opposite parietal bone, or "outer edge to inner edge." The parietal bones should measure less than 3 mm each. On the outer edge of the fetal head the soft tissue should not be included; measuring should begin from the skull bone. Gain settings should not be set too high because this can produce a false thickening and incorrect measurement. A reference curve should be applicable to the local population. BPD should not be used to date a pregnancy in cases of severe ventriculomegaly, which may alter the head size and produce macrocephaly, or when microcephaly or skull-altering

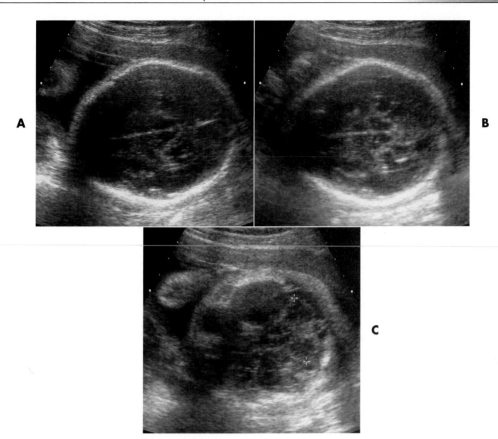

Figure 29-10   Transverse section through the fetal head taken at the level of the thalamus and the cavum septum pellucidi. **A,** The biparietal diameter (BPD) is measured from the outer border of the proximal skull to the inner border of the distal skull, or leading edge to leading edge. **B,** The head should be oval in shape, because too round or too flat of a head leads to overestimation or underestimation of fetal age. **C,** Inferior angulation from the BPD shows the posterior fossa with the cerebellum *(cross bars).*

head lesions are present. In these cases, other biometric parameters should be used.

If the fetus is too large for an accurate CRL but too early for a BPD with the proper landmarks identified, an approximation of the BPD can be obtained by incorporating the following landmarks: a smooth, symmetric head; visible choroid plexuses; and a well-defined midline echo that is an equal distance from both parietal bones (Figure 29-11).[11]

One technique to adjust for the biologic variability of fetal head growth uses the fetus as its own control.[19] Two separate BPD measurements are obtained, the first between 20 and 26 weeks and the second between 31 and 33 weeks. The growth interval was compared with average growth. This technique has been termed **growth-adjusted sonar age (GASA).**[19] The fetus is then categorized into a small, average, or large growth percentile. The developers of this method claim the use of GASA reduces the range in gestational age from ±11 days to ±3 days in 90% of fetuses and to ±5 days in approximately 97% of fetuses.[19] Although GASA compensates for the biologic variability in the individual fetus, it does not take into consideration other factors, such as dolichocephaly and brachycephaly or the standard error of measurement.

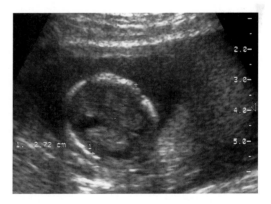

Figure 29-11   This represents a 14-week fetus that is too big for a crown-rump length measurement, yet too small to distinguish the proper biparietal landmarks in the fetal head. At this gestational age, it is acceptable to measure the fetal head at the level of the choroid plexus, which is echogenic and fills most of the head at this time. The same measurement criteria of outer border to inner border should be used.

Head Circumference.   Prenatal compression of the fetal skull is common. It occurs more often in fetal malpresentation, such as breech, or in conditions of intrauterine

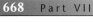

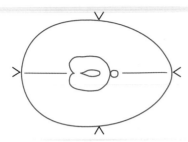

Figure 29-12 The head circumference should be taken at the level of the biparietal diameter; the calipers should be placed along the outer margin of the skull to obtain the measurement.

> **BOX HEAD CIRCUMFERENCE (HC)**
> **29-5 MEASUREMENT (FIGURE 29-12)**
>
> - Use the image of the BPD to calculate head circumference (HC).
> - Place area calipers along the outer margin of the skull to obtain circumference.
> - Accurate to ±2 to 3 weeks.

crowding, such as multiple pregnancies. The fetal skull can also be compressed in vertex presentations without any obvious reason or as a result of an associated uterine abnormality such as leiomyoma.[9] Head circumference (HC) is less affected than BPD by head compression; therefore HC is a valuable tool in assessing gestational age (Box 29-5, Figure 29-12).

The HC measurement is taken at the level of the BPD and can be calculated from the same frozen image. Most modern ultrasound equipment has built-in electronic calipers that open to the outline of the fetal head. If this feature is not available, the measurement can be obtained with a light pen, map reader, or electronic planimeter or by manually measuring with the electronic calipers. To manually measure the widest transverse diameter of the skull, the BPD level should be measured with the calipers on the outer border of each side (D1). The length of the occipital frontal diameter (OFD) should then be measured (D2). This is done by measuring from the outer border of the occiput to the outer border of the frontal bone (Figure 29-13). To obtain an accurate HC measurement, 60% to 70% of the skull outline should be displayed on the screen.[6] HC can then be calculated by the following formula:

$$\frac{HC = D1 + D2}{2} = \pi$$

Cephalic Index. The two most frequently noted alterations in head shape are **dolichocephaly** and **brachycephaly.** In dolichocephaly the head is shortened in the transverse plane (BPD) and elongated in the anteroposterior plane (OFD) (Figure 29-14). In brachycephaly the head is elongated in the transverse diameter (BPD) and

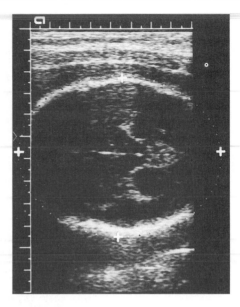

Figure 29-13 Transverse section of a fetal head demonstrating the ellipse method of measuring fetal head circumference (HC). The biparietal diameter and HC measurements can be taken from the same frozen image, because the same anatomic landmarks are used. The calipers should be placed outside the entire perimeter of the fetal skull *(dotted line)*. This measurement is not affected by head shape.

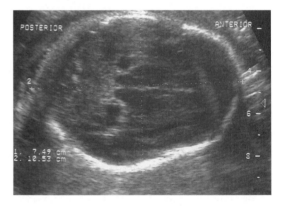

Figure 29-14 This represents a biparietal diameter (BPD) with dolichocephaly. The head is elongated in the anteroposterior diameter and falsely shortened in the transverse diameter. The BPD is mean for 29 weeks and the head circumference is mean for 30.3 weeks, but the actual gestational age is 32 weeks.

shortened in the anteroposterior diameter (OFD) (Figure 29-15).[11] One can underestimate gestational age from a dolichocephalic head or overestimate with brachycephaly. Because of these variations in fetal head shape, a cephalic index (CI) has been devised to determine the normality of the fetal head shape:

$$CI = BPD/OFD \times 100$$

A normal cephalic index is 80% ±1 standard deviation. The range of normal is 75% to 85%. A CI of greater than

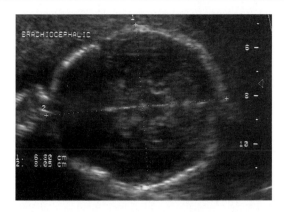

Figure 29-15   This biparietal diameter (BPD) is consistent with brachycephaly. The fetal head is falsely wider in the transverse diameter, yet shortened in the anteroposterior plane. The BPD overestimates the gestational age, but the head circumference (HC) remains unaffected. The BPD is mean for 26.7 weeks and the HC is mean for 24.9 weeks, but the actual gestational age is 23.5 weeks.

85% suggests brachycephaly and of less than 75% suggests dolichocephaly.[11] In one case report the CI changed from a high normal of 83% to a significantly abnormal index of 63% over a 2 ½-week period.[5] This change would normally take approximately 7 weeks. Fetal death resulted. The authors of the report claim that an abnormal CI can be the first indication of impending fetal death.[5]

Abdominal Circumference. The first description of the use of the fetal **abdominal circumference (AC)** in predicting fetal weight was in 1975.[2] The AC is very useful in monitoring normal fetal growth and detecting fetal growth disturbances, such as intrauterine growth restriction and macrosomia. It is more useful as a growth parameter than in predicting gestational age.

The fetal abdomen should be measured in a transverse plane at the level of the liver where the umbilical vein branches into the left portal sinus (Box 29-6, Figures 29-16 and 29-17). In this plane the left portal vein and the right portal vein form a J shape. The stomach bubble should be seen at this level on the left side of the fetal abdomen. The abdomen should be more circular than oval, because an oval shape indicates an oblique cut resulting in a false estimation of size. Fetal kidneys should not be seen when the proper plane is imaged. The AC may change shape with fetal breathing activity, transducer compression, or intrauterine crowding (as in multiple pregnancies or oligo-

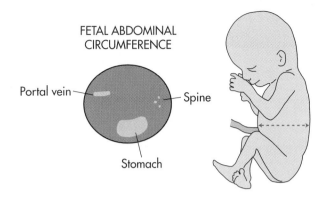

FETAL ABDOMINAL
CIRCUMFERENCE

Figure 29-16   The abdominal circumference should be taken from a round transverse image at the level of the umbilical vein as it joins the left portal vein within the liver.

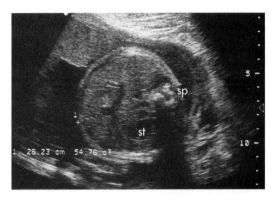

Figure 29-17   Transverse section of a fetal abdominal circumference (AC) at 30.3 weeks. The measurement should be taken at the level where the umbilical vein branches into the left portal sinus and forms a J shape. The fetal stomach *(st)* would be seen on the left at this level. One set of calipers should measure the distance from the fetal spine *(sp)* to the anterior abdominal wall. The other set should be placed perpendicular, measuring the widest transverse diameter. When tracing or using an ellipse to measure the AC the calipers should be placed along the external perimeter of the fetus to include the skin.

hydramnios) or secondary to fetal position, as in a breech presentation. When discrepancies do occur in AC measurements, multiple measurements should be taken and averaged to ensure accuracy. This is also true for other fetal measurements.

The AC can be measured with the same instruments used to measure the HC. The calipers should be placed along the external perimeter of the fetal abdomen to include subcutaneous soft tissue. The following formula can be used to calculate to AC:

$$AC = \frac{D1 + D2}{2} \times \pi$$

In this equation, *D1* is the diameter from fetal spine to anterior abdominal wall and *D2* is the transverse diameter perpendicular to *D1*. Unlike in the fetal head, there is no consistent relationship between the anteroposterior and transverse diameters.[11]

BOX 29-7 FEMUR MEASUREMENT

- Hyperechoic linear structure represents the ossified portion of the femoral diaphysis and corresponds to femoral length measurement from the greater trochanter to the femoral condyles (these are imaged as rounded hypoechoic masses at each end of the diaphysis called the epiphyseal cartilages; they should not be included in the femoral length measurement).
- The normal femur has a straight lateral border and a curved medial border.
- Femur length may be used with the same accuracy as BPD to predict gestational age.
- Femur length may indicate skeletal dysplasias or intrauterine growth restriction.

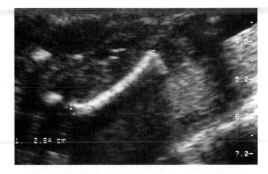

Figure 29-18 Longitudinal section through a fetal femur at 18.7 weeks. The longest section of bone should be obtained. The calipers should be placed from the major trochanter to the external condyle. Note the shadow cast posterior to the bone, appropriately demonstrating the absorption of the sound waves into the fetal bone.

Of the four basic gestational age measurements, AC has the largest reported variability and is more affected by growth disturbances than the other basic parameters.

BONE LENGTHS

Femur. The most widely measured and easily obtainable of all fetal long bones is the femur. It usually lies at 30 to 70 degrees to the long axis of the fetal body. **Femur length (FL)** is about as accurate as BPD in determining gestational age. Femur length is an especially useful parameter that can be used to date a pregnancy when a fetal head cannot be measured because of position or when there is a fetal head anomaly (Box 29-7).

The technique for measuring with real-time ultrasound is fairly simple. First, the lie of the fetus should be determined and the fetal body followed in a transverse section until the fetal bladder and iliac crests are identified. The iliac crests are echogenic and oblique to the fetal bladder. The transducer is moved slightly and rotated to visualize the full length of the femur. The ends of the femur should be distinct and blunt, not pointed, and an acoustic shadow should be cast because of the absorption of the sound waves into the bone (Figure 29-18).

Sonographers measure the femur from the major trochanter to the external condyle. The femoral head is not taken into account even when it is visible.[11] After 32 weeks the distal femoral epiphysis is seen, but it is not included in the femur length measurement One report claims that the fetal femur length can predict gestational age between 25 and 35 weeks to within fewer than 5 days' accuracy and within 6 days at 40 weeks.[22]

Overestimating the length of the femur by high gain settings or by including the femoral head or distal epiphysis in the measurement is possible. Underestimation can result from using incorrect plane orientation and not obtaining the full length of the bone.

In any routine obstetric evaluation, the femur is usually the only long bone measured, but if there is a 2-week or longer difference between femur length and all the other biometric parameters, all fetal long bones should be measured and a targeted examination of the fetal anatomy should be performed. Three studies found an association

BOX 29-8 TIBIA AND FIBULA MEASUREMENTS

- Tiba is longer than the fibula.
- Fibula is lateral to tibia and thinner.
- Measure length point to point.

between shortened femur and humerus lengths and trisomy.[1,6,18] Dwarfism is also a possibility. Constitutional hereditary growth factors should also be considered. Other bone lengths are sometimes valuable in assessing gestational age.

Distal Femoral and Proximal Tibial Epiphyseal Ossifications Centers. One report has correlated the distal femoral epiphyseal ossification (DFE) and the proximal tibial epiphyseal ossification (PTE) with advanced gestational age.[3] The DFE and PTE appear as a high-amplitude echo that is separate but adjacent to the femur or the tibia. The authors of the report found that the DFE can be identified in gestations greater than 33 weeks and that the PTE is identified in gestations greater than 35 weeks. It is not necessary to measure these ossifications—they are either present or absent. These assessments can be helpful when other growth parameters are compromised because of congenital anomalies or when differentiating an incorrectly dated fetus from a fetus with intrauterine growth restriction.

Tibia and Fibula. The tibia and fibula can be measured by first identifying the femur, then following it down until the two parallel bones can be identified. The tibia can be identified because the tibial plateau is larger than the fine, tapering fibula. The tibia is located medial to the fibula (Box 29-8, Figure 29-19).

Humerus. **Humerus length** is sometimes more difficult to measure than femur length. The humerus is almost always found very close to the fetal abdomen. The "up side" humerus, or the humerus closest to the transducer, falls in

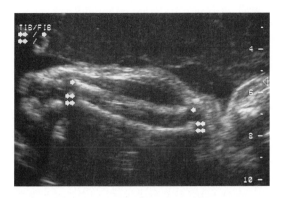

Figure 29-19 The tibia and fibula are demonstrated here at 21 weeks. The tibia can be distinguished from the fibula because the tibia is larger *(multiple arrows)* than the small tapering fibula *(single arrow)*.

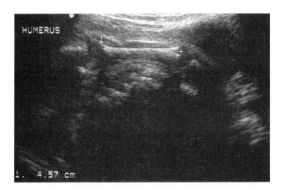

Figure 29-20 Longitudinal section through a fetal humerus at 26.7 weeks. The calipers should be placed at the most distal ends of the bone. The anterior, or "up side," humerus is measured here but does not cast an acoustic shadow because the fetal body is below and obscures it.

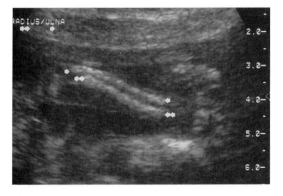

Figure 29-21 This represents a longitudinal section through the radius *(two arrows)* and ulna *(one arrow)* at 20.3 weeks of gestation. The calipers should be placed at the most distal portion of each individual bone. The ulna can be distinguished from the radius because the ulna is larger and penetrates much deeper into the elbow.

the near-field zone, where detail is not always focused and the acoustic shadow is less clear. The opposite, or "down side," humerus may be obscured because of the overlying fetal spine or fetal ribs (Box 29-9, Figure 29-20).

BOX 29-9 HUMERUS MEASUREMENT

- Image fetal spine in upper thoracic–lower cervical region.
- Identify scapula, then rotate transducer until long axis of humerus is seen.
- Only humeral shaft (diaphysis) is ossified and should be measured.

BOX 29-10 RADIUS AND ULNA MEASUREMENTS

- The ulna is longer than the radius proximally; distally they are the same.
- Measure length from point to point.

Radius and Ulna. The radius and ulna can be recognized by following the humerus down until two parallel bones are visualized and then rotating the transducer slightly until the full length of the bones is identified. The forearms are very commonly found by the fetal face. The ulna can be distinguished from the radius because it penetrates much deeper into the elbow (Box 29-10, Figure 29-21). The ulna is larger and anatomically medial.

USING MULTIPLE PARAMETERS

No single parameter is perfect in predicting gestational age. One report suggests that estimates of fetal age improve significantly when two or more parameters are used.[7] Use of multiple parameters in estimating fetal age is appropriate only when the fetus is growing normally. Congenital anomalies of the head, abdomen, and skeleton, as well as functional disturbances, must be taken into consideration before using multiple parameters.

A birth weight table has been developed based on measurements from a group of neonates who had accurate gestational dating by prenatal first-trimester ultrasonography in order to improve the accuracy of neonatal birth weight percentiles.[4] Prenatally, weight tables are used in conjunction with sonographically estimated fetal weight to help guide obstetric management decisions, especially those concerning the timing of delivery.[4] Fetal weight estimation is a useful parameter in following intrauterine growth restriction fetuses.

A study compared three-dimensional ultrasound (3DUS) birthweight predictions with two-dimensional methods and found a significant correlation existed between thigh volume and birth weight at term gestation.[12] Thigh volumes that included the soft tissue mass may represent important markers for fetal growth. The 3DUS may be an important predictor of growth-restricted fetuses, and the volume measurements may be able to be applied to each fetus to monitor growth.

One author used the technique of averaging the BPD, HC, AC, and FL to determine gestational age.[9] The value of using multiple parameters is that although any of the

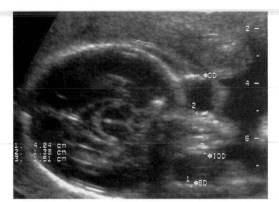

Figure 29-22 This sonogram represents a transverse section through the fetal head at the level of the orbits at 25.3 weeks. *OD* is the measure of a single fetal orbit. The binocular diameter *(BD)* is a measure of both the orbits at the same time, and the inner orbital diameter *(IOD)* is a measure of the distance between the two orbits. These measurements are especially useful when ruling out hypotelorism or hypertelorism.

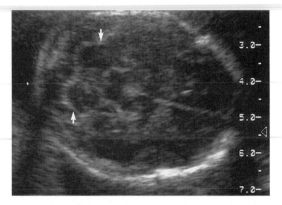

Figure 29-23 Transverse section through a fetal head demonstrating the fetal cerebellum. This image is obtained at the same anatomic level as the biparietal diameter, angling back into the posterior fossa of the fetal head. Note the classic dumbbell shape of the normal cerebellum. The widest diameter of the cerebellum should be measured *(arrows)*.

BOX 29-11   **ORBITAL MEASUREMENTS**

- Orbital diameter increases from 13 mm at 12 weeks to 59 mm or greater at term.
- Measure outer to outer diameter.
- Measure inner to inner diameter.

BOX 29-12   **CEREBELLAR DIMENSIONS**

- **Posterior fossa:** In the transaxial image of the head, obtain the BPD (cavum septi pellucidi and thalamus) and then angle the transducer inferior toward the base of the skull to image the posterior fossa.
- Obtain the length of the cerebellum at the level of the cerebellum, vermis, and fourth ventricle.
- Angle the transducer slightly more inferior from the cerebellum to record the cistern magnum and nuchal fold area.
- The depth of the cisterna magna is from the posterior aspect of the cerebellum to the occipital bone measured 5 mm ± 3mm; measurements >10 mm are abnormal.
- The nuchal fold should measure

---

measurements may be technically incorrect, it is very unlikely that all of the measurements are overestimated or underestimated.

OTHER PARAMETERS

Numerous other nomograms have been used to correlate almost every aspect of fetal anatomy with gestational age. Among the most interesting of these parameters are the orbits, the cerebellum, and the fetal epiphyseal ossification centers.

Orbits. Another parameter useful in predicting gestational age is the fetal orbit measurements. The ocular distance (OD), binocular distance (BD), and interocular distance (IOD) can be measured. Gestational age can best be predicted from the BDP[11]; this measure is more strongly related to the BPD and gestational age than are the other orbital parameters.[14] The fetal orbit should be measured in a plane slightly more caudal than the BPD. The orbits are accessible in every head position except the occipitoanterior position (i.e., face looking down). All measurements should be taken from outer border to outer border (Box 29-11, Figure 29-22). The OD measures a single fetal orbit. The BD includes both fetal orbits at the same time, whereas the IOD measures the length between the two orbits. One view states that (1) both eyes should have the same diameter, (2) the largest diameter of the eyes should be used, and (3) the image should by symmetric.[11] Care should be taken not to underestimate the measurement

when there is oblique shadowing from the ethmoid bone. This parameter is especially useful when other fetal growth parameters are affected, such as in ventriculomegaly or skeletal dysplasia. With careful sonographic examinations, the fetus with **hypotelorism, hypertelorism, anophthalmos,** or **microphthalmos** can be diagnosed.

Cerebellum. One study found the fetal cerebellum to be a more accurate reflection of gestational age than the BPD in cases of oligohydramnios, dolichocephaly, breech presentation, or twins or in the presence of a uterine anomaly.[15] The authors of the study claim this is true because the posterior fossa is not affected by any of these conditions. The cerebellum can be measured from the level at which the BPD is obtained, angling back into the posterior fossa to include the full length of the cerebellum. The cerebellum should have a dumbbell shape.

The widest diameter of the cerebellum should be measured (Box 29-12, Figure 29-23). Authors have described the **banana** and **lemon signs** that associate an abnormally shaped cerebellum with detection of fetal **spina bifida.**[16] In the presence of spina bifida the fetal cerebellum is

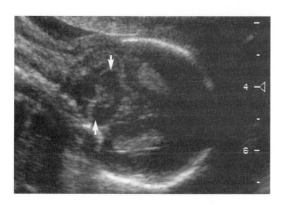

Figure 29-24   A coronal section of a fetal cerebellum, which can be used when the traditional views cannot be obtained.

pulled downward into the foramen magnum, altering its shape to appear oblong or banana shaped. The frontal bones of the fetal skull also give in to this pressure, collapsing and giving the fetal head a lemon shape.

The fetal cerebellum should not be used as a gestational dating parameter in the presence of a cerebellar or spinal abnormality. A more recent report states that the coronal view is just as accurate, especially in fetal heads when the traditional views are unobtainable (Figure 29-24).[21]

REVIEW QUESTIONS

1. Describe the earliest sonographic evidence of an intrauterine pregnancy, including the sonographic appearance, location, and biochemical laboratory values.
2. What is a yolk sac? Describe its purpose, sonographic appearance, and size.
3. What is the most accurate time to date a pregnancy? Why?
4. Describe the anatomic landmarks used to obtain a biparietal diameter and the technique used to accurately measure it.
5. Describe the techniques and formula to calculate a head circumference measurement.
6. What is a cephalic index and what is the range of normal?
7. What are the bony landmarks used when measuring a fetal femur length?
8. Discuss the various orbital measurements and how they are obtained. Which measurement is the most strongly related to the biparietal diameter and gestational age?
9. Describe the two techniques used to measure a fetal cerebellum. What is the classic shape and how is the shape important?

REFERENCES

1. Benacerraf B, Neuberg D, Frigoletto FD: Humeral shortening in second trimester fetuses with Down syndrome, *Obstet Gynecol* 77:223, 1991.

2. Campbell S, Wilkin D: Ultrasonic measurement of the fetal abdominal circumference in the estimation of fetal weight, *Br J Obstet Gynecol* 82:689, 1975.
3. Chinn D and others: Ultrasonic identification of fetal lower extremity epiphyseal ossification centers, *Radiology* 147:815, 1983.
4. Doubilet PM and others: Improved birth weight table for neonates developed from gestations dated by early ultrasonography, *J Ultrasound Med* 16:241, 1997.
5. Ford K, McGahan J: Cephalic index: its possible use as a predictor of impending fetal demise, *Radiology* 143:517, 1982.
6. Hadlock FP, Deter RL, Harrist RB: Sonographic detection of abnormal fetal growth patterns, *Clin Obstet Gynecol* 27:342, 1984.
7. Hadlock FP and others: Estimation of fetal weight with the use of head, body, and femur measurements: prospective study, *Am J Obstet Gynecol* 15:333, 1985.
8. Hobbins JC, Winsberg F, Berkowitz RL: *Ultrasonography in ob/gyn*, Baltimore, 1983, Williams and Wilkins.
9. Hohler CW: Ultrasonic estimation of gestational age, *Clin Obstet Gynecol* 27:2, 1984.
10. Hurwitz SR: Yolk sac sign: sonographic appearance of the fetal yolk sac in missed abortion, *J Ultrasound Med* 5:435, 1986.
11 Jeanty P, Romero R: *Obstetrical ultrasound*, New York, 1984, McGraw-Hill.
12. Lee W and others: Birthweight prediction by three-dimensional ultrasonographic volumes of the fetal thigh and abdomen, *J Ultrasound Med* 16:799, 1997.
13. Lyons E: Early pregnancy loss by endovaginal sonography. Proceedings of the State of the Art Ob/Gyn Imaging Course, San Diego convention, March 1992, American Institute of Ultrasound in Medicine.
14 Mayden K and others: Orbital diameters: a new parameter for prenatal diagnosis and dating, *Am J Obstet Gynecol* 144:289, 1982.
15. Mcleary R, Kuhns L, Barr M: Ultrasonography of the fetal cerebellum, *Radiology* 151:441, 1984.
16. Nicolaides KH and others: Ultrasound screening for spina bifida: cranial and cerebellar signs, *Lancet* 1:72, 1986.
17. Nyberg DA, Laing FC, Filly RA: Threatened abortion: sonographic distinction of normal and abnormal sacs, *Radiology* 158:397, 1986.
18. Rodis JF and others: Comparison of humerus length with femur length in fetuses with Down syndrome, *Am J Obstet Gynecol* 165:1051, 1992.
19. Sabbagha RE, Hughey M, Depp R: Growth-adjusted sonographic age (GASA) a simplified method, *Obstet Gynecol* 51:383, 1978.
20. Sabbagha RE, Tamura RK, Dal Campo S: Fetal dating by ultrasound, *Sem Roentgenol* 17:3, 1982.
21 Sarno AP, Rose GS, Harrington RA: Coronal transcerebellar diameter: an alternate view, *Ultrasound Obstet Gynecol* 2:158, 1992.
23 Yeh M and others: Ultrasonic measurement of the femur length as an index of fetal gestational age, *Am J Obstet Gynecol* 144:519, 1982.

BIBLIOGRAPHY

Goldberg BB, Kurtz AB: *Atlas of ultrasound measurements*, St Louis, 1990, Mosby.

CHAPTER 30

Fetal Growth Assessment by Ultrasound

Sandra L. Hagen-Ansert

Frank A. Chervenak

amniotic fluid index (AFI) - sum of the four quadrants of amniotic fluid

biophysical profile (BPP) - assessment of fetus to determine fetal well-being; includes evaluation of cardiac Non-Stress Test, fetal breathing movement, gross fetal body movements, fetal tone, and amniotic fluid volume

Doppler - the Doppler effect is a change in the frequency of a sound wave when either the source or the listener are moving relative to one another; the difference between the received echo frequency and the frequency of the transmitted beam is the Doppler shift; pulsed wave Doppler is used in most fetal examinations; this means the transducer has the ability to send and receive Doppler signals

estimated fetal weight (EFW) - incorporation of all fetal growth parameters (biparietal diameter, head circumference, abdominal circumference, femur and humeral length)

intrauterine growth restriction (IUGR) - decreased rate of fetal growth; may be symmetric (all growth parameters are small) or asymmetric (may be caused by placental problem; head measurements correlate with dates, body disproportionately smaller); formerly referred to as *intrauterine growth retardation*

large for gestational age (LGA) - fetus measures larger than dates (diabetic fetus)

macrosomia - birth weight greater than 4000 g or above the 90th percentile for the estimated gestational age

Non-Stress Test (NST) - utilizes Doptone to record the fetal heart rate and its reactivity to the stress of uterine contraction

placental grade - technique of grading the placenta for maturity

postterm - fetus born later than the 42-week gestational period

preterm - fetus born earlier than the normal 38- to 42-week gestational period

systolic to diastolic (S/D) ratio - Doppler determination of the peak systolic velocity divided by the peak diastolic velocity

small for gestational age (SGA) - fetus measures smaller than dates

---

Fetal growth assessment is very important to the perinatologist and obstetric physician. Before the availability of ultrasound determination of fetal growth, physicians had to rely on their physical assessment of the neonate to determine what occurred during fetal development. The physician's assessment would determine if the fetus was born **preterm** (before 38 menstrual weeks), at term (between 38 and 42 menstrual weeks), or **postterm** (later than 42 weeks). Further classification dictated whether the fetal birth weight was **small for gestational age (SGA),** appropriate for gestational age, or **large for gestational age (LGA).** This determination allowed the clinicians to recognize the increase in perinatal morbidity and mortality for the preterm or postterm and SGA or LGA fetus.

INTRAUTERINE GROWTH RESTRICTION

Intrauterine growth restriction (IUGR) is best described as a decreased rate of fetal growth. IUGR complicates 3% to 7% of all pregnancies. It is most commonly defined as a fetal weight at or below 10% for a given gestational age.[16] It often becomes difficult to differentiate the fetus that is constitutionally small (small for gestational age [SGA]) from one that is growth restricted. IUGR babies are at a greater risk of antepartum death, perinatal asphyxia, neonatal morbidity, and later developmental problems. Mortality is increased sixfold to tenfold, depending on the severity of the condition.

The most significant maternal factors for IUGR are the history of a previous fetus with IUGR, significant maternal hypertension or smoking, the presence of a uterine anomaly (bicornuate uterus or large leiomyoma), and significant placental hemorrhage (Box 30-1).

Before abnormal growth can be diagnosed it is necessary to accurately determine the gestational age of the pregnancy. In the prenatal period an accurate last menstrual period or a first-trimester ultrasound can be used. If a first-trimester ultrasound was not performed, then in the second or third trimester the standard biparietal diameter

(BPD), head circumference (HC), abdominal circumference (AC), and femur length (FL) should be used in conjunction with other tests of fetal well-being (e.g., biophysical profile [BPP] and fetal Doppler velocimetry).

In the postnatal period, several other body dimensions can be used. These include head circumference, crown-heel length, weight-height ratios, ponderal index (PI), and skinfold thickness. Other considerations include maternal size and race and the gender of the neonate.

The classification of IUGR is based on the morphologic characteristics of the fetuses studied. Symmetric IUGR is usually the result of a first-trimester insult such as a chromosomal abnormality or infection. This results in a fetus that is proportionally small throughout pregnancy.

Asymmetric IUGR begins late in the second or third trimester and results from placental insufficiency. This fetus usually shows head sparing at the expense of abdominal and soft tissue growth. The FL exhibits varying degrees of compromise. An early diagnosis of IUGR and close fetal monitoring (BPP, Doppler, and fetal growth evaluation) is of significant help in managing a pregnancy suspected of IUGR. Clinical observations and appropriate actions for IUGR are shown in Box 30-2.

SYMMETRIC INTRAUTERINE GROWTH RESTRICTION

Symmetric growth restriction is characterized by a fetus that is small in all physical parameters (e.g., BPD, HC, AC, and FL). This is usually the result of a severe insult in the first trimester. The causes may include low genetic growth potential, intrauterine infection, severe maternal malnutrition, fetal alcohol syndrome, chromosomal anomaly, or severe congenital anomaly.[38] One study demonstrated early IUGR in 9 of 11 fetuses with trisomy 13, in 2 of 5 fetuses with 45 XO, and in only 2 of 18 fetuses with

---

> **BOX 30-1 SIGNIFICANT MATERNAL FACTORS FOR INTRAUTERINE GROWTH RESTRICTION (IUGR)**
>
> - Previous history of fetus with IUGR
> - Significant maternal hypertension
> - History of tobacco use
> - Presence of uterine anomaly
> - Significant placental hemorrhage

> **BOX 30-2 CLINICAL OBSERVATIONS AND ACTIONS FOR INTRAUTERINE GROWTH RESTRICTION (IUGR)**
>
> - *Clinical Signs of IUGR:* Decreased fundal height and fetal motion
> - *Key IUGR sonographic markers:* Grade 3 placenta before 36 weeks or decreased placental thickness
> - *Sonographer action:* Alert the physician, determine the cause (maternal history, habits, environmental exposure, viruses, diseases, drug exposure), carefully evaluate placenta and fetal anatomy with ultrasound

trisomy 17.[22] Another report describes two cases of triploidy in association with early symmetric IUGR.[33] Because of the increased association of chromosomal abnormalities, prenatal testing to rule out aneuploidy should be considered (Figure 30-1).

ASYMMETRIC INTRAUTERINE GROWTH RESTRICTION

Asymmetric growth restriction is the more common form of IUGR and is usually caused by placental insufficiency. This may be the result of maternal disease such as diabetes (classes D to F), chronic hypertension, cardiac or renal disease, abruptio placentae, multiple pregnancy, smoking, poor weight gain, drug usage, or uterine anomaly. It should be noted that IUGR fetuses have been born to mothers that have no high-risk factors; therefore all pregnancies undergoing ultrasonic examinations should be evaluated for IUGR.

Asymmetric IUGR is characterized by an appropriate BPD and HC and a disproportionately small AC. This reinforces the brain-sparing effect, which states that the last organ to be deprived of essential nutrients is the brain. The BPD and HC may be slightly smaller, but this usually does not happen until the late third trimester.

A third type of IUGR has been described.[9] In the third type, it is proposed that fetuses with long FL (90th percentile or above) and small AC (at or below the 5th percentile) may be nutritionally deprived even though their estimated fetal weight (ETW) falls at least in the lowest 10%. The theory is that in asymmetric IUGR the fetal length is well preserved, whereas the soft tissue mass is deprived. The FL to AC ratio or PI would be abnormally low. The proponents of this theory claim this occurs in less than 1% of IUGR cases but stress the importance of detection because these cases of IUGR have an EFW within the limits of normal.[9]

ULTRASOUND DIAGNOSTIC CRITERIA

The IUGR multiple parameters are shown in Box 30-3.

BIPARIETAL DIAMETER

The BPD is not a very reliable predictor of IUGR, for many reasons. The first is the head-sparing theory, which is associated with asymmetric IUGR. Fetal blood is shunted away from other vital organs to nourish the fetal brain, giving the fetus an appropriate BPD (plus or minus 1 standard deviation) for the true gestational age.

The second problem is the potential alteration in fetal head shape secondary to oligohydramnios. Oligohydramnios is a decreased amount of amniotic fluid often associated with IUGR. Dolichocephaly or a falsely shortened BPD can lead to underestimation of the fetal weight, and brachycephaly or a falsely wider BPD can lead to overestimation of the EFW. The HC measurement is a more consistent parameter, but a combination of all growth parameters (BPD, HC, AC, and FL) should be used when diagnosing a fetal growth discrepancy.

ABDOMINAL CIRCUMFERENCE

Because of the variability of fetal proportion and size the AC is a poor predictor of gestational age but is very valu-

---

BOX 30-3 MULTIPLE PARAMETERS FOR INTRAUTERINE GROWTH RESTRICTION (IUGR)

- *BPD:* Imaged in the transverse plane using the cavum septi pellucidi, thalamic nuclei, falx cerebri, and choroid plexus as landmarks. The BPD can be misleading in cases associated with unusual head shapes. Used alone it is a poor indicator of IUGR.
- *HC/AC ratio:* High false-positive rate for use in screening general population. The HC/AC ratio is useful in determining type of IUGR.
- *FL/AC ratio:* Not dependent on knowing gestational age. The FL/AC ratio has a poor positive predictive value.
- *FL:* May decrease in size with symmetric IUGR.
- *AC:* Measure at level of portal-umbilical venous complex. When growth is compromised, AC is affected secondary to reduced adipose tissue and depletion of glycogen storage in liver. AC is the single most sensitive indicator of IUGR.

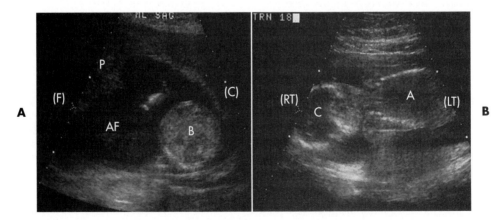

Figure 30-1 Second-trimester fetus with trisomy 18 shows symmetric intrauterine growth restriction. Both the head and abdomen measured well below expected growth curves. Echogenic bowel *(B)* is seen in image **A.** Image **B** shows the small cranium *(C)* and abdomen *(A). AF,* Amniotic fluid; *(LT),* Left; *P,* Placenta; *(RT),* Right.

able in assessing fetal size.[7] In IUGR the fetal liver is one of the most severely affected body organs, which alters the circumference of the fetal abdomen.[8]

HEAD CIRCUMFERENCE TO ABDOMINAL CIRCUMFERENCE RATIO

The HC to AC ratio was first developed to detect IUGR in cases of uteroplacental insufficiency.[5] The HC to AC ratio is especially useful in differentiating symmetric and asymmetric IUGR. For each gestational age, a ratio is assigned with standard deviations. In an appropriate-for-gestational-age (AGA) pregnancy the ratio should decrease as the gestational age increases.

In the presence of IUGR and with the loss of subcutaneous tissue and fat, the ratio increases. The HC to AC ratio is at least 2 standard deviations above the mean in approximately 70% of fetuses affected with asymmetric IUGR. The HC to AC ratio is not very useful, however, in predicting symmetric IUGR, because the fetal head and fetal abdomen are equally small. Another report also found the HC to AC ratio to be highly predictive of IUGR.[8]

ESTIMATED FETAL WEIGHT

The most reliable **estimated fetal weight (EFW)** formulas incorporate all fetal parameters, such as BPD, HC, AC, and FL. This is important because an overall reduction in the size and mass of these parameters naturally gives a below-normal EFW. An EFW below the 10th percentile is considered by most to be IUGR.

There are numerous formulas for estimating fetal weights. One method uses the BPD and AC to derive the fetal weight, with an accuracy of plus or minus 20%.[42] This formula does not take into consideration HC and FL, which contribute to fetal mass. It also ignores the fact that BPD can be altered slightly because of normal variations in head shape, such as brachycephaly or dolichocephaly. These variations can occur in association with oligohydramnios, which may found with IUGR.

Another method uses three basic measurements: HC, AC, and FL.[18] The use of the HC instead of the BPD has improved the predictive value to plus or minus 15%.

A third method defines three zones of EFW.[7] Each zone has a different prevalence of IUGR. In zone 1 the EFW is above the lower 20% confidence limit and IUGR is ruled out. In zone 3 the EFW is below the lower 0.5% confidence limit and yields an 82% prevalence of IUGR. Patients in this zone should be delivered as soon as lung maturity can be proven. If the EFW is between zone 1 and zone 3, it falls into zone 2, which has a 24% prevalence of IUGR. Patients in this zone should have serial sonograms and fetal heart rate monitoring.

Numerous other growth curves are available, but the one chosen must be appropriate for the population of patients (e.g., sea level versus below sea level). It is also important to remember that symmetric IUGR cannot be diagnosed in a single examination. The interval growth can be plotted on a graph to show the growth sequence. Eth-

nicity, previous obstetric history, paternal size, fetal gender, and the results of tests of fetal well-being must be considered before IUGR, rather than a healthy SGA, can be diagnosed.

A computer-generated antenatal chart is available that can be customized for individual pregnancies, taking the mother's characteristics and birth weights from previous pregnancies into consideration.[13] By review of 4179 pregnancies with ultrasound-confirmed dates, one study showed that in addition to gestation and gender, maternal weight at first antenatal visit, height, ethnic group, and parity were significant determinants of birth weight in the study population.[13] Correction factors were calculated and entered into a computer program to adjust the normal birth weight percentile limits. With adjusted percentiles the researchers found that 28% of babies that conventionally fit the criteria for SGA (less than the 10%), and 22% of those who were LGA (greater than the 90%) were in fact within normal limits for the pregnancy. Conversely, 24% and 26% of babies identified as small or large, respectively, with adjusted percentiles were missed by conventional unadjusted percentile assessment.[13]

AMNIOTIC FLUID EVALUATION

The association between IUGR and decreased amniotic fluid (oligohydramnios) is well recognized (Box 30-4). Oligohydramnios has also been associated with fetal renal anomalies, rupture of the intrauterine membranes, and postdate pregnancy. One method, developed for evaluating and quantifying amniotic fluid volume at different intervals during a pregnancy divides the uterine cavity into four equal quadrants by two imaginary lines running perpendicular to each other.[37] The largest vertical pocket of amniotic fluid, excluding fetal limbs or umbilical cord loops, is measured. The sum of the four quadrants is called the **amniotic fluid index (AFI)**.[37] Normal values have been calculated for each gestational age (plus or minus 2 standard deviations). Normal is 8 to 22 cm; decreased is less than 5 cm; and increased is greater than 22 cm (Figure 30-2).[37]

Not every laboratory has adapted the AFI technique, and it is still quite acceptable to use the "eyeball technique," which is simply a subjective survey to evaluate the overall amount of amniotic fluid. Various other criteria have been described for defining oligohydramnios, such as occurring when the largest vertical pocket is less than 3 cm,[19] less than 1 cm,[26] or less than 0.5 cm.[30] Whichever

---

BOX 30-4 POINTS TO REMEMBER FOR INTRAUTERINE GROWTH RESTRICTION (IUGR)

- Oligohydramnios occurs if the fetus cannot urinate.
- Polyhydramnios develops if the fetus cannot swallow.
- Amniotic fluid pocket less than 1 to 2 cm may represent IUGR.
- Not all oligohydramnios is associated with IUGR.

technique is chosen, co-workers should use it consistently. The AFI is very helpful in a busy laboratory where multiple sonographers evaluate patients and may have varying opinions on the appearance of normal, decreased, or increased amniotic fluid.

In the presence of oligohydramnios, care should be taken when evaluating fetal growth parameters, because they can be compressed. Because the fetus lacks the surrounding fluid protecting it, the circumferences can actually be changed by transducer pressure on the maternal abdomen. This in turn may alter the EFW.

PLACENTAL GRADE

The current accepted technique for determining **placental grade** (grade 0 to grade 3) for maturity has been described (see Chapter 34).[15] It should be noted that only 10% to 15% of term placentas are grade 3.[14] Early placental maturation and perinatal outcome have been compared, with report of the mean birth weight of the early maturation group significantly less than that of patients in the matched control group.[36]

Two key ultrasonic markers may help diagnose IUGR. They are a grade 3 placenta noted before 36 weeks or a decreased placental thickness (less than 1.5 cm).

TESTS OF FETAL WELL-BEING

Early diagnosis and estimation of fetal well-being are the main problems in managing IUGR. Fetal breathing motion and urine production were the first functional tests to be assessed. The fetal urine production rate was first de-

---

BOX 30-5   BIOPHYSICAL PROFILE (BPP)

To determine the BPP, assign a value of 2 points to each of the following:
- *Fetal breathing movement (FBM):* One episode for 30 seconds continuous during a 30-minute observation.
- *Gross body movement:* At least three discrete body or limb movements in 30 minutes, unprovoked. Continuous movement for 30 minutes should be counted as one movement.
- *Fetal tone:* Active extension and flexion of at least one episode of limbs or trunk.
- *Fetal heart rate (FHR):* Also known as the Non-Stress Test (NST). At least two episodes of fetal heart rate of >15 beats per minute and at least 15 seconds duration in a 20-minute period.
- *Amniotic fluid index (AFI):* One pocket of amniotic fluid at least 2 cm in two perpendicular planes or AFI total fluid measures of 5 to 22 cm.

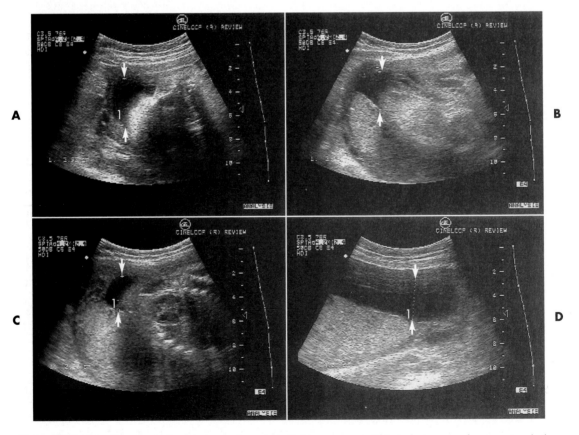

Figure 30-2   The four-quadrant technique of amniotic fluid assessment. This technique produces an amniotic fluid index (AFI). The uterus is divided into four equal parts, and the largest vertical pocket of amniotic fluid in each quadrant is measured, excluding fetal limbs or umbilical cord. The sum of the four quadrants is the AFI, which equals 14.2 cm at 31 weeks. This is within normal limits.

scribed in 1973.[6] The fetal bladder was measured in three dimensions and the volume was calculated. This was repeated hourly and the increase was calculated. Because of the time and cumbersome technique involved, this method has not been adopted for widespread use.[7]

BIOPHYSICAL PROFILE

The **biophysical profile (BPP)** was originally described in 1980.[27] Since then, numerous modifications and variations have been made by other authors. The BPP was adapted to form a linear relationship with the assessment of multiple fetal biophysical variables, such as the Apgar score in the newborn infant or vital signs in the adult. Five biophysical parameters were assessed individually and in combinations. Each test had a high false-positive rate that was greatly reduced when all five variables were combined.

The five parameters are as follows:

1. Cardiac Non-Stress Test (NST)
2. Observation of fetal breathing movements (FBM)
3. Gross fetal body movements (FM)
4. Fetal tone (FT)
5. Amniotic fluid volume (AFV)

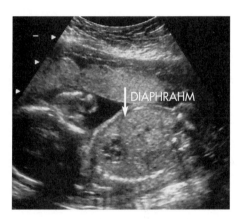

Figure 30-3 Fetal breathing may be seen as the chest wall moves inward and the anterior abdominal wall moves outward; or breathing may also be seen by watching the movement of the kidney in the longitudinal plane.

The fetus has a specified time limit (30 minutes) to perform these tasks (Box 30-5). Each variable is arbitrarily assigned a score of 2 when normal and 0 when abnormal. A BPP score of 8 to 10 is considered normal. A score of 4 to 6 has no immediate significance. A score of 0 to 2 indicates either immediate delivery or extending the test to 120 minutes.

Fetal Breathing Movements. A true breathing movement is described as simultaneous inward movement of the chest wall with outward movement of the anterior abdominal wall during inspiration (Figure 30-3). An alternative area to watch for breathing is the fetal kidney movement in the longitudinal plane. Two points are given if one episode of breathing lasting 30 seconds within a 30-minute period is noted by the practitioner. If this is absent, no points are given. The fetal central nervous system initiates and regulates the frequency of fetal breathing movements; these patterns vary with sleep-wake cycles.

Fetal Body and Trunk Gross Movements. At least three definite extremity or trunk movements must be observed within the 30-minute period to score 2 points (Figure 30-4). Less than three movements scores zero points. The intact nervous system controls gross fetal body movements; these patterns vary with sleep-wake cycles.

Fetal Tone. Fetal tone is characterized by the presence of at least one episode of extension and immediate return to flexion of an extremity or the spine (Figure 30-5). One active extension and flexion of an open and closed hand would be a good example of positive fetal tone (Figure 30-6). Such a movement would score 2 points. Abnormal fetal tone is noted by a partial extension or flexion of an extremity without a quick return and would score zero points.

Amniotic Fluid Volume. Amniotic fluid volume is related to the fetal-placental unit and is not influenced by the fetal central nervous system. Premature aging of the

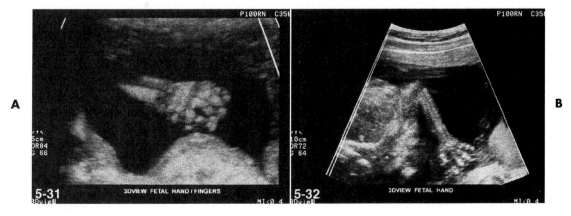

Figure 30-4 At least three definite extremity or trunk movements must be seen within the 30-minute period in a normal fetus. **A,** Open fetal hand and wrist. **B,** Elbow, forearm, and wrist.

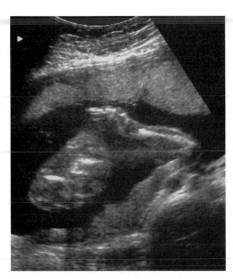

Figure 30-5   Fetal tone is characterized by the presence of at least one episode of extension and immediate return to flexion of an extremity or the spine. This view of the upper extremity is shown in flexion.

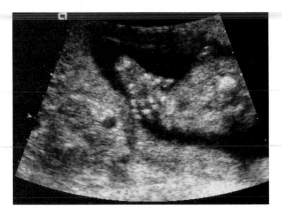

Figure 30-6   One active extension and flexion of an open and closed hand is a good example of positive fetal tone. This image shows the hand wide open with all fingers and thumb extended.

placenta (grade III) may contribute to oligohydramnios of IUGR syndrome. Evaluation of the four-quadrant amniotic fluid volume is considered normal if the pockets (quadrants) of fluid measure at least 2 cm or more in two planes and a score of two points is given. The transducer must be perpendicular to the center of the pocket of fluid in the center of the screen, and the uterine wall cannot be included as part of the fluid measurement.

Decreased amniotic fluid may represent IUGR or intrauterine stress, and serial growth parameters may need to be assessed. Fluid that is decreased near term indicates that the baby may need to be delivered earlier than planned. Decreased fluid means the blood is redistributed to the head and the heart; a decrease in blood to the kidneys causes the AFI to decrease.

NON-STRESS TEST

The **Non-Stress Test (NST)** is done using Doppler to record fetal heart rate and its reactivity to the stress of uterine contraction. The time expended for this portion of the examination is usually 40 minutes. Fetal motion is detected as a rapid rise on the recording of uterine activity or the patient noting fetal movements. The following conditions indicate a reactive, or normal, NST and score 2 points:

- Two fetal heart rate accelerations of 15 beats per minute or more
- Accelerations lasting at least 15 seconds
- Gross fetal movements noted over 20 minutes without late decelerations

These fetal heart accelerations with fetal movements are a positive sign of fetal well-being; late reductions in rate or decelerations indicate a poor prognosis. Zero points are awarded if two fetal heart rate accelerations with gross fe-

tal movements are not seen over a 40-minute period. Forty minutes is arbitrarily used to accommodate the fetal sleep-wake cycles.

According to a recent modification the test is considered normal when all the variables monitored by ultrasound imaging are normal (FBM, FM, FT, AFV) without the performance of the NST.[28]

The goal of the BPP is to find a way to predict and manage the fetus with hypoxia. One study analyzed the BPP variables based on the gradual hypoxia concept.[44] This concept states that dynamic biophysical activities (FT, FM, FBM, and fetal heart rate reactivity) are controlled by neural activity arising in distinct anatomic sites in the brain. These become functional at different stages of development, with the later-developing centers requiring higher oxygen levels. The fetal tone center develops at 7.5 to 8.5 weeks. The fetal movement center develops at 9 weeks, and regularized diaphragmatic motion develops by 20 to 21 weeks. Heart rate reactivity is the last to occur; it appears by the late second to early third trimester. This hypothesis further states that centers that develop later are more sensitive to acute hypoxia. It is therefore expected that the loss of cardiac reactivity and suppression of fetal breathing movements would occur with relatively mild hypoxia. Cessation of FM and eventually loss of FT would occur with progressively more profound hypoxemia.

DOPPLER ULTRASOUND

Obstetric **Doppler** velocimetry is one of the newest techniques to evaluate the fetal environment. Doppler is the study of reflections of blood flow. It was first described in 1842 by Christian Johann Doppler, an Austrian professor of mathematics and geometry.[11]

There are two basic types of Doppler. The simplest technique is continuous wave (CW) Doppler. The second is pulsed wave (PW) Doppler. With CW Doppler a single transducer has two separate piezoelectric crystals, one that continuously transmits signals and one that simultaneously receives signals. Because the crystals are either emit-

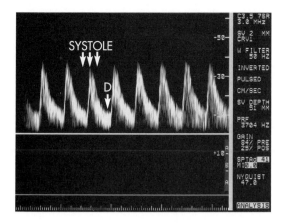

Figure 30-7 Typical umbilical artery Doppler waveform representing a normal systolic to diastolic ratio. The ratio measures peak-systolic to end-diastolic flow. The calipers should be placed at the top of the systolic peak and at the bottom of the diastolic trough. Note the normal amount of diastolic flow. *D*, Diastole.

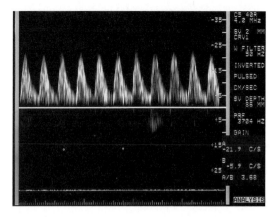

Figure 30-8 Umbilical artery Doppler waveform demonstrating increased vascular resistance (less diastolic flow) in the fetal umbilical circulation. The systolic to diastolic (S/D) ratio is 3.8. Some authors consider an S/D ratio over 3.0 after 30 weeks of gestation to be abnormal.

ting or receiving sound, CW Doppler measures no range or depth resolution. No intrauterine imaging is available with CW, but it may be used in conjunction with a real-time ultrasound system to locate or confirm a vessel sampling site. CW is limited to the study of superficial vessels because it cannot discriminate between signals arising from different structures along the beam path. CW Doppler is, however, portable, inexpensive, and simple to operate.

In pulsed wave (PW) Doppler, short bursts of ultrasound energy are emitted at regular intervals. The same piezoelectric crystal both sends and receives the signals. This allows for range or depth discrimination. The depth of the target is calculated from the elapsed time between transmission of the pulse and reception of its echoes, assuming a constant speed of sound in tissues. In PW Doppler a sonographer can electronically steer the insonating Doppler beam with the trackball or joystick on the keyboard. This permits sampling of vessels at specific anatomic locations.

In one study, CW and PW Doppler were compared using the patient as the control.[29] The systolic to diastolic (S/D or A/B) ratios were obtained from the umbilical artery and the maternal uterine arteries with both CW and PW Doppler systems. The results were comparable. Laboratories can use either a CW or PW Doppler system effectively.

Up to the present, Doppler, or real-time, ultrasound has not been associated with any ill effect to the mother or the fetus when used at the manufacturer's recommended safety level. Food and Drug Administration guidelines state that the spatial peak-temporal average intensity (SPTA, a unit used to measure ultrasound intensity) must be less than 94 milliwatts per square centimeter (mW/cm²) in situ. Most commercial equipment uses variable acoustic outputs between 1 and 46 mW/cm². The power output of a given unit should be known before the unit is used on a fetus.

Quantitative and Qualitative Measurements. Two main types of measurements can be taken from a Doppler waveform: quantitative and qualitative. Quantitative Doppler flow measurements include blood flow and velocity, whereas qualitative measurements look at the characteristics of the waveform that indirectly approximate flow and resistance to flow. Qualitative measurements include **systolic to diastolic ratio (S/D ratio),** resistance index (RI), and pulsatility index. The S/D ratio measures peak systole to end-diastolic blood flow. The RI is calculated as systole minus diastole divided by systole. The pulsatility takes the difference between peak-systole and end-diastole and divides this by the mean of the maximum frequency over the whole cardiac cycle.

Doppler ultrasound has shown that in fetuses with asymmetric IUGR, vascular resistance increases in the aorta and umbilical artery and decreases in the fetal middle cerebral artery. This reinforces the head-sparing theory, which describes the fetus ensuring blood flow to the fetal brain at the expense of the extremities.

Increased vascular resistance is reflected by an increased S/D ratio or pulsatility index. Some authors consider an S/D ratio over 3.0 in the umbilical artery after 30 weeks abnormal and demonstration of increased resistance in the fetal circulation.[40] The maternal uterine artery S/D ratio should be below 2.6 (Figures 30-7 and 30-8). A ratio above 2.6 suggests increased vascular resistance and indicates a decreased maternal blood supply to the uterus.

In the umbilical circulation, extreme cases of elevated resistance causing absent or reverse end-diastolic flow velocity waveforms are associated with high rates of morbidity and mortality.[37] One report demonstrated that an SGA fetus with an increased umbilical artery S/D ratio is at much higher risk for poor perinatal outcome than a small fetus with a normal S/D ratio (Figures 30-9 and 30-10).[43]

In one series a growth-restricted fetus with an abnormal S/D ratio was found to be at risk for early delivery, re-

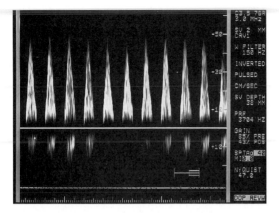

Figure 30-9   Umbilical artery waveform with absent end-diastolic velocity (AEDV). The S/D ratio cannot be measured in these cases because of the missing diastolic flow. The patient should be followed closely because AEDV has been associated with adverse perinatal outcome.

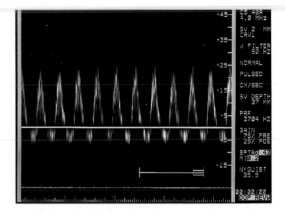

Figure 30-10   This umbilical Doppler waveform is the most severe Doppler finding and has been associated with adverse fetal outcomes. This finding is called *complete reversal of end-diastolic velocity.* Note how the diastolic flow dips below the baseline. These results should be reported immediately to the patient's physician.

duced birth weight, decreased amniotic fluid at birth, admission to the neonatal intensive care unit, neonatal complications associated with IUGR, and a prolonged hospital stay.[2] Other authors have reported similar results.[37,43]

Abnormal umbilical artery S/D velocity waveforms have been shown to improve with the patient on bed rest in the left lateral position.[41] The patients were closely monitored with serial Doppler, BPP, and fetal growth evaluation. Of 128 pregnant women, 66 (51.5%) reverted to normal flow in 4.5 ± 1.5 weeks. Another group (48.5%) exhibited persistent abnormal flow.[41] None of the improved group exhibited fetal distress or perinatal mortality, whereas in the abnormal flow group 24% experienced fetal distress and 13% experienced perinatal mortality. The report of the study proposes that a subset of patients with abnormal Doppler velocimetry improves with bed rest and has a better perinatal outcome, whereas patients with persistent abnormal flow are at risk for poor perinatal outcome.

In conclusion, the best method of solving the puzzle of whether a fetus has IUGR or is constitutionally small is to combine an evaluation of all parameters. Normal umbilical artery, maternal uterine artery, and fetal middle cerebral artery help evaluate the fetus that is well and normal but just small rather than small secondary to IUGR. The practitioner also must consider the family history of birth weights and ethnicity. For example, it is almost invalid to use the standard EFW growth curves when plotting the fetal growth of a constitutionally small ethnic group, such as Asians. A fetus could be labeled as SGA although its size might be totally appropriate for its heritage. Use of all the fetal surveillance tests (i.e., EFW, AFI, placental grading, BPP, NST) may allow better evaluation of the in utero environment.

MACROSOMIA

Macrosomia has classically been defined as a birth weight of 4000 g or greater or above the 90th percentile for esti-

mated gestational age. With respect to delivery, however, any fetus that is too large for the pelvis through which it must pass is macrosomic.[10] Macrosomia has shown to be 1.2 to 2 times more frequent than normal in women who are multiparous, 35 years or older, have a prepregnancy weight over 70 kg (154 lb), have a PI in the upper 10%, have pregnancy weight gain of 20 kg (44 lb) or greater, have a postdate pregnancy, or have a history of delivering an LGA fetus.[3,23]

Macrosomia is also a common result of poorly controlled maternal diabetes mellitus. The frequency of macrosomia in the offspring of mothers with diabetes ranges from 25% to 45%.[24] It is widely accepted that increased levels of glucose and other substrates result in fetal hyperinsulinemia, which promotes accelerated somatic growth. Macrosomic infants of insulin-dependent diabetic mothers are usually heavy and show a characteristic pattern of organomegaly. In addition to adipose tissue, the liver, heart, and adrenals are disproportionately increased in size.[31,32] Not all infants of diabetic mothers are overgrown; diabetic mothers with severe vascular disease may in fact be growth restricted.

Malformation syndromes in which fetal overgrowth, with or without organomegaly, is a feature include Beckwith-Wiedemann syndrome, Marshall-Smith syndrome, Sotos' syndrome, and Weaver's syndrome.[21]

The macrosomic fetus has an increased incidence of morbidity and mortality as a result of head and shoulder injuries and cord compression. One study found an increasing incidence of shoulder dystocia as birth weight increased.[1] The incidence was 10% in fetuses below 4500 g and increased to 22.6% in fetuses over 4500 g. Another study also found an increase, but the overall percentiles were less.[39] This study reported that shoulder dystocia occurred in 4.7% of study fetuses greater than 4000 g and 9.4% of fetuses greater than 4500 g.

Clavicular fractures, facial and brachial palsies, meconium aspiration, perinatal asphyxia, neonatal hypoglycemia, and other metabolic complications are significantly increased in macrosomic pregnancies.[3,35]

Timing and mode of delivery of the potential macrosomic fetus are of great concern to the obstetrician. One study demonstrated that the incidence of macrosomia increased from 1.7% at 36 weeks to 21% at 42 weeks.[3] A retrospective study evaluated 406 women by ultrasound late in the third trimester to see if the diagnosis of LGA altered the management of labor and delivery.[25] The sonographic prediction of LGA fetuses had a sensitivity, specificity, and positive predictive value of 50%, 90%, and 52%, respectively. Although there were no significant differences in the rate of induction, use of oxytocin, or use of forceps, women with an ultrasound diagnosis of an LGA fetus more frequently received epidural anesthesia and had more cesarean deliveries than women without that diagnosis. The sonographic prediction of EFW in this series was incorrect in half of the cases, with the EFW both underestimating and overestimating the actual birth weight.

Clinical considerations of macrosomia should include the genetic constitution (e.g., familial traits) and environmental factors (e.g., maternal diabetes or prolonged pregnancy).[10]

Two terms relating to macrosomic fetuses are *mechanical macrosomia* and *metabolic macrosomia*.[10] Three types of mechanical macrosomia have been identified: (1) fetuses that are generally large, (2) fetuses that are generally large but with especially large shoulders, and (3) fetuses that have a normal trunk but a large head. The first type can result from genetic factors, prolonged pregnancy, or multiparity. The second type is found in the diabetic pregnancy, and the third type can be caused by genetic constitution or pathologic process such as hydrocephalus.[10] One type of metabolic macrosomia has been identified, which is the group of LGA fetuses based on a standard weight curve appropriate for the population being studied and a normal range extending to 2 standard deviations above the mean.[10]

Ultrasound Findings

BIPARIETAL DIAMETER

Accurate sonographic prediction of macrosomia would be invaluable to the obstetrician in managing and delivering a fetus with macrosomia. The detection of fetal macrosomia by BPD was first described in 1979.[8] The authors found that all fetuses that were appropriate for gestational age (AGA) at delivery had normal antenatal BPD measurements, but 25 out of 26 fetuses with two or more BPD values above the 97th percentile were LGA at delivery.[8] Another study of the normal progression of fetal head growth in diabetic pregnancies found that, in contrast to the fetal liver, the fetal brain is not sensitive to the growth-promoting effects of insulin.[34] Most investigators believe, however, that BPD is not the optimal parameter for prediction of macrosomia.

ABDOMINAL CIRCUMFERENCE

As stated before, AC is useful as a parameter to assess fetal size. It is not very predictive of gestational age. It is probably the single most valuable biometric parameter used in

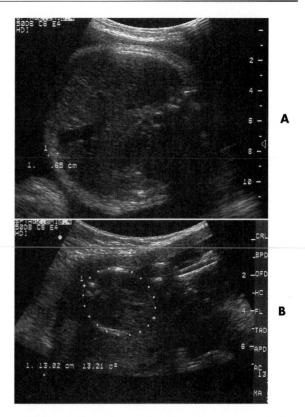

Figure 30-11 **A,** Transverse section through a macrosomic fetal abdomen. Note the fat rind *(calipers)* encircling the entire abdomen, compared with a severely intrauterine growth-restricted fetus **(B)** whose growth is 8 weeks behind. The fetal skin is almost transparent and difficult to differentiate from other surrounding organs.

assessing fetal growth (Figure 30-11). In one series the authors were able to predict 4 of 4 macrosomic fetuses when a change in the abdominal circumference was greater than or equal to 1.2 cm per week between the 32nd and 39th weeks of pregnancy (<4000 g), 17 out of 21 (81%) of the fetuses with birth weights between 4000 and 4499 g, and 5 out of 6 (83%) of the fetuses with birth weights exceeding 4500 g. [24] When the abdominal growth was less than 1.2 cm per week (between 32 and 39 weeks), normal fetal growth was correctly identified in 89.1% of cases.

One study found that in fetuses with birth weights less than 4000 g, both the BPD and AC were within the standard deviation for the gestational age.[34] In fetuses greater than 4000 g, normal BPD values were found but the AC values were greater than 2 standard deviations above the norm after 28 to 32 weeks.[34]

ESTIMATED FETAL WEIGHT

Sonographic estimation of fetal weight to determine macrosomia is of some value. According to one study, EFWs above the 90th percentile are considered macrosomic.[42] A significant number of false-positive and false-negative results can be expected unless the actual weight is either less than 3600 g or greater than 4500 g.[10] The reason for this may be that currently available formulas to estimate fetal weight assume a uniform density of tissue.[2] Because fat tissue is less dense than lean body mass, it can be hypothesized that sonographic overestimation of fetal weight, particularly in diabetic mothers, is the consequence of an elevated proportion of body fat. This results in a lower body density.

In one report, the PI and skinfold thickness were both significantly greater in infants whose sonograms overpredicted the fetal weight compared with those whose sonograms underpredicted the fetal weight.[2] The PI and skinfold thickness are indexes to directly measure fat. The study reported that estimating fetal fat would provide a correction to formulas predicting fetal weight and improve the accuracy of the estimation.

FEMUR LENGTH TO ABDOMINAL CIRCUMFERENCE

Another approach to detecting macrosomia is the femur length to abdominal circumference (FL/AC) ratio.[22] This is a time-independent proportionality index. A study of 156 fetuses within 1 week of delivery was done, using a cutoff of less than 20.5% (the 10th percentile).[17] Prenatal FL/AC values less than the 10th percentile and newborns with birth weights above the 90th percentile were classified as macrosomic, both prenatal and postnatal. The authors were only able to predict 63% of fetuses that were macrosomic, which suggests that this ratio has a limited clinical application. Current studies fail to show a significant increase in the length of the femur in the macrosomic infant.

CHEST CIRCUMFERENCE

Chest circumference has been described as a useful parameter in detecting the LGA fetus, with reported detection rates, respectively, of 80% and 47%, in relation to the 90th and 95th percentiles for macrosomic fetuses.[45] The sonographic technique of the study is unclear. It appears that fetal chest measurements were taken just below the area where cardiac pulsations were identified. The measurements were probably taken at the level of the upper fetal abdomen.

MACROSOMIA INDEX

Calculating a macrosomic index can be performed by subtracting the BPD from the chest diameter.[12] As in the previously described study on chest circumference, the chest circumference is measured at the level of the upper fetal abdomen.[45] In a study involving subtraction of the BPD from the chest diameter, 87% of infants weighing more than 4000 g had a macrosomic index of 1.4 cm or greater.[12] Fetal weight less than 4000 g was predicted accurately in 92% of infants who had a macrosomic index of 1.3 or less. Although this test appears to be quite sensitive, only 61% of those with a positive result were found to be macrosomic at birth.

OTHER METHODS

In addition to the numerous biometric parameters previously discussed as useful in diagnosing macrosomia, other ultrasound observations can alert to ruling out the possibility of fetal macrosomia. Mothers with diabetes may accumulate more amniotic fluid (polyhydramnios) than nondiabetic patients. The presence of polyhydramnios in the nondiabetic patient could alert the physician to the presence of undiagnosed maternal glucose intolerance. The possibility of a fetal anomaly should not be excluded; polyhydramnios has been associated with open neural tube defects.[20]

The placentas of the macrosomic fetus can become significantly large and thick because they are not immune to the growth-enhancing effects of fetal insulin. A placental thickness greater than 5 cm is considered thick when the measurement is taken at right angles to its long axis.[20]

REVIEW QUESTIONS

1. Describe the difference between symmetric and asymmetric IUGR.
2. What is the head-sparing theory?
3. How is an amniotic fluid index obtained? What are normal values?
4. What are the five parameters used when performing a biophysical profile? How are the scores assigned? What are normal values?
5. Describe the concept of gradual hypoxia?
6. What are the common indexes used to evaluate an obstetric Doppler waveform?
7. What are normal S/D values for the umbilical and maternal uterine arteries?
8. What is the definition of macrosomia?
9. Why is the diagnosis of macrosomia of great concern to the obstetrician?

REFERENCES

1. Acker DB, Sachs BP, Freidman EA: Risk factors for shoulder dystocia, *Obstet Gynecol* 66:762, 1985.
2. Bernstein I, Catalano P: Influence of fetal fat on the ultrasound estimation of fetal weight in diabetic mothers, *Obstet Gynecol* 79:561, 1992.
3. Boyd ME, Usher RH, Mclean FH: Fetal macrosomia: prediction, risks, proposed management, *Obstet Gynecol* 61:715, 1983.
4. Bracero L et al: Umbilical artery velocimetry waveform in diabetic pregnancy, *Obstet Gynecol* 68:654, 1986.
5. Campbell S, Thoms A: Ultrasonic measurement of the fetal head to abdominal circumference ratio in the assessment of growth retardation, *Br J Obstet Gynecol* 84:165, 1977.
6. Campbell S, Wladimiroff JW, Dewhurst CJ: The antenatal measurement of fetal urine production, *J Obstet Gynaecol Br Common W* 80:680, 1973.
7. Chervenak FA, Jeanty P, Hobbins JC: Current status of fetal age and growth assessment, *Clin Obstet Gynecol Pec* 10:424, 1983.
8. Crane JP, Kropa MM: Prediction of intrauterine growth retardation via ultrasonically measured head/abdominal circumference ratios, *Obstet Gynecol* 54:597, 1979.
9. Dal Compo S, Sabbagha RE: Intrauterine growth retardation. In Berman M, editor: *Obstetrics and gynecology*, New York, 1991, JB Lippincott.

10. Deter RL, Hadlock FP: Use of ultrasound in the detection of macrosomia: a review, *J Clin Ultrasound* 13:519, 1985.

11. Doppler CJ: Uber das farbige Licht der Doppler-sterne, *Abhand Lungen der Koniglishen Bohmischen Gesellschaft der Wissenchaften* 2:465, 1842.

12. Elliott JP and others: Ultrasound prediction of fetal macrosomia in diabetic patients, *Obstet Gynecol* 60:159, 1982.

13. Gardosi J et al: Customized antenatal growth charts, *Lancet* 339:283, 1992.

14. Grannum P, Hobbins JC: The placenta. In Callen PW, editor: *Ultrasonography in obstetrics and gynecology,* Philadelphia, 1983, WB Saunders.

15. Grannum PA, Berkowitz RL, Hobbins JC: The ultrasonic changes in the maturing placenta, *Am J Obstet Gynecol* 133:915, 1979.

16. Hadlock FP, Deter RL, Harrist RB: Sonographic detection of abnormal fetal growth patterns, *Clin Obstet Gynecol* 27:342, 1984.

17. Hadlock FP and others: Estimation of fetal weight with the use of head, body, and femur measurements: a prospective study, *Am J Obstet Gynecol* 15:333, 1985.

18. Hadlock FP and others: Use of the femur length/abdominal circumference ratio in detecting the macrosomic fetus, *Radiology* 154:503, 1985.

19. Halpern ME and others: Reliability of amniotic fluid volume estimation from ultrasonograms: intraobserver and interobserver variation before and after the establishment of criteria, *Am J Obstet Gynecol* 153:264, 1985.

20. Hobbins JC, Winsberg F, Berkowitz RL: *Ultrasonography in ob/gyn,* Baltimore, 1983, Williams and Wilkins.

21. Jones KL, Smith S: *Recognizable patterns of human malformation,* ed 4, Philadelphia, 1988, WB Saunders.

22. Joupilla P and others: Ultrasonic abnormalities associated with the pathology fetal karyotype results during the early second trimester of pregnancy, *J Ultrasound Med* 7:218, 1988.

23. Klebanoff MA, Klebanoff MA: Mother's birthweight as a predictor of fetal macrosomia, *Am J Obstet Gynecol* 153:253, 1985.

24. Landon M and others: Sonographic evaluation of fetal abdominal growth: predictor of the large-for-gestational-age infant in pregnancies complicated by diabetes mellitus, *Am J Obstet Gynecol* 160:115, 1989.

25. Levine AB and others: Sonographic diagnosis of the large for gestational age fetus at term: does it make a difference? *Obstet Gynecol* 79:55, 1992.

26. Manning FA, Hill LM, Platt LD: Qualitative amniotic fluid volume determination by ultrasound: antepartum detection of intrauterine growth retardation, *Am J Obstet Gynecol* 139:254, 1981.

27. Manning FA, Platt LP, Sypus L: Antepartum fetal evaluation: development of a biophysical profile, *Am J Obstet Gynecol* 136:787, 1980.

28. Manning FA and others: Fetal assessment based on biophysical scoring, *Am J Obstet Gynecol* 162:703, 1990.

29. Mehalek K and others: Comparison of continuous wave and pulsed wave S/D ratios of umbilical and uterine arteries, *Am J Obstet Gynecol* 72:603, 1988.

30. Mercer LJ and others: A survey of pregnancies complicated by decreased amniotic fluid, *Am J Obstet Gynecol* 149:355, 1984.

31. Morris FH: Infants of diabetic mothers: fetal and neonatal pathophysiology, *Perspect Pediatr Pathol* 8:223, 1984.

32. Naeye RL: Infants of diabetic mothers: quantitative morphologic study, *Pediatrics* 35:980, 1965.

33. Nicolaides KH, Rodeck CH, Goslen CM: Rapid karyotyping in non-lethal fetal malformations, *Lancet* 1:283, 1986.

34. Ogata ES and others: Serial ultrasonography to assess evolving fetal macrosomia, *JAMA* 243:2405, 1980.

35. Ott WJ, Doyle S: Ultrasonic diagnosis of altered fetal growth by use of a normal ultrasonic fetal weight curve, *Obstet Gynecol* 63:201, 1984.

36. Patterson RM, Hayashi RH, Cavazos D: Ultrasonically observed placental maturation and perinatal outcome, *Am J Obstet Gynecol* 147:773, 1983.

37. Phelan JP and others: Amniotic fluid volume assessment with the four quadrant technique at 36-42 weeks gestation, *J Reprod Fertil* 32:540, 1987.

38. Sabbagha RE: Intrauterine growth retardation: avenues of future research in diagnosis and management by ultrasound, *Sem Perinatol* 8:31, 1984.

39. Sandmire MF, O'Halloin TJ: Shoulder dystocia: its incidence and associated risk factors, *Int J Gynecol Obstet* 26:65, 1988.

40. Schulman H and others: Umbilical velocity wave ratio in human pregnancy, *Am J Obstet Gynecol* 148:985, 1984.

41. Sengupta S and others: Perinatal outcome following improvement of abnormal umbilical artery velocimetry, *Obstet Gynecol* 78:1062, 1992.

42. Shephard MJ and others: An evaluation of two equations for predicting fetal weight by ultrasound, *Am J Obstet Gynecol* 142:47, 1982.

43. Trudinger BJ and others: Flow velocity waveforms in the material uteroplacental and fetal umbilical placental circulations, *Am J Obstet Gynecol* 152:155, 1985.

44. Vintzileos AM and others: The fetal biophysical profile and its predictive value, *Obstet Gynecol* 62:271, 1983.

45. Wladimeroff JW, Bloemsma CA, Wallenberg HCS: Ultrasonic diagnosis of the large-for-dates infant, *Obstet Gynecol* 52:285, 1978.

Ultrasound and High-Risk Pregnancy

Sandra L. Hagen-Ansert

OBJECTIVES

- List the different types of multiple gestations and the effect the gestations may have on the pregnancy
- Differentiate between monozygotic and dizygotic twins
- Describe twin-twin transfusion syndrome
- List what the sonographer should include in the ultrasound examination in multiple pregnancies
- Differentiate between immune and nonimmune hydrops and the sonographic findings
- Discuss how maternal diabetes may affect the pregnancy
- Describe the effect hypertension has on pregnancy
- Describe the sonographic findings in a patient with systemic lupus erythematosus
- Describe the sonographic findings in fetal demise
- List the complications of premature labor on the fetus

MULTIPLE PRENANCY
DIZYGOTIC TWINS
MONOZYGOTIC TWINS
TWIN-TWIN TRANSFUSION SYNDROME
SONOGRAPHIC APPROACH

IMMUNE AND NONIMMUNE HYDROPS
IMMUNE HYDROPS
ALLOIMMUNE THROMBOCYTOPENIA
NONIMMUNE HYDROPS

MATERNAL DISEASES OF PREGNANCY
DIABETES
HYPERTENSION

SYSTEMIC LUPUS ERYTHEMATOSUS
OTHER MATERNAL DISEASE

FETAL DEATH

ULTRASOUND IN LABOR AND DELIVERY
PREMATURE LABOR
EXTERNAL CEPAHLIC VERSION
DELIVERY OF THE SECOND TWIN

REVIEW QUESTIONS

KEY TERMS

caudal regression syndrome - lack of development of the lower limbs (may occur in the fetus of a diabetic mother)

conjoined twins - occurs when the division of the egg occurs after 13 days

dizygotic - twins that arise from two separately fertilized ova

eclampsia - coma and seizures in the second- and third-trimester patient secondary to pregnancy induced hypertension

erythroblastosis fetalis - hemolytic disease marked by anemia, enlargement of liver and spleen, and hydrops fetalis

fetus papyraceous - fetal death that occurs after the fetus has reached a certain growth that is too large to resorb into the uterus

hydrops fetalis - fluid occurs in at least two areas: pleural effusion, pericardial effusion, ascites, or skin edema

hyperemesis gravidarum - excessive vomiting that leads to dehydration and electrolyte imbalance

hypertension - elevation of maternal blood pressure that may put fetus at risk

maternal serum alpha-fetoprotein (MSAFP) - an antigen present in the fetus; the maternal serum is tested between 16 and 18 weeks of gestation to detect abnormal levels

monozygotic - twins that arise from a single fertilized egg that divides to produce two identical fetuses

nonimmune hydrops (NIH) - term that describes a group of conditions in which hydrops is present in the fetus but not a result of fetomaternal blood group incompatibility

oligohydramnios - too little amniotic fluid

polyhydramnios - too much amniotic fluid

preeclampsia - complication of pregnancy characterized by increasing hypertension, proteinuria, and edema

premature rupture of the membranes (PROM) - may lead to premature delivery or infection

Rh blood group - system of antigens that may be found on the surface of red blood cells. When the Rh factor is present, the blood type is Rh positive; when the Rh antigen is absent, the blood type is Rh negative. A pregnant woman who is Rh negative may become sensitized by the blood of an Rh positive fetus. In subsequent pregnancies, if the fetus is Rh positive, the Rh antibodies produced in maternal blood may cross the placenta and destroy fetal cells, causing erythroblastosis fetalis.

Spaulding's sign - overlapping of the skull bones; occurs in fetal death

systemic lupus erythematosus (SLE) - inflammatory disease involving multiple organ systems; fetus may develop heart block and pericardial effusion

twin-to-twin transfusion - monozygotic twin pregnancy with single placenta and arteriovenous shunt within the placenta; the donor twin becomes anemic and growth restricted with oligohydramnios; the recipient twin may develop hydrops and polyhydramnios

---

Ultrasound has come to play an important role in the management of obstetric patients. It can provide a "window" through which the physician can "see" inside the uterus and look at the fetus. The information that ultrasound can provide regarding pregnancy is extensive. For example, when a mother presents with vaginal bleeding, a common obstetric complication, placental location can easily be determined. Gestational age can be determined and fetal growth can be monitored to assess whether the fetus is growing appropriately. Twins and triplets can be diagnosed early in pregnancy to provide necessary information that physicians use in providing prenatal care.

Ultrasound has also improved patient care. With ultrasound guidance, amniocentesis no longer must be done blindly. The physician can see that the tip of the needle is in the pocket of amniotic fluid and not in the fetus. Ultrasound has changed the method of intrauterine transfusions in Rh disease. Whereas intrauterine transfusion was formerly performed using fluoroscopic guidance, it can now be done using ultrasound guidance, with less radiation to the fetus and mother.

There are many more examples of how ultrasound can influence obstetric management of the pregnant patient. This chapter deals with the interaction between high-risk obstetrics and ultrasound.

MULTIPLE PREGNANCY

The mother who has just been told that she is pregnant with twins is usually very excited. Having twins is an unusual event. The physician providing medical care for the patient, however, now views her not as routine but as a high-risk patient. The mother with a multiple gestation is at increased risk for obstetric complications, such as **preeclampsia,** third-trimester bleeding, and prolapsed cord.[27] The fetuses are at increased risk of premature delivery and congenital anomalies.[14,24] As a result, a twin has a five times greater chance of perinatal death than a singleton fetus.[11] Physicians follow multiple gestations closely with ultrasound.

Before ultrasound was used routinely, as many as 60% of twins were not diagnosed before delivery.[14] With routine use of ultrasound, most multiple gestations are diagnosed before the onset of labor. During the first trimester, multiple pregnancy can be identified by visualizing more than one gestational sac within the uterus (Figure 31-1). A firm diagnosis should not be made unless a fetal pole can be seen within each sac, regardless of the number of sacs that are seen (Figure 31-2).

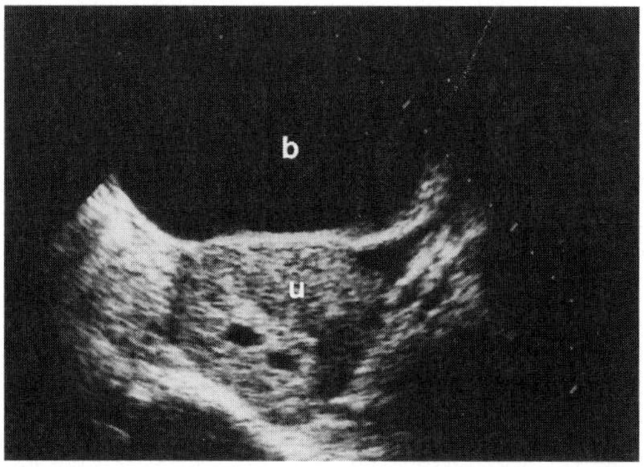

Figure 31-1   Early twin pregnancy manifested by two echolucent gestational sacs. Fetal poles are not yet seen. *b,* Bladder; *u,* uterus.

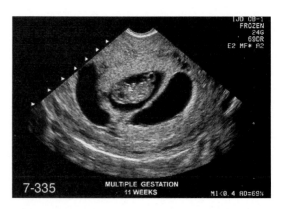

Figure 31-2   Early triplet pregnancy showing three gestational sacs and one fetal pole in the middle sac. In other views, the second and third fetal poles were seen.

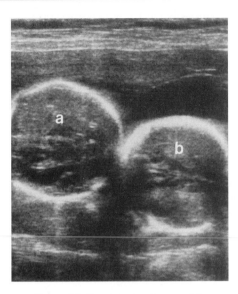

Figure 31-3 Twin heads, *a* and *b*.

In the second and third trimesters, several clinical findings may prompt an ultrasound examination. The patient's uterus may be larger on examination than expected for dates. **Maternal serum alpha-fetoprotein (MSAFP)** screening is performed routinely to detect neural tube defects. Twin pregnancies, by virtue of having two fetuses rather than one, are associated with elevations of MSAFP. Therefore a patient with elevated MSAFP may present for a scan to rule out neural tube defects and be found to be carrying twins. The physician may detect two fetal heart beats or palpate two heads, prompting an ultrasound examination. Finally, the twins may be unsuspected and found serendipitously (Figure 31-3).

Once a multiple gestation has been identified, a detailed ultrasound examination should be performed specifically looking for fetal anomalies, because twins are at increased risk for anomalies. To understand why this is so, the etiology of twinning must be reviewed (Box 31-1).

The number of chorions and amnions in a twin pregnancy depends on the number of zygotes and, in monozygotic twinning, the timing of zygotic division.[21]

DIZGOTIC TWINS

There are two types of twins, monozygotic (identical) and dizygotic (fraternal). **Dizygotic** twins arise from two separately fertilized ova. Each ovum implants separately in the uterus and develops its own placenta, chorion, and amniotic sac (diamniotic, dichorionic). The placentas may implant in different parts of the uterus and be distinctly separate or may implant adjacent to each other and fuse. Although the placentas are fused, their blood circulations remain distinct and separate from each other (Figure 31-4).

MONOZYGOTIC TWINS

Monozygotic twins (identical) arise from a single fertilized egg, which divides, resulting in two genetically identical fe-

tuses. Depending on whether the fertilized egg divides early or late, there may be one or two placentas, chorions, and amniotic sacs. If the division occurs early, 1 to 3 days postconception, there will be two amnions and two chorions (diamniotic, dichorionic). If the division occurs at 4 to 8 days, there will be one chorion and two amniotic sacs (diamniotic, monochorionic) (Figures 31-5 to 31-7). If the division occurs after 8 days, two fetuses will be present but only one amniotic sac and one chorion (monoamniotic, monochorionic) (Figure 31-8). If the division occurs after 13 days, the division may be incomplete and conjoined twins may result. The twins may be joined at a variety of sites, including head, thorax, abdomen, and pelvis (Figures 31-9 and 31-10).

One twin may die in utero and the other one continue to grow. One ultrasound study showed that 70% of pregnancies that began with twins ended with a singleton.[18] Many of these losses occur very early and are never detected. Others are detected early when the patient presents with vaginal bleeding in the second trimester and two sacs are visualized, one with a healthy fetus and one with a demise (Figure 31-11). If the demise occurs very early, complete resorption of both embryo and gestational sac or early placenta may occur. If the fetus dies after reaching a size too large for resorption, the fetus is markedly flattened from loss of fluid and most of the soft tissue. This is termed **fetus papyraceous** (Figure 31-12).

TWIN-TWIN TRANSFUSION SYNDROME

Monozygotic twins present a very high-risk situation. Besides being associated with an increased incidence of fetal anomalies, if there is only one amniotic sac, the twins may entangle their umbilical cords, cutting off their blood supply. In these monochorionic diamniotic pregnancies only the two layers of amnion separate the twins. Because the circulations of the monozygotic twins communicate through a single placenta, they are at increased risk for a syndrome known as **twin-to-twin transfusion.** This exists when there is an arteriovenous shunt within the placenta. The arterial blood of one twin is pumped into the venous system of the other twin (Figure 31-13). As a result, the donor twin becomes anemic and growth restricted. This twin has less blood flow through its kidneys, urinates less, and develops **oligohydramnios.** The recipient twin, however, gets too much blood flow. The twin may be normal or large in size. This fetus has excess blood flow through

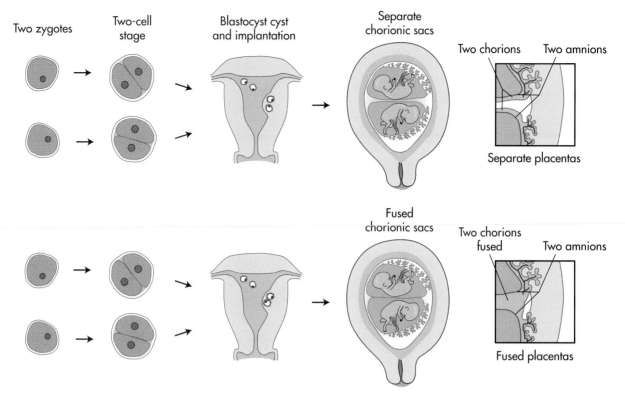

Figure 31-4   The dichorionicity and diamnionicity of dizygotic twins.

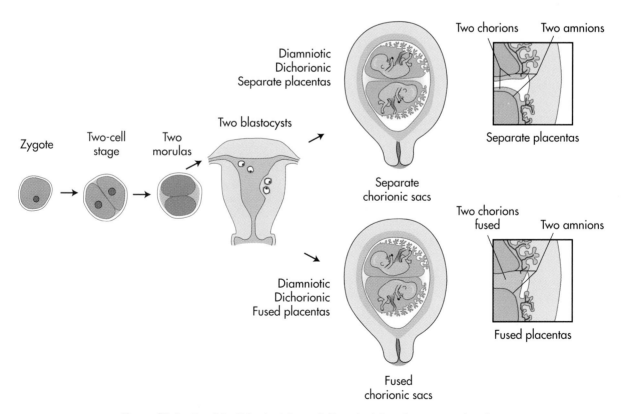

Figure 31-5   Possible dichorionicity and diamnionicity of monozygotic twins.

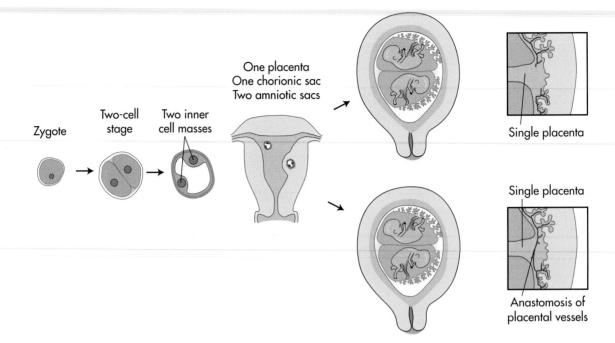

Figure 31-6   A monochorionic, diamniotic monozygotic twin gestation.

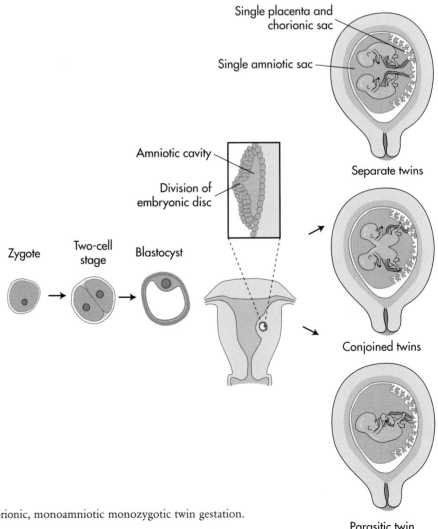

Figure 31-7   A monochorionic, monoamniotic monozygotic twin gestation.

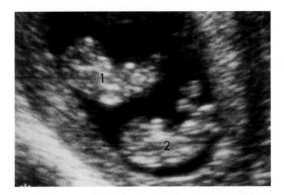

Figure 31-8 Monoamniotic pregnancy showing twin fetuses *(1, 2)* within the same sac. Note the absence of the amnion. This pregnancy is at risk for twin-to-twin transfusion.

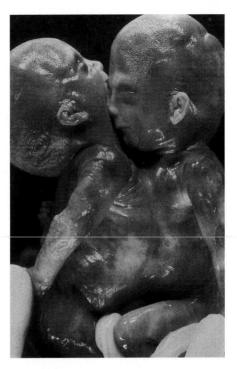

Figure 31-10 Conjoined twins.

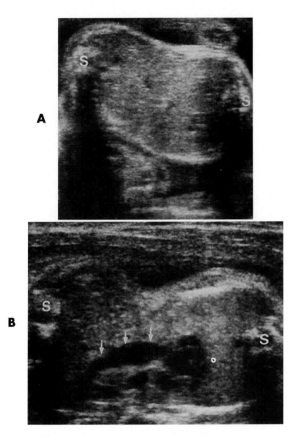

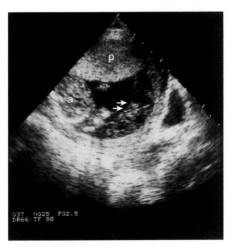

Figure 31-9 **A,** Conjoined twins, seen through cross-sections of abdomen. *S,* Spine. **B,** Conjoined twins on cross-section sharing a common heart *(arrows). S,* Spine.

Figure 31-11 Early twin pregnancy with intrauterine demise of second twin in sac to right *(arrows). a,* Surviving fetus; *p,* placenta.

its kidneys and urinates too much, leading to **polyhydramnios.** This twin may even go into heart failure and become hydropic (Figures 31-14 and 31-15).

When oligohydramnios exists in one sac and polyhydramnios in the other, the small twin may appear stuck in position within the uterus, hence the term "stuck twin." In the event that twin-to-twin transfusion exists, the growth of the twins will be discordant, with the donor twin falling

off the growth curve. If twin-to-twin transfusion exists, both twins are at risk of dying, the smaller one because it is starving to death and the larger one because of heart failure. Depending on the gestational age, the obstetrician may be forced to deliver the fetuses early if it appears one or both of the twins are at risk of dying in utero. Fetal surveillance is increased when growth discordance, oligohydramnios, or polyhydramnios is discovered.[31]

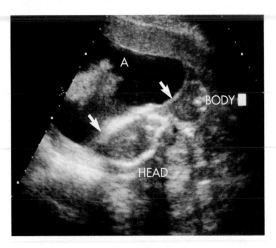

Figure 31-12 Arrows demonstrate a fetus papyraceus, a result of the demise of one twin, with the other surviving. *A*, Amniotic fluid normal sac.

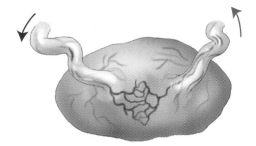

Figure 31-13 The placenta of a pregnancy complicated by the twin-twin transfusion syndrome.

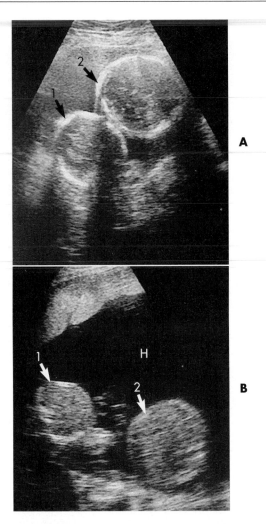

Figure 31-14 Ultrasound demonstrating the discordant growth of twins in the case of a twin-to-twin transfusion syndrome. **A,** The difference in the size of the heads of the twins *(1, 2)*. **B,** The difference in the size of the abdominal circumferences *(1, 2). H*, Hydramnios.

Not all growth discordance results from twin-to-twin transfusion syndrome. Multiple gestations have a high rate of anomalies, and a careful search must be performed to rule out birth defects. Chromosome abnormalities, such as trisomy 18, can also cause growth restriction, and genetic amniocentesis should be considered. Occasionally, if the twins are dizygotic, the growth potential of one may be less than that of the other, which may explain the difference in size.

SONOGRAPHIC APPROACH
Multiple gestations have many potential risks; therefore the sonographer must do a complete job of scanning the fetuses and include the following information in the report: number of sacs, number and location of placentas, gender of the fetuses, biometric data, and whether any anomalies are present.

During the first trimester, the sonographer must be careful to analyze the uterine contents for the presence of multiple gestations. One article reports that multiple gestations were initially undercounted in early pregnancies under 6 weeks performed with transvaginal ultrasound.[8] The report states that an important role of first-trimester sonography is to determine pregnancy number (i.e., whether the pregnancy is singleton, twin, or higher-order multiple gestation).[8] After 6 weeks of gestational age, determining pregnancy number is easily accomplished by counting embryos in the uterus. Before 6 weeks the embryo is not consistently visualized and the sonographer must count the gestational sacs and small yolk sacs. The article reported that the frequency of undercounting multiple gestations on a 5.0- to 5.9-week sonogram was highest for monochorionic twins (86%), followed by higher-order gestations (16%), and last by dichorionic twins (11%).[8] The authors of the report reasoned that some of the gestational sacs may differ in size or the yolk sac may be too small to adequately image so early. This may account for the "vanishing twin" or "appearing twin" phenomenon.

When scanning multiple gestations, the sonographer should always attempt to determine whether there are one or two amniotic sacs by locating the membrane that separates the sacs (Figures 31-16 and 31-17). If two sacs are seen, the pregnancy is known to be diamniotic, but sonography will not be able to indicate whether the twins are identical. As mentioned before, both monozygotic and dizygotic twins may have two amniotic sacs.

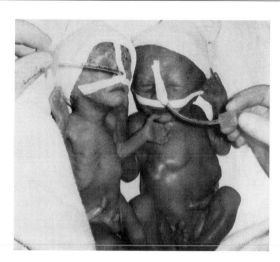

Figure 31-15   Twins from a pregnancy complicated by twin-to-twin transfusion syndrome. Note the lack of subcutaneous fat and smaller size of the twin on the left.

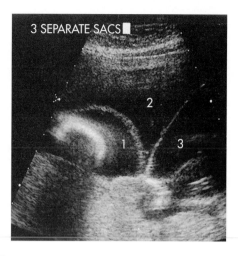

Figure 31-17   Triplet pregnancy showing three distinct amniotic sacs *(1, 2, 3).*

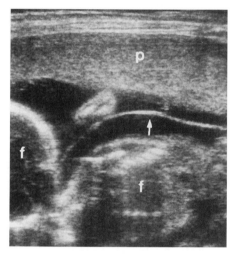

Figure 31-16   Twin pregnancy with membrane *(arrow)* separating the two sacs. *f,* Fetus; *p,* placenta.

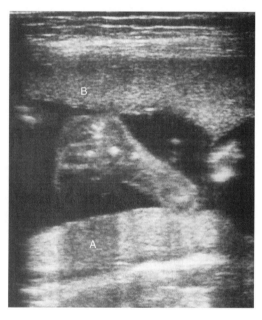

Figure 31-18   Two separate placentas of a twin pregnancy. *A,* Posterior; *B,* anterior.

Documentation of a membrane separating the fetuses confirms the presence of a diamniotic pregnancy. The membrane, composed of amnion with or without chorion, exhibits a characteristic appearance that permits distinction from other membranes of pregnancy. In a twin pregnancy with two separate placentas the membrane extends between the fetuses obliquely across the uterus from the edge of the placenta to the contralateral edge of the other placenta.[21] If only one placental site exists, the membrane extends between the fetuses away from the central portion of the placental site.[21] The fetus may touch the membrane but does not cross it, and the membrane does not adhere to entrap the fetus.[21] The membrane has no free edge within the amniotic fluid. These features distinguish the normal membrane separating twins from other membranes or membranelike structures within the amniotic fluid (i.e., uterine synechiae, partial uterine septations, or amniotic bands.[21]

Failure to image the membrane separating the twin fetuses does not reliably predict the presence of a monoamniotic pregnancy.[21] If only one placenta is seen and a membrane cannot be visualized, other features may assist in the prediction of amnionicity, chorionicity, and zygosity. A male and female fetus is dizygotic, diamniotic, and dichorionic. A twin pregnancy with intertwined umbilical cords, **conjoined twins,** or greater than three vessels in the umbilical cord is found in a monozygotic pregnancy that is monoamniotic and monochorionic.[21]

The location of the placenta should be determined. An attempt also should be made to determine the number of placentas. Occasionally, clearly separate placentas may be identified (Figure 31-18). If two placentas are implanted immediately adjacent to each other and fuse, it may be dif-

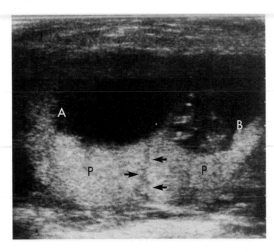

Figure 31-19 Twin pregnancy with two separate but adjacent placentas. *Arrows* show line of demarcation. *P,* Placenta.

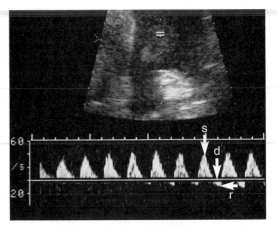

Figure 31-21 Reverse end-diastolic umbilical cord blood flow with pulsed Doppler. *Arrow* indicates reverse diastolic flow *(r)*. *d,* Absent diastolic phase; *s,* systolic phase.

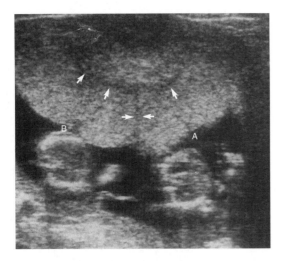

Figure 31-20 Early twin pregnancy showing separation between the two placentas *(horizontal arrows)* and also a small uterine contraction *(vertical arrows)*.

ficult to determine whether there are one or two placentas. The placentas appear to be one large placenta. The body of the placenta should be scanned to determine whether a line of separation can be seen (Figures 31-19 and 31-20).

The twins should each then be scanned for corroboration of dates and size, measuring parameters that include biparietal diameter (BPD), head circumference (HC), abdominal circumference (AC), and femur length (FL).

Dolichocephaly can be common in twin pregnancies as a result of crowding. In dolichocephaly the BPD is shortened and the occipitofrontal diameter (OFD) is lengthened because of compression. Therefore the BPD underestimates gestational age with dolichocephaly. The sonographer should always determine the cephalic index (CI) (CI = BPD/OFD $\times$ 100). CI of less than 75% suggests dolichocephaly. The normal CI is 75% to 85%.

Because the growth of twins is similar to that of singletons early in pregnancy, singleton growth charts are gener-

ally used. It is important to keep in mind that a fetus from a multiple gestation is usually smaller than a singleton fetus. It is known that twins are smaller in size at birth than singleton fetuses of comparable gestational age. Of concern is the ability to detect growth restriction in one or both fetuses. When attempting to determine whether only one twin is growth restricted, differences between the measurements of the two twins must be examined. A difference in estimated fetal weight of more than 20%, a difference in BPD of 6 mm, a difference in AC of 20 mm, and a difference in femur length of 5 mm have been reported as predictors of discordance of growth between twins.[32]

The gender of the fetuses is important to determine. If there is growth discordance between the twins but one is a male and one is a female, then twin-to-twin transfusion cannot exist. If both twins are of the same sex, however, and growth discordance exists, twin-to-twin transfusion syndrome may be a possibility.

Umbilical cord Doppler may be useful for fetal surveillance. During the fetal cardiac cycle, there is umbilical blood flow during both the pumping (systole) and filling (diastole) phases of the heartbeat. No flow (absent end-diastolic flow) (Figure 31-21) or reverse flow during diastole (reverse end-diastolic flow) are signs of fetal jeopardy and may prompt the obstetrician to do further fetal well-being testing or even deliver the fetuses.

One report suggests that most cases of twin transfusion syndrome are identified in the second semester.[28] Abnormal Doppler studies in twin pregnancies should prompt a search for other findings seen in this syndrome, such as polyhydramnios, stuck twin, or hydrops. When Doppler flow patterns are abnormal, careful follow-up should be used to determine if shunting exists.

The multifetal pregnancy reduction method has been used on pregnancies with greater than four fetuses to improve the survival chances of the remaining fetuses. The procedure is performed toward the end of the first trimester by ultrasonographically guided injection of

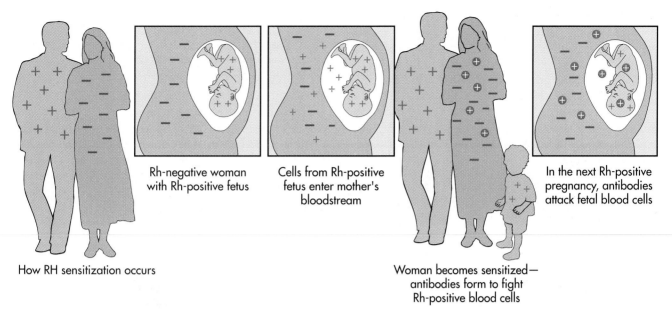

How RH sensitization occurs

Rh-negative woman
with Rh-positive fetus

Cells from Rh-positive
fetus enter mother's
bloodstream

Woman becomes sensitized—
antibodies form to fight
Rh-positive blood cells

In the next Rh-positive
pregnancy, antibodies
attack fetal blood cells

Figure 31-22   Diagram illustrating the concept of Rh sensitization.

potassium chloride into the thoraxes of the fetuses to be aborted.[1]

IMMUNE AND NONIMMUNE HYDROPS

Hydrops fetalis can be classified according to immune and nonimmune causes. By ultrasound evaluation, both types are characterized by extensive accumulation of fluids in fetal tissues or body cavities, reflecting a massive disturbance of fetal water balance.[34] Knowledge of the etiology of hydrops and the fetal karyotype will dictate whether aggressive management is appropriate.[34]

IMMUNE HYDROPS

Erythroblastosis fetalis, whether the result of ABO, Rh, or irregular blood group antigen incompatibility, is a problem of which the sonographer must be aware. Isoimmunization because of blood group incompatibility results when fetal red blood cells obtain entry into the maternal blood system. The fetal red cells possess antigens to which the mother, lacking that antigen, mounts an immune response (Figure 31-22). The resulting antibody can cross the placenta because of its small size. It attaches to the fetal red blood cell and destroys it (hemolysis). This hemolysis then results in fetal anemia, and the fetal bone marrow must then replace the destroyed red blood cells. If the bone marrow cannot keep up with the destruction, extramedullary sites of red blood cell production, such as the liver and spleen, are recruited into erythropoiesis (production of red blood cells). If the production of red blood cells cannot keep up with the destruction, the anemia can become severe and congestive heart failure and edema of fetal tissues may occur.

An isoimmunized fetus may be very sick. If the severely anemic fetus does not receive a blood transfusion, it may die in utero. If a transfusion is not performed in utero and the fetus is delivered prematurely, complications resulting from prematurity, such as respiratory distress syndrome and intracranial hemorrhage, may threaten the life of the infant.

The perinatal death rate for Rh-sensitized pregnancies was 25% to 35% before intrauterine transfusions were performed.[24] With the institution of aggressive treatment and modern intensive neonatal care, the perinatal death rate has decreased significantly. The death rate depends on the severity of the hydrops. The more severe the disease, the greater the chance of fetal death. In 45% to 50% of cases of Rh sensitization the disease is mild, whereas 25% of the time the disease is severe.[30]

Blood group isoimmunization is diagnosed by maternal ABO and Rh determination and antibody screening during pregnancy. Once an antibody known to cause hydrops fetalis has been identified, the antibody titer must be determined. If the antibody titer is less than 1:16, experience at most centers shows that intrauterine death is unlikely. If the antibody titer is greater than 1:16, the pregnancy should be monitored.

The severity of fetal anemia can be determined by two methods, amniocentesis, the older method, and cordocentesis, the newer method. Because hemolysis results in breakdown of red blood cells, a by-product, bilirubin, stains the amniotic fluid. Bilirubin absorbs light at the 450-nm wavelength. A spectrophotometric analysis of the fluid to check light absorption of this level indirectly measures the amount of bilirubin present in the fluid and therefore gives a measure of the degree of hemolysis.

Amniotic fluid can be obtained by amniocentesis. The gestational age at which the first amniocentesis is performed depends on past obstetric history. For example, if the current pregnancy is the first sensitized pregnancy, the first amniocentesis is performed at 26 to 28 weeks of gestation. If the mother has had prior affected infants or fetuses requiring intrauterine transfusions, the physician may need to perform the first amniocentesis earlier than 26 to 28 weeks.

Once the amniocentesis is performed and the amniotic fluid is sent for spectrophotometric analysis, the ΔOD450 is categorized into three zones on the Liley curve (Figure 31-23).[19]

1. *Low zone:* Rh-negative and mildly affected fetuses are found in the low zone. They should be followed expectantly and delivered at term.
2. *Mid-zone:* A downward trend within the mid-zone indicates the fetus is probably affected but will survive, and delivery should occur at 38 weeks of gestation. A horizontal or rising trend indicates that the fetus is in danger of intrauterine or neonatal death and that preterm delivery or intrauterine transfusion and preterm delivery are indicated.
3. *High zone:* Fetal death zone. The fetus in the high zone requires immediate treatment or death will result.

Amniocentesis has been abandoned by some in favor of cordocentesis, a technique in which the umbilical cord is punctured (using ultrasound guidance) by a 22-gauge spinal needle to obtain a fetal blood specimen (Figure 31-24). The fetal hemoglobin level can be checked and if necessary a blood transfusion can be performed immediately.

Ultrasound findings.   The ultrasound team plans an important role in managing the isoimmunized pregnancy. Early in pregnancy, ultrasound confirmation of dates is important in aiding the clinician to decide when the first examination will be performed. During the pregnancy the fetus can be monitored for signs of hydrops up until delivery regardless of whether the pregnancy is being monitored solely by amniocentesis or whether the fetus is undergoing cordocentesis and transfusion.

In examining a fetus for signs of hydrops the sonographer is looking for signs of edema. Scalp edema may be present. The fetus may have ascites (Figures 31-25 and 31-26), pleural effusions, or pericardial effusion (Figures 31-27 and 31-28). Polyhydramnios is generally present if

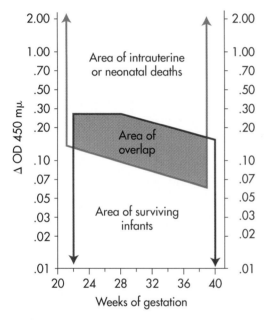

Figure 31-23   The Liley curve, illustrating perinatal outcome based on ΔOD450 values.   (From Queenan JT: *Modern management of the Rh problem*, ed 2, Hagerstown, Pa, 1977, Harper & Row.)

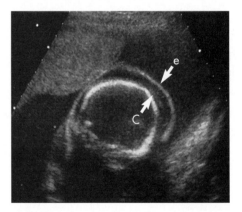

Figure 31-25   Ultrasound of a fetus demonstrating scalp edema. *C,* Head; *e,* edema of the scalp.

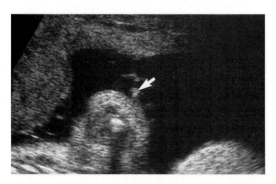

Figure 31-24   Arrow indicates a needle within the umbilical vein during cordocentesis.

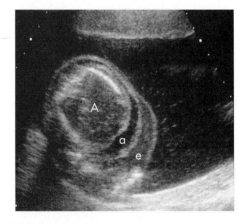

Figure 31-26   Ultrasound demonstrating massive skin edema *(e)* and ascites *(a)* in a fetal demise. *A,* Abdomen.

the fetus is hydropic. The placenta will be large and thick. Because the liver and spleen are involved in producing red blood cells, they will be large. The size of the liver has been measured in isoimmunized fetuses to see whether the severity of the disease can be predicted.[33]

Ultrasound also plays a key role in transfusion of the fetus. Before ultrasound was available for use in transfusion, intrauterine transfusion was performed using fluoroscopic guidance. Now transfusions are done exclusively using ultrasound guidance.

There are two methods of transfusing a fetus. The first, intraperitoneal, was the original method and is not used as often anymore. Using ultrasound guidance, a catheter is placed in the peritoneal cavity of the fetus. The blood is then transfused into the peritoneal space through the catheter. The fetus slowly absorbs the red blood cells from the peritoneal cavity. The second and currently more popular method is direct intravascular transfusion via the umbilical vein (cordocentesis).[6] Using ultrasound guidance, a fine needle is directed through the maternal abdomen toward the umbilical vein where it enters the placenta (Figure 31-29). The red blood cells are transfused directly into the umbilical vein. This method is preferred, because a specimen of fetal blood can be obtained before transfusion to confirm that the fetus is isoimmunized and that it is indeed anemic, requiring transfusion. A specimen can be obtained after transfusion to document that the fetal hematocrit is adequate.

ALLOIMMUNE THROMBOCYTOPENIA

In a rare circumstance a mother may develop an immune response to fetal platelets in a manner similar to that of red blood cells. When this occurs, she develops antibodies to the fetal platelets. The result can be a fetus with a danger-

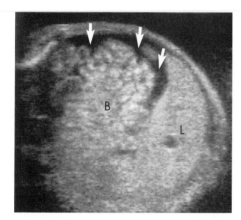

Figure 31-27   Cross-section of fetal abdomen showing ascites *(arrows)* in a fetus with severe hemolytic disease. *B,* bowel, *L,* liver.

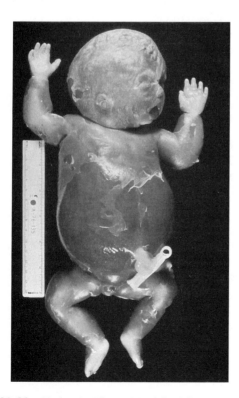

Figure 31-28   Hydropic, Rh-sensitized fetal demise. Note the edema of the extremities and the protuberant abdomen.

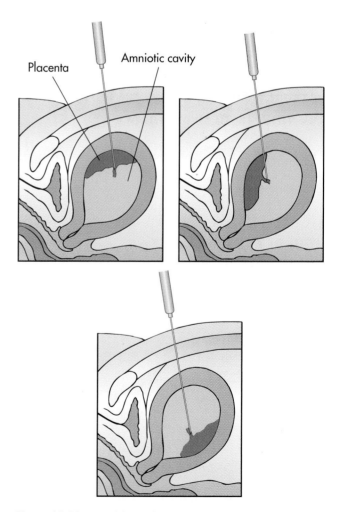

Figure 31-29   Possible needle paths in cordocentesis depending on placental position.

ously low platelet count (thrombocytopenia). There fetuses can have spontaneous bleeding. Babies have been born with this condition, having had intracerebral hemorrhage in utero. Cordocentesis is performed in these cases to document fetal platelet counts before vaginal delivery is attempted. Ultrasound can also be useful to look for evidence of in utero fetal intracerebral hemorrhage.

NONIMMUNE HYSROPS

Nonimmune hydrops (NIH) describes a group of conditions in which hydrops is present in the fetus but is not a result of fetomaternal blood group incompatibility. Numerous fetal, maternal, and placental disorders are known to cause or be associated with NIH, including cardiovascular, chromosomal, hematologic, urinary, and pulmonary problems, as well as twin pregnancies, malformation syndromes, and infectious diseases (Box 31-2).[16]

The incidence of NIH is approximately 1 in 2500 to 1 in 3500 pregnancies, but NIH accounts for about 3% of fetal mortality.[18,19] In the past, 46% to 80% of hydrops fetalis cases resulted from Rh isoimmunization. With the widespread use of Rh immune globulin, the incidence of hydrops fetalis resulting from Rh isoimmunization has steadily declined to the point where the ratio of nonimmunologic to immunologic cases of hydrops fetalis is rising.

The exact mechanism of why NIH occurs is unclear. A variety of maternal, fetal, and placental problems are known to cause or have been found in association with NIH, some of which are listed in Box 31-2. Although the causes of NIH are varied, certainly the same processes described for the hydrops associated with Rh sensitization may apply to NIH.

Cardiovascular lesions are often the most frequent causes of NIH.[16] Congestive heart failure may result from functional cardiac problems, such as dysrhythmias, tachycardias, and myocarditis, as well as from structural anomalies, such as hypoplastic left heart and other types of congenital heart disease. Obstructive vascular problems occurring outside of the heart, such as umbilical vein thrombosis, and pulmonary diseases, such as diaphragmatic hernia, can cause NIH. Large vascular tumors functioning as arteriovenous shunts can also result in NIH.

Severe anemia of the fetus is another well-recognized etiology for NIH.[16] Although the anemia is not caused by isoimmunization, the result is the same. Severe anemia may occur in a donor twin of a twin-to-twin transfusion syndrome causing hydrops. Anemia may result from (-thalassemia or significant fetomaternal hemorrhage. To make the diagnosis of NIH, Rh, or irregular blood group antibody (e.g., Kell or Duffy) isoimmunization is ruled out with an antibody screen.

BOX 31-2 DISORDERS ASSOCIATED WITH NONIMMUNE HYDROPS

CARDIOVASCULAR PROBLEMS
Tachyarrhythmia
Complex dysrhythmia
Congenital heart block
Anatomic defects
Cardiomyopathy
Myocarditis
Intracardiac tumors

CHROMOSOMAL PROBLEMS
Trisomy 21
Turner's syndrome
Other trisomies
XX/XY mosaicism
Triploidy

TWIN PREGNANCY
Twin-to-twin transfusion

HEMATOLOGIC PROBLEMS
α-Thalassemia
Arteriovenous shunts
In utero closed-space hemorrhage
Glucose-6-phosphate deficiency

URINARY PROBLEMS
Obstructive uropathies
Congenital nephrosis
Prune belly syndrome
Ureterocele

RESPIRATORY PROBLEMS
Diaphragmatic hernia
Cystic adenomatoid malformation of the lung
Tumors of the lung

GASTROINTESTINAL PROBLEMS
Jejunal atresia
Midgut volvulus
Meconium peritonitis

LIVER PROBLEMS
Hepatic vascular malformations
Biliary atresia

INFECTIOUS PROBLEMS
Cytomegolovirus
Syphilis
Herpes simplex, type I
Rubella
Toxoplasmosis

PLACENTA/UMBILICAL CORD PROBLEMS
Chorioangioma
Fetomaternal transfusion
Placental and umbilical vein thrombosis
Umbilical cord anomalies

Ultrasound findings. Ultrasonically the fetus may appear very similar to a sensitized baby. Scalp edema, as well as pleural and pericardial effusions, may be present along with ascites (Figures 31-30 and 31-31). Other findings may be present in addition, indicating the cause of the hydrops. If the hydrops is a result of a cardiac tachyarrhythmia, a heart rate in the range of 200 to 240 is common. If a diaphragmatic hernia is present, bowel will be visible in the chest cavity.

If twin-to-twin transfusion is causing hydrops of one twin, there should be a discordance in the size of the two twins. The twin supplying the blood should be growth restricted, whereas the recipient will be normal or large for gestational age. A thorough examination of the fetus, along with fetal echocardiography, must be carried out because, as shown in Box 31-2, abnormalities of almost every organ system have been described with NIH. In addition to the ultrasound examination, genetic amniocentesis for karyotype is indicated, because chromosomal abnormalities have been described as etiologies for NIH.

Many times an etiology for NIH cannot be determined. If an etiology is found, treatment depends on the cause. As an example, if hydrops results from a tachycardia, medicine can be given to the mother in an attempt to slow the fetal heart rate. Ultrasound can be useful in monitoring the progress of the fetus. Resolution of ascites and gross edema has been documented after the fetal heart was converted to a normal rhythm. If the fetus is anemic because of twin-to-twin transfusion, intrauterine transfusion will not solve the anemia problem, because most of the fetus' blood is being shunted away. Ultrasound can help the clinician assess how sick the fetus is by indicating the severity of the hydrops and by biophysical profile (discussed later). The clinician can then make an informed choice about when to deliver the fetus.

MATERNAL DISEASES OF PREGNANCY

DIABETES

The ultrasound team is often called on to perform multiple examinations of pregnant diabetics. Diabetic pregnancies are at high risk. There is an increased risk of unexplained stillbirth and congenital anomalies among insulin-dependent pregnant diabetics (IDDM).[25,35] Diabetic pregnancies may be

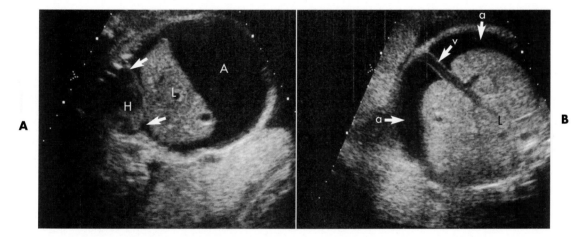

Figure 31-30   Transverse sections of fetal abdomen showing ascites in a fetus with nonimmune hydrops. **A,** Sagittal plane. *A,* Acites; *H,* heart; *L,* liver. **B,** Tranverse plane. *a,* Acites; *L,* liver; *v,* ductus venosus.

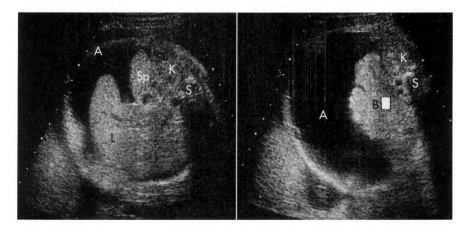

Figure 31-31   Cross-section of fetal abdomen showing ascites. *A,* Ascites; *Sp,* spleen; *B,* bowel; *K,* kidney; *L,* liver; *S,* spine.

complicated by frequent hospitalizations for glucose control, serious infections such as pyelonephritis, and problems at the time of delivery (Box 31-3).

Glucose is the primary fuel for fetal growth. If glucose levels are very high and uncontrolled (as happens in diabetes resulting from an inability to produce enough insulin), the fetus may have many problems. The fetus may become macrosomic. A macrosomic infant (Figure 31-32) may become too large to fit through the mother's pelvis, making cesarean section necessary. If delivery is accomplished vaginally, however, the physician may have difficulty delivering the shoulders of the baby after the head has delivered. This is termed *shoulder dystocia.* Brachial plexus nerve injuries may result from the traction placed on the head and neck in attempts to get the remainder of the baby delivered.

Once delivered, an infant of a diabetic mother may have many problems, including glucose control in the nursery necessitating intravenous glucose administration. If maternal glucose control is good, these problems can be avoided. This is why glucose control in a diabetic pregnant patient is very important.

There are two kinds of diabetes, type 1 (immune-mediated) and type 2. A diabetic pregnant patient may have diabetes antedating her pregnancy. Some pregnant diabetics, however, may manifest signs of diabetes only during pregnancy and have normal glucose levels when they are not pregnant (i.e., gestational diabetics). Gestational diabetics may be diet-controlled or require insulin.

Ultrasound findings. Pregnancy dates should be confirmed with ultrasound. Because of unexplained stillbirth and pregnancy complications, the physician may elect to deliver the diabetic patient at 38 to 40 weeks or when fetal lung maturity is demonstrated. Correct dating is very important. A diabetic baby delivered preterm may have respiratory distress syndrome and require placement in the high-risk nursery.

Scans may give the clinician information about glucose control in the diabetic. Polyhydramnios is associated with poor glucose control (Figure 31-33). A fetus measuring large for gestational age also raises concerns about the diabetic compliance. Increased adipose tissue may be seen on the fetus in utero (Figures 31-34 and 31-35). If the estimated fetal weight is greater than 4500 g at term, the clin-

BOX 31-3 CONGENITAL ANOMALIES IN INFANTS OF DIABETIC MOTHERS

SKELETAL AND CENTRAL NERVOUS SYSTEM
Caudal regression syndrome
Neural tube defects excluding anencephaly
Anencephaly with or without herniation of neural elements
Microcephaly

CARDIAC
Transposition of the great vessels with/without ventricular septal defect
Ventricular septal defect
Atrial septal defect
Coarctation of the aorta with/without ventricular septal defect
Cardiomegaly

RENAL
Hydronephrosis
Renal agenesis
Ureteral duplication

GASTROINTESTINAL
Duodenal atresia
Anorectal atresia
Small left colon syndrome

OTHER
Single umbilical artery

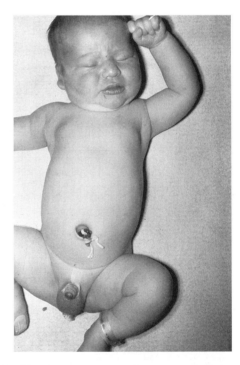

Figure 31-32 A 5280-g (11-lb) infant of a diabetic mother.

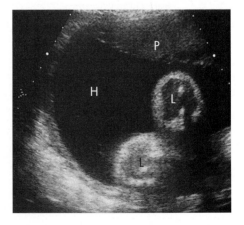

Figure 31-33 Ultrasound demonstrating polyhydramnios *(H)* associated with diabetes. *L,* limb; *P,* placenta.

ician will be alert to the problems of dystocia with a vaginal delivery and may prefer cesarean delivery.

Ultrasound plays a very important role in scanning for fetal anomalies. **Caudal regression syndrome** (lack of development of lower limbs) is seen almost exclusively in diabetic individuals.[25] Commonly seen anomalies are congenital defects of the heart and neural tube defects.[25,35] Finally, ultrasound assists the clinician with amniocentesis for lung maturity studies. When the fetal lung profile (tests that indicate maturity of fetal lungs: lecithin/sphingomyelin [L/S] ratio and phosphatidylglycerol [PG]) is mature, the fetus can safely be delivered.

One study found that mean Doppler values were higher in diabetic patients with vasculopathy than in nondiabetic control patients or in diabetic patients without vasculopathy.[32] The third-trimester systole to diastole ratio (S/D) was greater than 3.0 in almost 50% of patients with vasculopathy. A tendency toward adverse outcomes was observed at S/D ratios approaching 4.0. Statistically significant correlations were found between elevated Doppler indexes and maternal vasculopathy associated with hypertension and worsening renal insufficiency. Intrauterine growth restriction and neonatal metabolic complications were also significantly correlated with elevated Doppler indexes. There was no correlation between Doppler indexes and glucose values.

HYPERTENSION

Hypertension is a medical complication of pregnancy that occurs frequently in high-risk populations. Hypertension places both mother and fetus at risk. Hypertensive pregnancies may be associated with small placentas because of the effect of the hypertension on the blood vessels. If the placenta develops poorly, the blood supply to the fetus may be restricted and growth restriction may result. Growth-restricted fetuses are at increased risk of fetal distress and death in utero.

There are various forms of hypertensive disease during pregnancy. In the past, the term *toxemia* was used to describe hypertensive disorders, because it was believed that a "toxin" in the mother's bloodstream caused the hypertension. Currently, pregnancy-induced hypertension is considered to be caused by prostaglandin abnormalities.

The terminology currently used in clinical practice to describe hypertensive states during pregnancy includes (1) pregnancy-induced hypertension (which includes preeclampsia, severe preeclampsia, and eclampsia) and (2) chronic hypertension, which was present before the woman was pregnant. Preeclampsia is a pregnancy condition in which high blood pressure develops with proteinuria (protein in the urine) or edema (swelling). If the hypertension is neglected, the patient may develop seizures that can be life threatening to both mother and fetus. Severe preeclampsia may develop in some cases and refers to the severity of hypertension and proteinuria. Severe preeclampsia generally indicates that the patient must be delivered immediately. **Eclampsia** represents the occurrence of seizures or coma in a preeclamptic patient. Chronic hypertension is diagnosed in patients in whom high blood pressure is found before 20 weeks of gestation. Chronic hypertension can result from primary essential hypertension or from secondary hypertension (renal, endocrine, or neurologic causes).

Ultrasound findings. The ultrasound team may be called on to perform serial scans for fetal growth and to monitor for the adequacy of amniotic fluid. If fetal growth

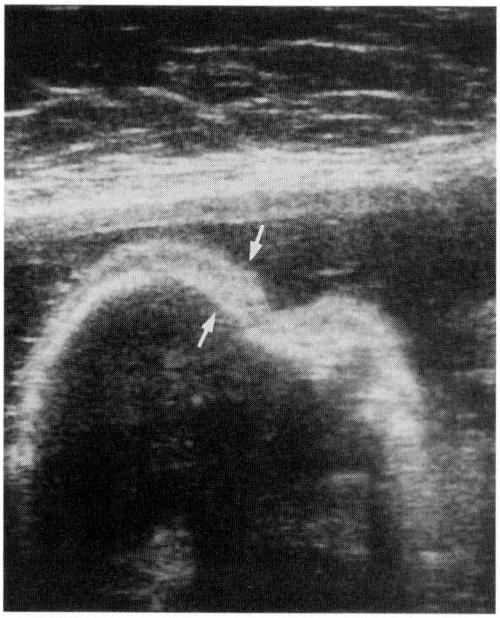

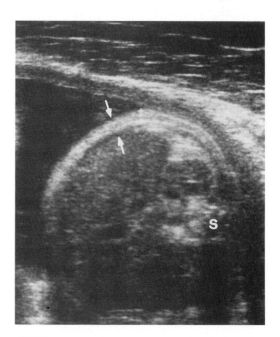

Figure 31-34   Fetus of a diabetic mother showing increased subcutaneous fat on scalp. *Arrows,* Adipose tissue.

Figure 31-35   Fetus of diabetic mother with increased subcutaneous fat. *Arrows,* Subcutaneous adipose tissue; *S,* spine on cross-section of abdomen.

is falling off the normal growth curve or oligohydramnios occurs, the obstetrician may intervene and deliver the fetus, fearing that intrauterine fetal demise is imminent. Hypertensive pregnancies are also associated with abruptio placenta.

SYSTEMIC LUPUS ERYTHEMATOSUS

Systemic lupus erythematosus (SLE) is a chronic autoimmune disorder that can affect almost all organ systems in the body. It is most common in women of childbearing age and may cause multiple peripartum complications. The incidence of spontaneous abortion and fetal death is 22% to 49% in patients with SLE.[6] The placenta is affected by the immune complex deposits and inflammatory responses in the placental vessels and may account for the increased number of spontaneous abortions, stillbirths, and intrauterine growth restricted fetuses.[14] The fetus must be monitored to rule out congenital heart block and pericardial effusion.

OTHER MATERNAL DISEASE

Hyperemesis. Ultrasound can be useful in the workup of vomiting in the pregnant woman. Nausea and vomiting are common symptoms associated with pregnancy. **Hyperemesis gravidarum** exists when a pregnant woman vomits so much that she develops dehydration and electrolyte imbalance. When this occurs, hospitalization with intravenous fluid administration is usually necessary. The physician must ensure that the vomiting results strictly from pregnancy and not other disease, such as gallstones, peptic ulcers, or trophoblastic disease. Trophoblastic disease can easily be ruled out by demonstrating a viable intrauterine pregnancy. Gallstones can be ruled out by careful sonographic examination of the gallbladder.

Urinary Tract Disease. Ultrasound can also be useful in the workup of urinary tract disease. Approximately 4% to 6% of pregnant women have asymptomatic bacteriuria. If the bacteriuria is not treated, 25% of these women develop pyelonephritis.[17] Although pyelonephritis usually presents with flank pain, fever, and white blood cells in the urine, hydronephrosis is another condition that presents with flank pain. Pregnancy is normally associated with mild hydronephrosis.[7] The hydronephrosis may result from a combination of effects. First, progesterone has a dilatory effect on the smooth muscle of the ureter.[10] Second, the enlarging uterus also compresses the ureters at the pelvic brim, causing a hydronephrosis or obstruction.[13] If a woman presents with more than one episode of pyelonephritis or has continued flank pain, ultrasound examination may provide information as to the etiology.

Adnexal Cysts. Physiologic ovarian cysts may be associated with early pregnancy. These cysts may be large,

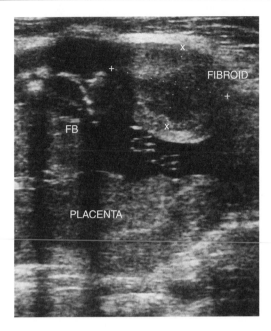

Figure 31-36 Ultrasound of a pregnant uterus showing a uterine fibroid. *FB,* Fetal body.

ranging from 8 to 10 cm. The cyst should shrink as the pregnancy progresses. If the cyst does not resolve, surgical exploration may be necessary to rule out ovarian cancer. Periodic ultrasound examinations are necessary for follow-up of a cyst.

Obesity. Maternal obesity has been associated with an increased incidence of neural tube defects and may be attributed to a deficiency in diet.[26] More women who are obese than women who are of normal weight start their pregnancy with chronic hypertension, and obese women are at an increased risk for pregnancy-induced hypertension.[26] Likewise, obese women are at an increased risk for severe eclampsia. Multiple births and urinary tract infections have also been reported higher in obese women.

Uterine Fibroids. Finally, pregnant women may periodically present with problems related to uterine fibroids. Fibroids are actually benign tumors or uterine smooth muscle that may be stimulated to excessive growth by the hormones of pregnancy, specifically estrogen. If the growth is very rapid, the fibroid may outgrow its blood supply and undergo necrosis. This in turn may cause pain and premature labor (Figure 31-36). Ultrasound examination of the uterus in a pregnant woman may detect uterine fibroids. This is important information for the clinician.

FETAL DEATH

Intrauterine fetal death accounts for roughly one half of all perinatal mortality. Although the cause of death can-

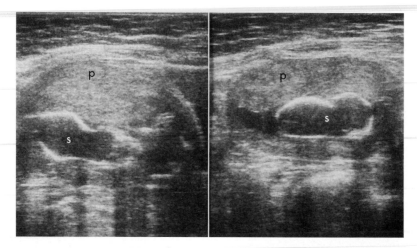

Figure 31-37   Fetal death with compression of fetal skull and overlapping of skull bones. *P,* Placenta; *s,* skull.

not be determined in approximately half of the cases, known causes are infection (usually associated with premature rupture of membranes), congenital or chromosomal abnormalities, preeclampsia, placental abruption, diabetes, growth restriction, and blood group isoimmunization.

Fetal death may occur in any trimester of pregnancy. The incidence of pregnancy loss in the first trimester is 15 to 20 per 100 pregnancies, with most of the losses resulting from cytogenetic abnormalities.[3] As pregnancy progresses, the incidence decreases to 5 to 10 per 1000 pregnancies (one half the perinatal mortality rate), and factors other than cytogenetic causes play a more important role.

Clinically, first-trimester pregnancy wastage may be diagnosed when the patient presents to her physician with vaginal bleeding, cramping, or passage of tissue. Ultrasound examination may reveal a blighted ovum or a fetus with no heart motion. As the pregnancy progresses into the second trimester, pregnancy landmarks become important in determining whether the pregnancy is proceeding normally. Fetal heart tones should be heard with Doppler at approximately 12 weeks of gestation. At 20 weeks of gestation the uterine fundal height should have risen to the umbilicus and the uterus should measure approximately 20 cm above the symphysis pubis. The mother should also perceive fetal movements on a daily basis beginning between 16 and 20 weeks of gestation. Failure to achieve any one of these landmarks may prompt the clinician to obtain an ultrasound examination.

As the pregnancy progresses, the clinician will follow the pregnant woman at regular intervals, listening to fetal heart tones and measuring the uterine fundal height at each visit. The mother will be questioned about fetal movements. The absence of a fetal heart rate usually prompts the clinician to obtain an ultrasound examination. Cessation of fetal movements should prompt an immediate search for fetal heart tones. If none are present, ul-

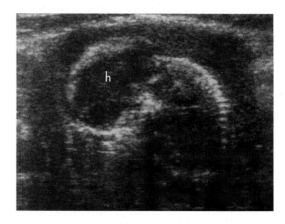

Figure 31-38   Fetal death with exaggerated curvature of spine. *h,* Head.

trasound examination will confirm or rule out intrauterine fetal demise.

Ultrasound findings. The presence or absence of fetal heart motion can be easily determined with real-time ultrasound. Historically the physician could rely on radiologic signs of fetal death, including (1) overlap of skull bones **(Spalding's sign)** caused by liquefaction of the brain (Figure 31-37), (2) an exaggerated curvature of the fetal spine (Figure 31-38), and (3) gas in the fetus (Figure 31-39).[29] These signs require several days to develop and, if present, indicate that the baby has been dead for more than 48 hours. In addition to these signs, which are signs of death, there may be other ultrasound findings that may indicate the cause of death. As an example, the presence of severe oligohydramnios may indicate that intrauterine growth restriction or renal anomalies may have been present. Fetal ascites may indicate the presence of blood group isoimmunization or NIH. Lack of fetal heart motion, however, with real-time ultrasound will make the definitive diagnosis of death.

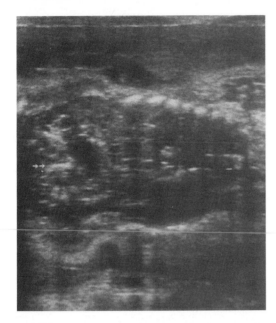

Figure 31-39 Intrauterine fetal death. *Arrows,* Gas within the bowel.

BOX
31-4 WARNING SIGNS OF PRETERM LABOR

- Menstrual-like cramps (constant or intermittant)
- Low, dull backache
- Pressure (feels like baby is pushing down)
- Abdominal cramping (with or without diarrhea)
- Increase of change in vaginal discharge (contains mucus or is watery, light, or bloody)
- Fluid leaking from the vagina
- Feeling poorly
- Uterine contractions

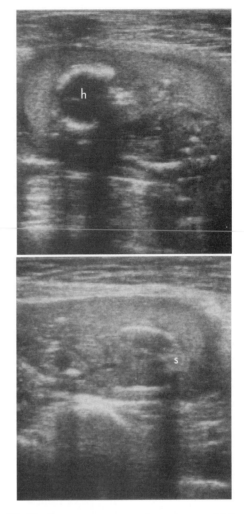

Figure 31-40 Premature rupture of membranes at 16 weeks of gestation with marked oligohydramnios. *h,* Head; *s,* spine.

ULTRASOUND IN LABOR AND DELIVERY

PREMATURE LABOR

Premature labor is the onset of labor before 37 weeks of gestation (Box 31-4). Premature labor is a very common obstetric complication occurring in 15% to 20% of all pregnancies.[29] Often, if the contractions are perceived early enough, that is, before significant cervical dilation has occurred, an attempt can be made to stop the labor with various medications. Sometimes tocolysis (the inhibition of labor) is not successful or is not indicated, and a preterm infant is born. These babies can have a multitude of problems. The earlier they are born, the greater the risk of problems, such as respiratory distress syndrome, intracranial hemorrhage, bowel immaturity, and feeding problems.

The etiologies of preterm labor are myriad. Common causes include premature rupture of membranes, intrauterine infection, bleeding, fetal anomalies, polyhydramnios, multiple pregnancy, growth restriction, maternal illness such as diabetes or hypertension, incompetent cervix, and uterine abnormalities.[12,29]

Epidemiologic factors such as socioeconomic class; maternal age, weight, and height; poor antenatal care; smoking; coitus; and a poor previous obstetric history are presumed etiologies also.[12] In about 50% of cases, no cause or association can be identified as being responsible for the preterm labor.

Ultrasound findings. Ultrasound can provide the health care team with important information regarding the pregnancy. It can document whether the amniotic fluid is normal, increased, or decreased. Increased amniotic fluid may be idiopathic (no identifiable cause) or may be a result of maternal diabetes or fetal anomalies. Decreased amniotic fluid may be associated with growth restriction or ruptured membranes (Figure 31-40). The fetal measurements may indicate that the fetus is growth restricted. The dates may be incorrect, and the fetus may be older or younger than previously thought. The estimated fetal weight may be very important. The obstetric and neonatal team may consider fetuses weighing less than 500 g as non-

viable, for example. The obstetric team may not perform a cesarean section for a breech fetus that weighs less than 650 g. The ultrasound-predicted estimated fetal weight may give critical information to the obstetrician.

In addition to any abnormalities that may be identified, ultrasound may assist the clinician if an amniocentesis is performed. Amniocentesis may be performed to obtain amniotic fluid to determine fetal lung maturity and to culture for infection of the amniotic cavity.

Premature rupture of membranes (PROM) may be a common cause of preterm labor.[29] The clinical management of PROM is controversial, ranging from conservative (expectant) management to active intervention. Conservative management consists of observing the patient without induction of labor, intervening to deliver the fetus only if there is evidence of infection or fetal distress. The conservative viewpoint holds that keeping the baby inside the mother is safer and less expensive than a bed in a neonatal unit. Active management consists of delivering the fetus soon after rupture of membranes because of concern that infection may jeopardize both the mother and fetus.

Ultrasound findings. Ultrasound can play an important role in the management of PROM. Amniocentesis can be difficult after the membranes have ruptured because less amniotic fluid is present. Ultrasound-guided amniocentesis is safer for the fetus. Fluid can be obtained for culture for infection and for lung maturity studies. If the fetal lungs are mature or if infection is present, labor can be induced. Estimated fetal weights may guide decisions regarding vaginal versus operative deliveries. Caution must be taken at this point. When decreased amniotic fluid is present, fetal weights may be underestimated. Ultrasound plays an integral role in the management of preterm labor and premature rupture of membranes.

EXTERNAL CEPHALIC VERSION
Breech deliveries account for 4% of all deliveries at term. Early in pregnancy the fetus is small and there is a lot of amniotic fluid. The fetus can move around a lot and may assume a vertex, breech, or transverse position.

As the pregnancy progresses, fetal movement is more restricted. The fetus grows in size and the amniotic fluid decreases. The heaviest portion of the fetus, the head, is drawn by gravity into the pelvic inlet. The incidence of breech presentation decreases gradually to the point that at term approximately 4% of all fetuses are in a breech or transverse presentation.

Breech presentation at the time of delivery is associated with multiple pregnancies, congenital abnormalities, prematurity, uterine anomalies, and placenta previa. Breech vaginal deliveries are associated with an increased perinatal mortality rate, prolapsed cord, lower Apgar scores, fetal distress, and higher complication rates.[4] For these reasons, obstetricians are more inclined to perform cesarean section for delivery of a breech baby rather than allow it to deliver vaginally.

Cesarean section rates have increased significantly over the past 10 to 15 years, and breech presentation has accounted for some of that increase.[2] Nationwide interest has focused on this increase in cesarean section rates. Ways of reducing the number of cesarean sections have been suggested, one of which is converting a breech presentation to a vertex presentation by applying pressure to the baby through the mother's abdomen (external cephalic version).[36] This procedure is performed preferably before the onset of labor and at greater than 38 weeks of gestation. The patient is placed supine and the fetus is scanned for position. Placing one hand in the area of the head and one around the buttocks of the fetus, pressure is applied through the maternal abdomen in an attempt to turn the fetus within the uterus to a cephalic presentation. Ultrasound is used to observe whether version has been successful. The fetal heart rate can also be monitored so that, if slowing occurs, the version can be halted to allow for recovery of the fetal heart rate. The location of the fetal head, body, and limbs must be known, the head must be flexed, and the location of the placenta determined.

Contraindications to performing this procedure do exist. In general, this procedure is not attempted if the mother has had prior cesarean section or if the membranes have ruptured. The placenta should not be anterior, because the operator wants to avoid manipulation of the placenta. Obesity, decreased amniotic fluid, and a tight abdominal wall may limit the success of the version attempt.

The version attempt should be performed in a hospital setting so that tocolytic (uterine relaxation) agents can be used to help prevent uterine contractions. Also, to manage possible complications successfully, the patient should be in a labor and delivery suite equipped to handle those problems. Finally, if the version is successful and the patient is at term, labor can be induced while the fetus is in vertex presentation. Fetuses have been known to convert from vertex back to breech presentation (and vice versa) rather quickly.

The success rates of external cephalic version vary, depending on the week of gestation and the experience of the operator. The version attempt will be more successful at 30 weeks of gestation, for example, than at 39 weeks because the baby is smaller and there is more fluid. Many of these fetuses may spontaneously convert to cephalic on their own, and version may not be necessary. If complications occur during the version, however, the term fetus will have fewer problems in the nursery than the preterm fetus.

DELIVERY OF THE SECOND TWIN
The delivery of twins is always an exciting event, not only for the family but for the health care team. When there is only one fetus, it can present either as a vertex or a breech for delivery. When there are two fetuses, however, there are four possible combinations of presentation: (1) twin A is vertex and twin B is vertex, (2) twin A is vertex and twin B is breech, (3) twin A is breech and twin B is vertex, and (4) twin A is breech and twin B is breech.

Because of a variety of factors, including the medicolegal climate and studies showing that there is more morbidity when delivering a breech baby vaginally, most obstetricians deliver a breech baby by cesarean section. Management of twins is therefore fairly straightforward. If both twins are vertex, they are both likely to deliver vaginally. If both are breech, or if the first baby is breech, regardless of the presentation of the second twin, a cesarean section will be performed.

If the first twin is vertex and the second twin is breech, management is not so straightforward. In the past, after the first twin was delivered, the obstetrician would deliver the second twin as a breech. Some physicians still manage vertex or breech twins in this manner; however, more physicians are moving toward cesarean delivery of the breech twin. This results in an increase in cesarean section rates. An alternative is to use external cephalic version to convert a breech second twin to a vertex presentation.[5] Ultrasound can be helpful in the delivery room for this procedure.

After the first twin has delivered, ultrasound can be used to demonstrate the position of the second twin and assess the fetal heart rate. The physician can then attempt to move the baby as described previously. Ultrasound can be used to monitor the progress of the version and can also monitor the fetal heart rate.

ACKNOWLEDGMENTS

The author acknowledges the contribution of Kara L. Mayden-Argo and Laura J. Zuidema to this chapter in the last edition of this book.

REVIEW QUESTIONS

1. What are the differences between monoamniotic and diamniotic pregnancies?
2. Which sonographic features help to distinguish between these types of twinning?
3. What is the physiologic reason for twin-twin transfusion syndrome?
4. Which sonographic parameters are useful in diagnosing this condition?
5. What is the physiology of Rh sensitization and the effect of anemia on the fetus?
6. What testing is employed to screen, diagnose, and treat the affected fetus?
7. What are the causes of nonimmune hydrops (NIH)?
8. How is ultrasound used to monitor the pregnant diabetic patient?
9. When will ultrasound information affect pregnancy management?
10. What should the sonographer expect to see when maternal diseases are present (e.g., hypertension, premature rupture of the membranes [PROM], preterm labor, renal disease)?

REFERENCES

1. Benson CM and others: Multifetal pregnancy reduction of both fetuses of a monochorionic pair by intrathoracic potassium chloride injection of one fetus, *J Ultrasound Med* 17:447, 1998.
2. Bottoms SF, Rosen MG, Sokol RJ: The increase in the cesarean birth rate, *N Engl J Med* 302:559, 1980.
3. Boue J, Boue A, Lazar P: Retrospective and prospective epidemiological studies of 1500 karyotyped spontaneous human abortions, *Teratology* 12:11, 1975.
4. Brenner WE, Bruce RD, Hendricks CH: The characteristics and perils of breech presentation, *Am J Obstet Gynecol* 118:700, 1974.
5. Chervenak FA and others: Intrapartum external version of the second twin, *Obstet Gynecol* 62:160, 1983.
6. Classen SR, Paulson PR, Zacharias SR: Systemic lupus erythematosus: perinatal and neonatal implications, *J Obstet Gynecol Neonat Nurs* 27:493, 1998.
7. Daffos F, Capella-Pavlovsky M, Forestier F: A new procedure for fetal blood sampling in utero: preliminary results of fifty three cases, *Am J Obstet Gynecol* 146:985, 1983.
8. Doubilet PM, Benson CB: "Appearing twin": undercounting of multiple gestations on early first trimester sonograms, *J Ultrasound Med* 17:199, 1998.
9. Fainstat T: Ureteral dilatation in pregnancy: a review, *Obstet Gynecol Surv* 18:845, 1963.
10. Ferguson WF: Perinatal mortality in twins, *Obstet Gynecol* 23:861, 1964.
11. Gravett M: Causes of preterm delivery, *Sem Perinatol* 8:246, 1984.
12. Harrow B, Sloane JA, Salhanick L: Etiology of hydronephrosis of pregnancy, *Surg Gynecol Obstet* 119:1042, 1964.
13. Harvey CJ, Verklan T: Systemic lupus erythematous: obstetric and neonatal complications, *NAACOG Clin Issues Perinat Women Health Nurs* 1:177, 1990.
14. Holzgreve W and others: Investigation of nonimmune hydrops fetalis, *Am J Obstet Gynecol* 150:805, 1984.
15. Kass EH: Bacteriuria and pyelonephritis of pregnancy, *Trans Assoc Am Phys* 72:257, 1959.
16. Levi S: Ultrasonic assessment of the high rate of human multiple pregnancy in the first trimester, *J Clin Ultrasound* 4:3, 1976.
17. Liley AW: Liquor amnii analysis in management of pregnancy complicated by rhesus sensitization, *Am J Obstet Gynecol* 82:1359, 1961.
18. Mahony BS, Filly RA, Callen, PW: Amnionicity and chorionicity in twin pregnancies: prediction using ultrasound, *Radiology* 155:205, 1985.
19. Medearis AL and others: Perinatal deaths in twins, *Am J Obstet Gynecol* 134:413, 1979.
20. Mills JL, Baker L, Goldman AS: Malformation in infants of diabetic mothers occurring before the seventh gestational week: implications for treatment, *Diabetes* 28:292, 1979.
21. Morin KH: Perinatal outcomes of obese women: a review of the literature, *J Obstet Gynecol Neonat Nurs* 27:431, 1998.
22. Newton ER, Cetrulo SL: Management of twin gestation. In Cetrulo CL, Sbaria AJ, editors: *The problem-oriented medical record for high risk obstetrics*, New York, 1984, Plenum.
23. Pretorius DH and others: Doppler ultrasound of twin transfusion syndrome, *J Ultrasound Med* 7:117, 1988.

24. Pritchard JA, MacDonald PC: Obstetric hemorrhage. In *Williams' obstetrics,* ed 16, New York, 1980, Appleton Century-Crofts.

25. Queenan JT: Intrauterine transfusion. In Queenan JT, editor: *Modern management of the Rh problem,* Hagerstown, Md, 1977, Harper & Row.

26. Ray M and others: Clinical experience with the oxytocin challenge test, *Am J Obstet Gynecol* 114:1, 1972.

27. Reece EA, Hobbin JC: Diabetic embryopathy: pathogenesis, prenatal diagnosis and prevention, *Obstet Gynecol Surv* 41:325, 1986.

28. Reece EA and others: Diabetes mellitus in pregnancy and the assessment of umbilical artery waveforms using pulsed Doppler ultrasonography, *J Ultrasound Med* 13:73, 1994.

29. Santolaya J and others: Antenatal classification of hydrops fetalis, *Obstet Gynecol* 79:254, 1992.

30. Soler NG, Walsh CH, Malins JM: Congenital malformations in infants of diabetic mothers, *J Med* 178:303, 1976.

31. Spellacy WN: Cesarean section: update 1983, *Postgrad Obstet Gynecol* 3:1, 1983.

BIBLIOGRAPHY

Evertson LR, Gauthier RJ, Schifrin BS: Antepartum fetal heart rate testing. I. Evaluation of the nonstress test, *Am J Obstet Gynecol* 133:29, 1979.

Hendricks CH: Twinning in relation to birth weight, mortality and congenital anomalies, *Obstet Gynecol* 27:47, 1966.

Macafee CAJ, Fortune DW, Beischer NA: Nonimmunologic hydrops fetalis, *Br J Obstet Gynaecol* 77:226, 1970.

Maidman JR and others: Prenatal diagnosis and management of non-immunologic hydrops fetalis, *Obstet Gynecol* 56:571, 1980.

Manning FA, Platt LD, Sipos L: Antepartum fetal evaluation: development of fetal biophysical profile, *Am J Obstet Gynecol* 136:787, 1980.

Storlazzi E and others: Ultrasonic diagnosis of discordant fetal growth in twin gestations, *Obstet Gynecol* 69:363, 1987.

Vintzileos AM and others: Fetal liver ultrasound measurements in isoimmunized pregnancies, *Obstet Gynecol* 68:162, 1986.

CHAPTER 32

Prenatal Diagnosis of Congenital Anomalies

Charlotte Henningsen

alpha-fetoprotein (AFP) - protein manufactured by the fetus, which can be studied in amniotic fluid and maternal serum. Elevations of alpha-fetoprotein may indicate fetal anomalies (neural tube, abdominal wall, gastrointestinal), multiple gestations, or incorrect patient dates. Decreased levels may be associated with chromosomal abnormalities.

amniocentesis - transabdominal removal of amniotic fluid from the amniotic cavity using ultrasound. Amniotic fluid studies are performed to determine fetal karyotype, lung maturity, and Rh condition.

cystic hygroma - dilation of jugular lymph sacs (may occur in axilla or groin) because of improper drainage of the lymphatic system into the venous system. Large, septated hygromas are frequently associated with Turner's syndrome, congestive heart failure, and death of the fetus in utero; isolated hygromas may occur as solitary lesions at birth.

hypertelorism - abnormally wide-spaced orbits usually found in conjunction with congenital anomalies and mental retardation.

hypotelorism - abnormally closely spaced orbits; association with holoprosencephaly, chromosomal and central nervous system disorders, and cleft palate.

intrauterine growth restriction (IUGR) - a decreased rate of fetal growth, usually a fetal weight below the tenth percentile for a given gestational age.

micrognathia - abnormally small chin; commonly associated with other fetal anomalies.

omphalocele - anterior abdominal wall defect in which abdominal organs (liver, bowel, stomach) are atypically located within the umbilical cord; highly associated with cardiac, central nervous system, renal, and chromosomal anomalies.

polydactyly - anomalies of the hands or feet in which there is an addition of a digit; may be found in association with certain skeletal dysplasias.

ALPHA-FETOPROTEIN AND CHROMOSOMAL DISORDERS

A major congenital anomaly is found in 3 of every 100 births, and an additional 10% to 15% of births are complicated by minor birth defects. Since prenatal ultrasound has become the investigative tool for the obstetrician to access the developing fetus, it is likely that the fetus with an anomaly will be subjected to ultrasound at some time during pregnancy. The role of the sonographer is to screen for the unsuspected anomaly and to study the fetus at risk for an anomaly. The benefits of the examination are greatest when the sonographer is adept at detecting congenital anomalies and understands the cause, progression, and prognosis of the common congenital anomalies.

When a fetal anomaly is found antenatally, a multidisciplinary team approach to managing the fetus, mother, and family is preferable because the fetus may need special monitoring (e.g., serial ultrasound), delivery, and postnatal care, as well as surgery. This multidisciplinary team includes the perinatologist (maternal-fetal medicine specialist), neonatologist (specialist for the critically ill infants), sonologist, perinatal sonographer, pediatric surgeon and other pediatric specialists, geneticist, obstetrician, perinatal and pediatric social workers, and other support personnel. Consultation with specialists is recommended when diagnosis is uncertain. Once an anomaly is found, these specialists can work as a team to optimize clinical manage-ment, to prepare the patient and family for possible surgery, to provide the patient and family with emotional support, and to plan for delivery. Most fetuses with major birth defects are delivered in perinatal regional centers where the specialized physicians, nurses, equipment, treatment, and postnatal surgery are available.

This chapter discusses chorionic villus sampling, amniocentesis, maternal serum alpha-fetoprotein (MSAFP), other similar testing, and basic medical genetics. Included is a discussion of common chromosomal abnormalities.

GENETIC TESTING

CHORIONIC VILLUS SAMPLING

Chorionic villus sampling (CVS) is an ultrasound-directed biopsy of the placenta or chorionic villi (chorion frondosum). The chorion frondosum is the active trophoblastic tissue that becomes the placenta. Because the chorionic villi are fetal in origin, chromosomal abnormalities may be detected when cells from the villi are grown and analyzed. Other conditions, such as biochemical or metabolic disorders, thalassemia, and sickle cell disease (hemoglobinopathies), may also be diagnosed using chronic villi.[30]

CVS is an alternative test used to obtain a fetal karyotype by the culturing of fetal cells, similar to amniocentesis. The advantage of CVS includes the following: (1) it is performed early in pregnancy (10 to 12 weeks), (2) results are available within 1 week, and (3) earlier results allow more options for parents.

CVS is performed transcervically or transabdominally (Figure 32-1). Ultrasound performed before the actual pro-

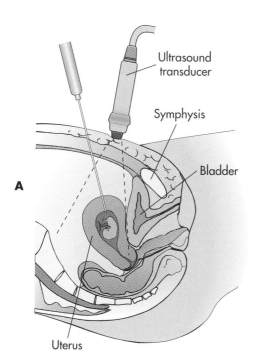

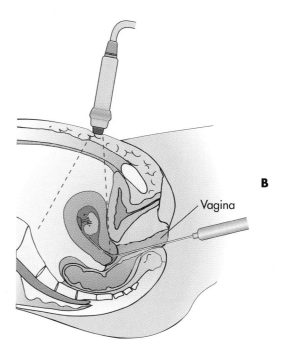

Figure 32-1   **A,** Transabdominal chorionic villus sampling. **B,** Transcervical chorionic villus sampling.

cedure should aid in the following ways: (1) Determine the relationship between the lie of the uterus and cervix and path of the catheter. Bladder fullness influences this relationship. Filling or emptying of the bladder may be necessary to facilitate the catheter route. (2) Assess the fetus in terms of life, normal morphology, and age. (3) Identify uterine masses or potential problems that may interfere with passage of the catheter.

Transvaginal CVS is performed in the dorsolithotomy position (pelvic examination position). The sonographer aids the obstetrician in determining the correct route to pass the catheter through the cervix to the placenta. A guiding stylet is initially introduced to check uterine and placental position. A flexible catheter is then introduced and directed into the placental tissue (Figure 32-2). The placental cells are aspirated through the catheter. The villi are collected in media-prepared syringes and immediately transported to the cytogenetics technician for analysis. Additional retrievals often are necessary. The sonographer should monitor the fetal heart rate and check for procedural bleeding.

The transabdominal CVS approach entails using a special apparatus attached to the needle hub to permit adequate suction to withdraw the villi. The procedure is performed in a manner similar to amniocentesis (see discussion of amniocentesis).

The risk of fetal loss because of CVS is approximately 1% to 3%.[29] There has been some association with limb-reduction defects when CVS is performed before 10 weeks of gestation.[24] $Rh_o(D)$ immune globulin (RhoGam) should be administered to Rh-negative unsensitized women to prevent sensitization problems in subsequent pregnancies.

EMBRYOSCOPY

Embryoscopy is a specialized prenatal test that permits the direct viewing of the developing embryo using a transcervical endoscope inserted into the extracoelomic cavity during the first trimester of pregnancy. With this method, fetal anomalies may be detected or samples of blood aspirated and checked for various blood disorders. Investi-

gators are optimistic that this technique will permit gene therapy in the future.[20]

AMNIOCENTESIS

Amniocentesis was first used as a technique to relieve polyhydramnios, to predict Rh isoimmunization, and to document fetal lung maturity.[3,10,25] In the mid-1960s, amniocentesis was used to study fetal cells from amniotic fluid, which allowed the analysis of fetal chromosomes (see Figure 32-3). Normal and abnormal chromosomal patterns (see Figures 32-4 through 32-5) could be identified.[8]

Amniocentesis is a test offered to expectant patients who are at risk for a chromosomal abnormality or biochemical disorder that may be prenatally detectable. Advanced maternal age is a common reason for performing amniocentesis. All pregnant women are at risk for having a child with a chromosomal defect, but the risk is greater in a woman of advanced maternal age. The risk of having a fetus with Down syndrome is 1 in 365 in a woman who is 35 years of age, whereas the risk for a woman who is 21 years of age is only about 1 in 2000. The risk of having a fetus with any chromosomal anomaly is 1 in 180 in the woman who is 35 years of age versus 1 in 500 for the woman who is 21 years of age.

Other indications for genetic amniocentesis include a history of a balance rearrangement in a parent or previous child with a chromosomal abnormality, a history of an unexplained abnormal AFP level or an abnormal triple screen, and a fetus with a congenital anomaly.

Amniocentesis for genetic reasons is ideally performed between 15 and 18 weeks of gestation. Amniocentesis may be done as early as 12 weeks but may lead to the development of fetal scoliosis or clubfoot secondary to the reduced amount of amniotic fluid. The rate of miscarriage in early amniocentesis is unknown. Amniocentesis performed beyond 20 weeks of gestation is possible but may be associated with poor cell growth.

The amniocentesis procedure should include a fetal survey to exclude congenital anomalies. A fetal examination

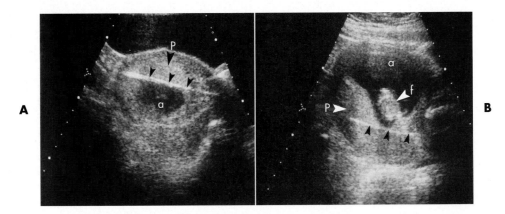

Figure 32-2 **A,** Transcervical chorionic villus sampling at 10 weeks of gestation demonstrating the placement of the sampling catheter *(arrowheads)* within an anterior placenta *(p)* or chorion frondosum. *a,* Amniotic cavity. **B,** Transcervical chorionic villus sampling at 11 weeks of gestation showing the placement of the sampling catheter *(arrowheads)* within a posterior placenta *(p)*. Note the fetal abdomen *(f)* within the amniotic cavity *(a)*.

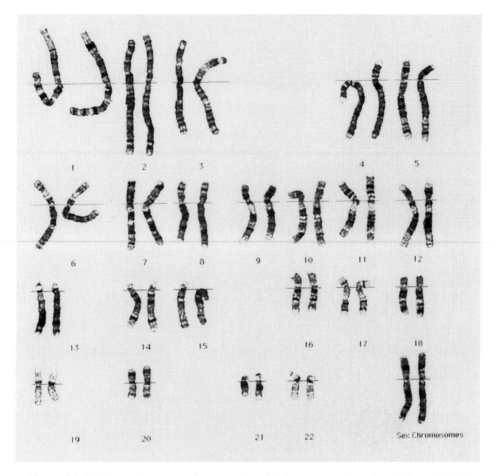

Figure 32-3   Normal karyotype demonstrating 46 chromosomes in a female fetus (46, XX).

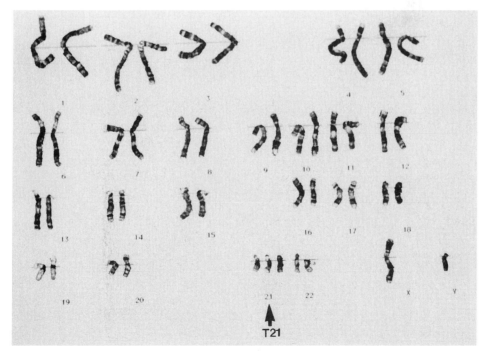

Figure 32-4   Karyotype of trisomy 21 (Down syndrome) in a male fetus (47, XY, +21). Note the extra chromosome at the twenty-first position *(arrow)*. Note the sex chromosomes indicating a male fetus.

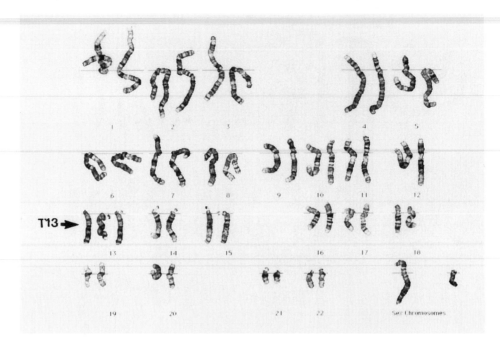

Figure 32-5   Karyotype of trisomy 13 (47, XY + 13) *(arrow)* male fetus.

should be performed, and targeted areas of anatomy should be documented to exclude the physical features that would suggest a chromosomal anomaly (e.g., hand clenching, hypoplasia of the fifth middle phalanx, choroid plexus cysts, ventriculomegaly, thickened nuchal fold, cardiac anomalies, omphalocele, spina bifida, or foot anomalies).

The sonographer will also assist the physician in the amniocentesis procedure. The optimal collection site for amniotic fluid should be away from the fetus, away from the central portion of the placenta, away from the umbilical cord, and near the maternal midline to avoid the maternal uterine vessels.

TECHNIQUE OF GENETIC AMNIOCENTESIS

Ultrasound-monitored amniocentesis is a technique that allows the continuous monitoring of the needle during the amniocentesis procedure.[14] Using this technique, the maternal skin is prepared with a povidone-iodine solution.

The transducer is placed in a sterile cover or sterile glove to allow monitoring on the sterile field during the procedure. Sterile coupling gel may be applied to the maternal skin to ensure good transmission of the sound beam. The amniocentesis site is rescanned to confirm the amniotic pocket, and then the site and pathway for the introduction of the needle is determined. The distance to the amniotic fluid may be measured with electronic calipers, which may be useful in obese patients in whom a longer needle may be necessary. In many instances, a new site is chosen as a result of fetal movement or a myometrial contraction in the proposed site, and the transducer is moved to a new sterile area. On successful identification of the amniocentesis site, a finger is placed between the transducer and the skin to produce an acoustic shadow. The needle is then inserted under continuous ultrasound ob-

servation (Figure 32-6). Inserting the needle in a plane perpendicular to the transducer will allow for a bright reflection of the needle tip, so that it can be easily observed (Figure 32-7) at the edge of the uterine wall and then as it punctures the uterine cavity. When incorrectly directed, the needle may be repositioned.

Amniotic fluid is aspirated through a syringe connected to the needle hub. The first few millimeters of fluid should be discarded to avoid contamination. Between 20 and 30 ml of amniotic fluid will be collected for chromosomal analysis and AFP evaluation. In advanced pregnancies, additional amniotic fluid may be required. When amniocentesis is performed because of a known fetal anomaly, acetylcholinesterase and viral studies (TORCH titers) may be ordered. Following aspiration of amniotic fluid, the needle is removed under sonographic guidance from the uterus.

After the amniocentesis has been completed, fetal cardiac activity should be identified and documented. If the placenta has been traversed, the site should be monitored for bleeding. The use of videotaping can allow for continuous recording and documentation of the fetal examination and the amniocentesis and postamniocentesis ultrasound evaluation.

The continuous monitoring with ultrasound during amniocentesis is invaluable in cases of oligohydramnios, anterior placental position, and premature rupture of membranes. Ultrasound imaging can help achieve a successful amniocentesis when only small pockets of fluid are available.

GENETIC AMNIOCENTESIS AND MULTIPLE GESTATIONS

Amniocentesis in multiple gestations warrants special consideration. Preliminary sonographic examination for each fetus should be performed to include a survey of fetal

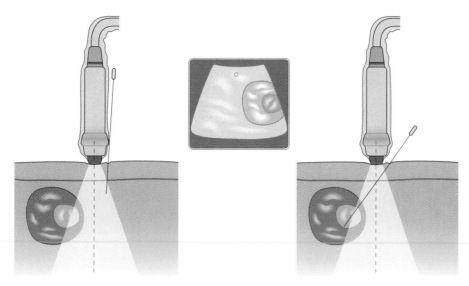

Figure 32-6 If the needle is inserted parallel to the transducer, only the tip will be represented. If the needle is inserted at an angle with the transducer, the beam will intersect the needle, but it will not demonstrate its tip, which could be in a harmful position. Notice that in both cases the image on the screen is the same. Angling the needle is a dangerous procedure that should be avoided.

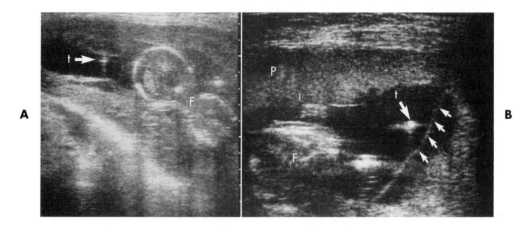

Figure 32-7 **A,** Genetic amniocentesis at 15.6 weeks of gestation using direct visualization method. The needle tip *(t)* is identified within the amniotic cavity. *F,* Fetus. **B,** Genetic amniocentesis at 16 weeks of gestation in a twin pregnancy. The needle tip *(t)* is identified within the sac above the amniotic membrane *(arrows)*. *F,* Fetus; *P,* placenta. *1,* Umbilical cord insertion into placenta.

anatomy and growth profiles. Monozygocity or dizygocity should be determined, and the amniotic fluid within each sac, if there are multiple sacs, should be assessed.

The amniocentesis technique for multiple gestations is similar to the singleton method, except that each fetal sac is entered. To be certain that amniotic fluid is obtained from each sac, indigo carmine dye can be injected into the first sac. The presence of clear amniotic fluid indicates that the second sac has been penetrated when the second pass is made. If dye-stained fluid is visible, it indicates that the first sac has been penetrated a second time. Documentation of each amniocentesis and meticulous labeling of fluid samples is recommended. It is desirable to avoid the placenta in patients who are Rh-negative. In all Rh-negative patients, RhoGAM is administered within 72 hours of the procedure.

CORDOCENTESIS
Cordocentesis is another method in which chromosomes are analyzed. Fetal blood is obtained through needle aspiration of the umbilical cord. Karyotype results can be processed within 2 to 3 days. This rapid assessment may be beneficial for patients with an equivocal amniocentesis result or when a fetal anomaly is detected later in pregnancy.

MATERNAL SERUM MARKERS

ALPHA-FETOPROTEIN
Alpha-fetoprotein (AFP) is the major protein in fetal serum and is produced by the yolk sac in early gestation and later by the fetal liver. AFP is found in the fetal spine, gastrointestinal tract, liver, and kidneys. This protein is transported into the amniotic fluid by fetal urination and

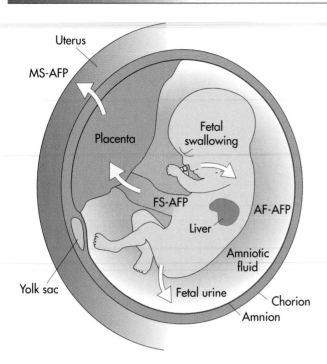

Figure 32-8 Schematic drawing showing the production and distribution of alpha-fetoprotein (AFP) into its three components: fetal tissues, amniotic fluid, and maternal serum. *AF-AFP,* Amniotic fluid AFP; *FS-AFP,* fetal serum AFT; *MS-AFP,* maternal serum AFP.

reaches maternal circulation or blood through the fetal membranes (Figure 32-8). AFP may be measured in the maternal serum (MSAFP) or from amniotic fluid (AFAFP).

AFP levels are considered abnormal when elevated or low. Neural tube defects, such as anencephaly and open spina bifida are common reasons for high AFP levels. In both instances, AFP leaks from the defect to enter the amniotic fluid and then diffuses into the maternal bloodstream (see Figure 32-8). AFP elevations will not be found when there is closed spina bifida (occulta), because there is no opening to allow leakage.

Monitoring of AFP is a screening test for neural tube defects and other conditions (see Box 32-1). MSAFP screening detects approximately 88% of anencephalics and 79% of open spina bifida cases when 2.5 multiples of the median (MOM) are used.[27]

MSAFP levels increase with advancing gestational age and peak from 15 to 18 weeks of gestation (the ideal sampling time). AFAFP, in contrast, decreases with fetal age. A common reason for elevations is incorrect dates. Because AFP levels vary with gestational age, if the fetus is older or younger than expected, AFP levels will be reported as increased or decreased.

Other reasons for elevations are acrania and encephalocele (which may occur in association with Meckel-Gruber syndrome), with AFP leakage from the exposed membranes and tissues. The concentration of AFP correlates with the size of the defect. AFP levels tend to be significantly higher in fetuses with anencephaly than with spina bifida, because more tissue is exposed. It is important to remember that approximately 20% of spina bifida lesions are covered by skin, so AFP elevations will not de detected in serum or amniotic fluid. Sacrococcygeal teratomas are also known to be associated with high AFP levels.

Two common abdominal wall defects, omphalocele and gastroschisis, produce elevations of AFP. With an **omphalocele,** AFP leaks through the membrane encasing the herniated bowel or liver. In gastroschisis, AFP diffuses directly into the serum and amniotic fluid from the herniated bowel, which lacks a covering membrane; thus AFP levels are higher in a fetus with gastroschisis than in a fetus with an omphalocele.

Other abdominal wall defects cause leakage in the same manner. Bladder or cloacal exstrophy, ectopia cordis (herniation of the heart out of the chest), limb-body wall complex, and amniotic band syndrome are examples of other anomalies that may present with an elevated AFP level.

It is expected that the AFP level in a twin pregnancy will be twice that of a singleton pregnancy because two fetuses make twice the AFP. In multiple gestations in which there is death of a co-twin (fetus papyraceous) or when one twin is an acardiac twin, AFP may be higher than normal.

Obstructions of the gastrointestinal tract may cause reduced clearance of AFP. This may explain elevations with anomalies such as an annular pancreas, esophageal atresia, and duodenal atresia.

A fetus with a kidney lesion may produce increased AFP. In congenital nephrosis, extremely high levels of AFP are excreted by the kidneys. Polycystic kidneys and urinary tract obstruction may also lead to AFP rises, because there is abnormal clearance or filtration of AFP because of kidney maldevelopment and urinary tract leakage.

Placental lesions, such as chorioangiomas, hemangiomas, and hematomas, are known to be responsible for AFP elevations. Placental problems in general may explain the prevalence of growth restriction, fetal death, and abruption in patients with unexplained AFP elevations.[6]

In heart failure, faulty diffusion of AFP may lead to abnormal AFP increase when hydrops, ascites, or lymphangiectasia are present. Severely sensitized fetuses with Rh isoimmunization may have heart failure because of severe anemia. In the fetus with a **cystic hygroma,** obstructed lymph sacs lead to AFP diffusion through the hygroma into the blood stream and amniotic fluid.

Liver disease in the mother or fetus may cause high AFP levels. Hepatitis, maternal herpes virus and resultant fetal liver necrosis, skin lesions, hepatocellular carcinoma, and fetal liver tumors (hamartoma) are rare causes of elevated AFP.

Other causes include chromosomal abnormalities associated with fetal anomalies or placental problems that per-

---

BOX 32-1   REASONS FOR ELEVATIONS OF ALPHA-FETOPROTEIN AND ACETYLCHOLINESTERASE

Neural tube defects
  Anencephaly
  Exencephaly (acrania)
  Encephalocele (including Meckel-Gruber syndrome)
  Spina bifida
  Sacrococcygeal teratoma
Abdominal wall defects
  Omphalocele
  Gastroschisis
  Limb-body wall complex
  Amniotic band syndrome
  Bladder or cloacal exstrophy
  Ectopia cordis
Multiple gestation
  Twin with a co-twin death
  Acardiac twin
  Fetus papyraceous
Gastrointestinal obstruction
  Annular pancreas
  Duodenal atresia
  Esophageal atresia
Renal anomalies
  Congenital nephrosis
  Hydronephrosis
  Polycystic kidney disease (including Meckel syndrome)
  Urinary tract obstruction
  Prune-belly syndrome
  Urethral atresia
Placental and cord abnormalities
  Chorioangioma
  Placental or cord hematoma
  Umbilical cord hemangioma
  Hydatidiform mole

Fetal heart failure
  Hydrops and/or ascites
  Lymphangiectasia
  Rh isoimmunization
Neck masses
  Cystic hygroma
  Noonan's syndrome (with hygroma)
Liver disease
  Hepatitis
  Maternal herpes virus (fetal liver necrosis and skin lesions)
  Hepatocellular carcinoma
  Hamartoma of liver
Miscellaneous causes
  Incorrect dates
  Fetal demise
  Oligohydramnios
  Unexplained
  Hereditary overproduction of alpha-fetoprotein
  Blood in amniotic fluid
  Chromosome abnormalities
      (trisomies 18 and 13, Turner's syndrome, triploidy)
  Cystadenomatoid malformation
  Epignathus
  Intracranial tumor
  Pilonidal cyst
  Skin defects
  Hydrocephalus
  Congenital heart defects
  Viral infections (cytomegalovirus [CMV], parvovirus)

Modified from Milunsky A, editor; *Genetic disorders and the fetus, diagnosis, prevention and treatment*, ed 3, Baltimore: Johns Hopkins University Press, 1992; Nyberg DA, Mahony BS, Pretorius DH, editors: *Diagnostic ultrasound of fetal anomalies*, text and atlas, St Louis, Mosby, 1990.

---

mit the abnormal passage of AFP. Fetuses with trisomy 13 or trisomy 18 may also have renal anomalies, neural tube defects, ventral wall defects, or skin lesions that cause elevations in the AFP level. Fetuses with Turner's syndrome often present with cystic hygromas. In triploidy, abnormal placental molar degeneration leads to increased AFP diffusion.

Cystic adenomatoid malformations cause rises in AFP because of excessive leakage from the lungs. Pilonidal cysts of the back and various skin disorders and tumors, such as epignathus and intracranial lesions, are also associated with high AFP levels. Rarely, the fetus manufactures excessive amounts of AFP as a hereditary condition.

Fetal death is a frequent cause of a high MSAFP level. Pregnancies complicated by oligohydramnios may have higher concentrations of AFP because there is less amniotic fluid to diffuse the protein.

Contamination of an amniotic fluid specimen by blood may also falsely increase the level of AFP.

In utero viral infections (cytomegalovirus and parvovirus) are reported to permit excessive AFP leakage, because the maternal-fetal surface may be irritated and disrupted by inflammation.

Unexplained elevations in MSAFP suggest that the pregnancy is at increased risk for complications and poor outcomes, including low birth weight and stillbirth.[6] Preeclampsia, hypertension, and abruptio placentae are other third-trimester complications associated with these elevations.

Mothers with elevated MSAFP values and normal AFAFP values are potentially at risk for other fetal anomalies unrelated to neural tube defects. Hydrocephalus, without a spinal defect (increased cerebrospinal fluid allows increased diffusion), and congenital heart disease (probable altered perfusion of blood flow through placenta) are reported in conjunction with unexplained, non–neural tube defect problems.

Low AFP levels (Box 32-2) have been found with chromosomal abnormalities such as trisomy 21, trisomy 18, and trisomy 13. Other causes include incorrect patient dates (fetus younger that expected), fetal death, hydatidiform moles, spontaneous abortion, and a non-pregnant state. In some cases, the cause may remain unknown.

Amniocentesis may be offered when MSAFP levels are elevated and ultrasound reveals no obvious explanation. Amniotic fluid tests usually include karyotyping for chromosomal abnormalities, AFAFP levels, and acetylcholinesterase. AFAFP is more specific for detecting levels of AFP. Acetylcholinesterase is specific for detecting an open neural tube.[16] Beyond 20 weeks of gestation, acetylcholinesterase is the preferred test, because AFP analysis is no longer sensitive.

When AFP is elevated (greater than 3 MOM) and the cranium (ventricles and cisterna magna) and spine appear normal, the risk of the fetus actually having a small spinal defect is approximately halved. The overall risk of miscarriage from an amniocentesis is 1 in 200, so it important to weigh the risk of complication with the possible yield of identifying an abnormality.

Prenatal scanning and amniocentesis are used to evaluate the fetus with a low AFP value to exclude any physical features that may suggest a chromosomal abnormality. Such findings might include choroid plexus cysts, hand anomalies, or cardiac defects.

TRIPLE SCREEN

Another biochemical screening test known as the triple test or triple screen evaluates AFP, human chorionic gonadotropin (hCG), and unconjugated estriol. This blood test improves the detection rate for trisomy 21 over MSAFP testing alone. Biochemical screening in trisomy 21 fetuses reveals high hCG levels and decreased AFP and estriol levels.[9,22] Additionally, biochemical screening may suggest trisomy 18 when hCG, AFP, and estriol levels are all decreased. The risk for a neural tube defect or chromosomal problem is calculated for each mother. A patient may elect to undergo ultrasound with or without amniocentesis, based on the risk for chromosomal or neural tube defects.

PREGNANCY-ASSOCIATED PLASMA PROTEIN A

A first-trimester serum marker used to detect anomalies is pregnancy-associated plasma protein A (PAPP-A). PAPP-A is a glycoprotein derived from the trophoblastic tissues that is then diffused into the maternal circulation. PAPP-A levels increase in maternal serum throughout pregnancy. PAPP-A levels have been found to be decreased in pregnancies affected by aneuploidy.[31]

MEDICAL GENETICS

A normal karyotype consists of 46 chromosomes, 22 pairs of autosomes and a pair of sex chromosomes (see Figure 32-3). Aneuploidy is an abnormality of the number of chromosomes. One of the most common aneuploid conditions is Down syndrome, in which an individual has an extra chromosome number 21 (see Figure 32-4). The cause of trisomy is usually nondisjunction, the failure of normal chromosomal division at the time of meiosis. The etiology of nondisjunction is unknown, although there is strong association with maternal age.[26]

A chromosomal disorder is caused by too much or too little chromosome material. A dominant disorder is a condition caused by a single defective gene (autosomal dominant). It is usually inherited from one parent (who is also affected) but may arise as a new mutation (spontaneous gene change). An inherited dominant disorder carries a 50% chance that each time pregnancy occurs, the fetus will have the condition. An example of an autosomal-dominant condition is osteogenesis imperfecta (types 1 and 4).

A recessive disorder (autosomal recessive) is caused by a pair of defective genes, one inherited from each parent. With each pregnancy, the parents have a 25% chance of having a fetus with the disorder. An example of an autosomal-recessive condition is infantile polycystic kidney disease.

X-linked disorders are inherited by boys from their mothers. Affected males do not transmit the disorder to their sons, but all of their daughters will be carriers for the disorder. The sons of female carriers each have a 50% chance of being affected, and the daughters each have a 50% chance of being a carrier. Whereas an X-linked gene is located on the female sex chromosome (the X), an autosomal gene is located on one of the numbered chromosomes.[26] An example of an X-linked condition, occurring in male fetuses, is aqueductal stenosis. Aqueductal stenosis, however, may also occur in females.

BOX 32-2 COMMON SONOGRAPHIC FEATURES OF CHROMOSOMAL ANOMALIES

TRISOMY 21	TRISOMY 18	TRISOMY 13	TRIPLOIDY	TURNER'S SYNDROME
Nuchal thickness	Heart defects	Holoprosencephaly	Hydatidiform placental degeneration	Cystic hygroma
Heart defects	Choroid plexus cysts	Heart defects	Heart defects	Heart defects
Duodenal atresia	Clenched hands	Cleft lip and palate	Renal anomalies	Hydrops
Shortened femurs	Micrognathia	Omphalocele	Omphalocele	Renal anomalies
Mild pyelectasis	Talipes	Polydactyly	Cranial defects	
Mild ventriculomegaly	Renal anomalies	Talipes	Facial defects	
Echogenic bowel	Cleft lip and palate	Echogenic chordae tendineae		
	Omphalocele	Renal anomalies		
	CDH	Meningomyelocele		
	Cerebellar hypoplasia	Micrognathia		

A multifactorial condition is an abnormal event that arises because of the interaction of one or more genes and environmental factors. Anencephaly is an example of a multifactorial disorder.

Mosaicism is the occurrence of a gene mutation or chromosomal abnormality in a portion of an individual's cells. It is difficult to predict the types of problems that will occur when mosaicism is found.

CHROMOSOMAL ABNORMALITIES

Chromosomal abnormalities are found in 1 of every 180 live births.[17] There is a high prevalence of chromosomal abnormalities in patients referred for second-trimester amniocentesis because of advanced maternal age, abnormal AFP, abnormal triple screen (hCG, AFP, and estriol), or ultrasound detection of multiple fetal anomalies. It is important to become familiar with and to search for the physical features (see Box 32-2) that would suggest trisomies 13, 18, and 21, triploidy, and Turner's syndrome.

NUCHAL TRANSLUCENCY

An abnormal fluid collection behind the fetal neck has been strongly associated with aneuploidy.[15,18,19] This nuchal translucency has been reported as a late first-trimester finding identified between 10 and 14 weeks of gestation.[19] A nuchal translucency of 3 mm or greater has been associated with chromosomal abnormalities such as trisomies 13, 18, and 21, as well as triploidy and Turner's syndrome.[19] This first-trimester finding is not a precursor to the development of a cystic hygroma or second-trimester edema.[19]

Ultrasound findings. Transvaginal technique is recommended, and scanning in two planes perpendicular to each other can help to avoid error. Care should be taken to avoid confusing amnion with a nuchal translucency. The translucency should be oriented perpendicular to the ultrasound beam, and the measurement should be taken from inside the fetal neck to inside the nuchal membrane.

Nuchal translucency is viewed as an early, noninvasive means of assessing the risk of aneuploidy. Using a measurement of 3 mm increases the risk of aneuploidy four times, and nuchal translucencies of 4 mm and greater carry an even greater risk. There has also been documentation of resolution of this abnormality with a normal outcome.[18] Even in fetuses with normal chromosomes, an increased nuchal translucency has been associated with an increased incidence of structural defects such as cardiac, diaphragmatic, renal, and abdominal wall anomalies. In addition to the increased risk of chromosomal abnormality and other anomalies, an increased nuchal translucency has also been associated with spontaneous miscarriage and perinatal death.[19]

TRISOMY 21

Trisomy 21, also known as Down syndrome, occurs in 1 in 660 births.[4] It is one of the most common chromosomal disorders and is characterized by an extra chromosome number 21.[11] There is an association with advanced maternal age; however, this anomaly may affect infants born to women of all ages. Trisomy 21 is associated with an abnormal triple screen.

Infants with trisomy 21 may present with a variety of physical features (Figure 32-9) including brachycephaly; epicanthal folds (a fold of skin that covers the inner corner of the eye); a flattened nasal bridge, round, small ears; broad neck with extra skin (nuchal fold); and a protruding tongue.[4] Other anomalies that have been associated with Down syndrome include heart defects (septal defects, endocardial cushion defect, tetralogy of Fallot), duodenal atresia, esophageal atresia, anorectal atresia, and omphalocele (Figure 32-10). Cystic hygroma, nonimmune hydrops, and hydrothorax may also be observed. Skeletal anomalies may be present, including shortened extremities, space between the first and second toes, hypoplasia of the middle fifth phalanx (Figure 32-11), and clinodactyly of the fifth finger (inward curving).[2] A single palmar (hand) crease is found in approximately 30% of affected infants.[13]

The prognosis for survival depends on associated anomalies, with heart anomalies a major cause of mortality in infancy. Mental retardation is always present, with IQ ranges between 25 and 50 in childhood.[23] In addition to heart failure, alimentary defects can also be life threat-

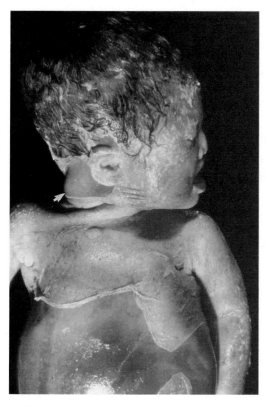

Figure 32-9   Postmortem photograph of a neonate with trisomy 21 (Down syndrome). Duodenal atresia was found. Note the nuchal thickening *(arrow)*.

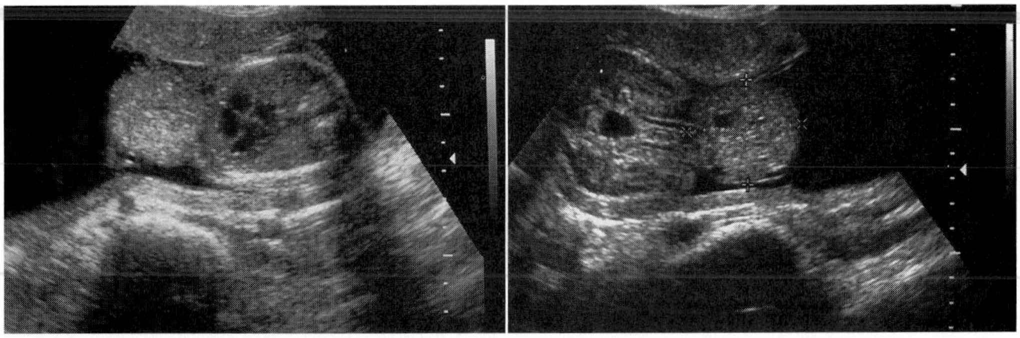

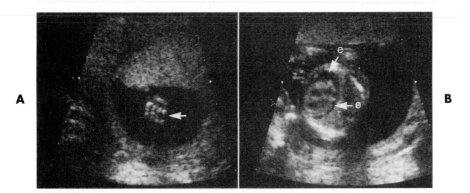

Figure 32-10 **A,** A 22-week fetus with tetralogy of Fallot (ventricular septal defect [VSD], overriding aorta, pulmonary stenosis, right ventricular hypertrophy). Only the VSD is appreciated in this four-chamber view. **B,** Omphalocele in same fetus. These findings together are highly suggestive of a chromosomal anomaly.

Figure 32-11 **A,** Absent fifth middle phalanx *(arrow)* in a chromosomally normal fetus. **B,** In the same fetus, pericardial effusion *(e)* is observed. Other anomalies were right atrial hypertrophy and outflow abnormalities.

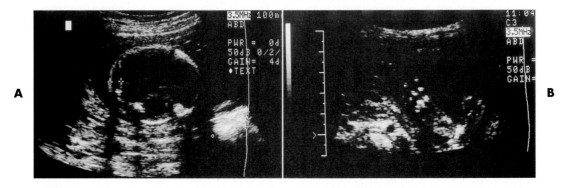

Figure 32-12 A fetus presenting at 21 weeks. **A,** Ultrasound identified an increased nuchal fold measuring 7.7 mm. **B,** Widely spaced toes in same fetus. Amniocentesis confirmed trisomy 21.

ening. Respiratory problems, eye problems, and premature aging are common.

Ultrasound findings. Ultrasound diagnosis of trisomy 21 is limited because of the subtleness and infrequency of some of the phenotypic expressions.[4] Anomalies that may be identified with Down syndrome include the following:

- Nuchal fold of 6 mm or greater (see Figure 32-12).
- Extremity anomalies (hypoplasia of the middle phalanx or clinodactyly of the fifth finger, space between first and second toes)
- Shortened femurs

- Duodenal atresia (Figure 32-13) (observed in 30% but may not be identified before 22 to 24 weeks of gestation)[7]
- Shortened ear length
- Heart defects (Figure 32-14) (present in approximately 40% to 50% of fetuses)[28]
- **Intrauterine growth restriction (IUGR)**
- Mild pyelectasis (4 mm in anteroposterior diameter)[7,28]
- Echogenic bowel (Figure 32-15)[28]
- Mild ventriculomegaly (Figure 32-16)[7]

TRISOMY 18

Trisomy 18, also known as Edward's syndrome, is the second most common chromosomal trisomy, occurring in 3 of

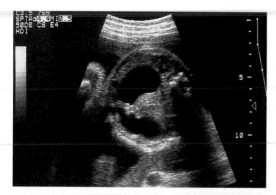

Figure 32-13 The double bubble sign is identified in this case of duodenal atresia. This is a significant finding associated with trisomy 21.

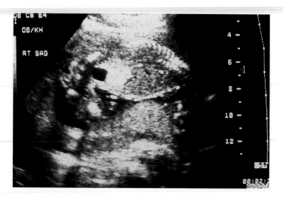

Figure 32-15 Echogenic bowel, bowel with the same echogenicity as fetal bone, is a subtle finding associated with trisomy 21.

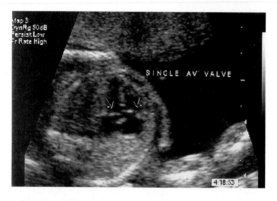

Figure 32-14 This endocardial cushion defect (atrioventricular canal) presented with an atrial septal defect, ventricular septal defect, and common valve. (Courtesy Ginny Goreczky, RDMS, Maternal Fetal Center at Florida Hospital, Orlando, Fla.)

10,000 live births.[1,5] This karyotype demonstrates an extra chromosome 18. Trisomy 18 is associated with an abnormal triple screen.

Physical features that have been identified in fetuses with trisomy 18 (Figure 32-17) include cardiac anomalies, which are present in approximately 90% of fetuses and most commonly have associated ventricular septal defects.[23] Cranial anomalies that have been identified are dolichocephaly, microcephaly, hydrocephalus, agenesis of the corpus callosum, cerebellar hypoplasia, a strawberry-shaped head, and choroid plexus cysts (Figure 32-18). Facial abnormalities include low-set ears, **micrognathia,** and cleft lip (Figure 32-19) and palate. Abnormal extremities identified with trisomy 18 include persistently clenched hands, talipes, rocker-bottom feet, and radial aplasia (Figure 32-20). Other anomalies associated with Edward's syndrome include omphalocele, congenital diaphragmatic hernia (Figure 32-21), neural tube defects, cystic hygroma, and renal anomalies.

The fetus with trisomy 18 will often spontaneously abort. Infants are profoundly retarded. It is considered a lethal anomaly, with 90% of infants dying within the first year of life.[1,23]

Ultrasound findings. Sonographic features of trisomy 18 are evident in 80% of affected fetuses,[1] and, in addition to the feature listed above, may also include polyhydramnios, IUGR, single umbilical artery, and nonimmune hydrops.

TRISOMY 13

Trisomy 13, also known as Patau's syndrome, occurs in 1:5000 births.[1] Is it the result of an extra chromosome 13. This extremely severe anomaly consists of multiple anomalies, many of which involve the brain.[7]

The physical features (Figure 32-22) characteristic of trisomy 13 include holoprosencephaly (Figure 32-23), which affects 40% of fetuses with trisomy 13.[23] Other cranial anomalies include agenesis of the corpus callosum and microcephaly. Facial anomalies may be associated with the presence of holoprosencephaly and include **hypotelorism,** proboscis (Figure 32-24), cyclopia, and nose with a single nostril. Cleft lip and palate, microphthalmia, and micrognathia may also be present. Heart defects are present in 90% of fetuses and may include ventricular septal defect, atrial septal defect, and hypoplastic left heart.[7] Other anomalies associated with trisomy 13 include omphalocele, renal anomalies (Figure 32-25), and meningomyelocele. Associated limb anomalies (Figure 32-26) include **polydactyly,** talipes, rocker-bottom feet, and overlapping fingers.[23] Cystic hygroma and echogenic chordae tendineae (Figure 32-27) may also be identified.

The prognosis for trisomy 13 is extremely poor, with 85% of infants dying within the first year. It is considered a lethal anomaly. Survivors are profoundly retarded, with multiple deficits and problems.[23]

Ultrasound findings. Sonographic features are evident in 90% of fetuses with trisomy 13.[1] In addition to the features listed above, trisomy 13 may also be associated with IUGR. Trisomy 13 and Meckel-Gruber syndrome (encephalocele, cystic kidneys, polydactyly) may have a similar sonographic appearance.

TRIPLOIDY

Triploidy is the result of a complete extra set of chromosomes. It often occurs as the result of an ova being fertilized by two sperm. It is estimated to occur in approxi-

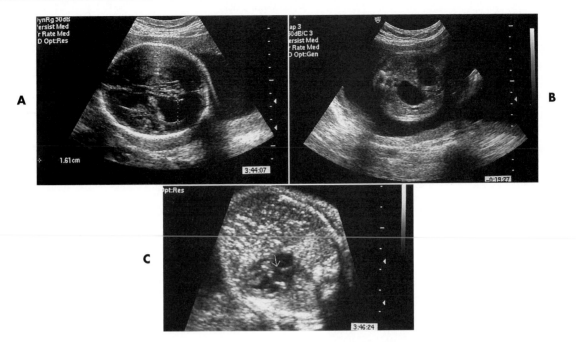

Figure 32-16 A fetus presented at 26 weeks of gestation with an uncertain last menstrual period. Ultrasound revealed ventriculomegaly **(A)** and duodenal atresia **(B). C,** Subsequent ultrasound examination also identified an atrial septal defect. The fetus demised in utero at 35 weeks of gestation.

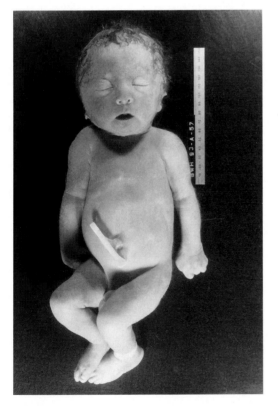

Figure 32-17 Neonate with trisomy 18. Note the clenched hands and rocker-bottom feet. Prenatal ultrasound revealed a supratentorial cyst confirmed after autopsy.

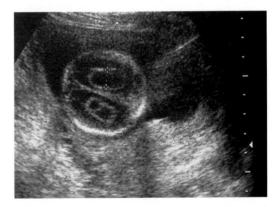

Figure 32-18 Bilateral choroid plexus cysts were identified in a pregnancy referred for triple screen suggestive of trisomy 18. Amniocentesis confirmed Edward's syndrome.

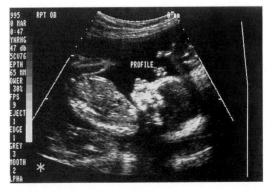

Figure 32-19 Cleft lip and palate are associated with aneuploidy. Bilateral clefts, as in this example, and median clefts carry a greater risk than a unilateral cleft.

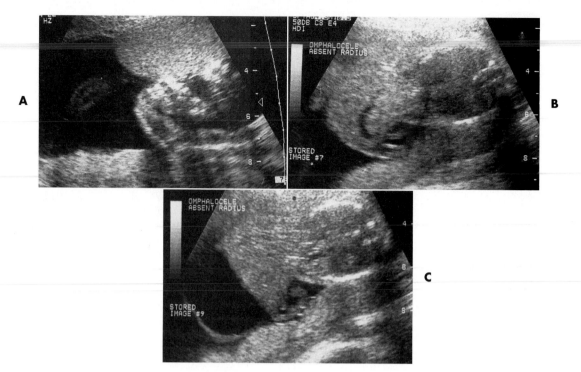

Figure 32-20 This fetus with trisomy 18 presented with radial aplasia and the ultrasound appearance of a clubbed hand **(A)** and an omphalocele **(B). C,** Note the ascites present in the defect.

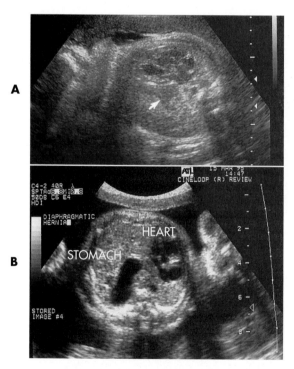

Figure 32-21 Congenital diaphragmatic hernia (CDH) is associated with aneuploidy. **A,** This is an unusual presentation of CDH in that the stomach was not identified in the thorax, even though it was a left-side defect. Note the malposition of the heart. There is bowel adjacent to the heart. Karyotype revealed normal chromosomes. The baby died shortly after birth because of respiratory complications. **B,** A common ultrasound presentation of CDH with the stomach evident within the thorax. Note the displacement of the heart. (Courtesy of Ginny Goreczky, RDMS, Maternal Fetal Center at Florida Hospital, Orlando, Fla.)

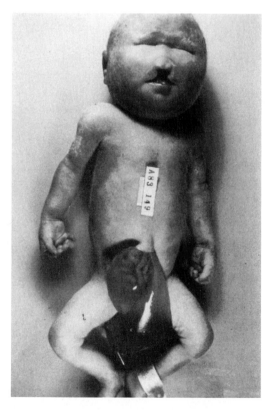

Figure 32-22 Neonate with trisomy 13. Note the hypotelorism, bilateral cleft lip and palate, bowel-filled omphalocele, and polydactyly of the hands. (From Nyberg DA, Mahony BS, Pretorius DH, editors: *Diagnostic ultrasound of fetal anomalies: text and atlas,* St Louis, 1990, Mosby.)

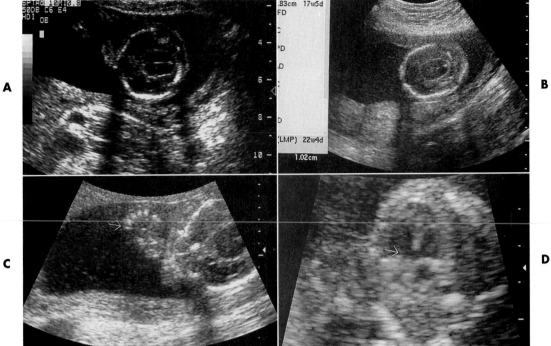

Figure 32-23 This pregnancy presented at 18 weeks and 4 days. Multiple anomalies were identified consistent with alobar holoprosencephaly. Amniocentesis confirmed trisomy 13. Ultrasound findings included a proboscis **(A)**, fused thalamus and thickened nuchal fold **(B)**, polydactyly **(C)**, and a ventricular septal defect **(D)**. A single umbilical artery and cyclopia were also evident.

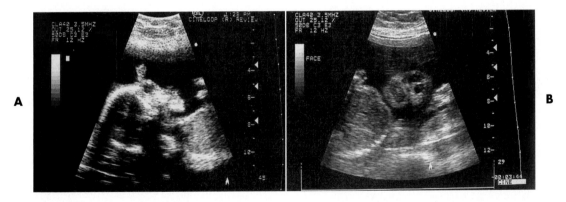

Figure 32-24 The facial anomalies associated with trisomy 13 include a proboscis **(A)** and hypotelorism (closely-spaced eyes) **(B)**.

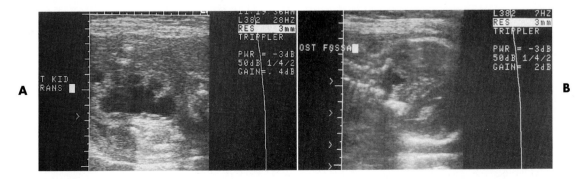

Figure 32-25 A fetus with trisomy 13 presents with hydronephrosis **(A)** and Dandy-Walker malformation **(B)**.

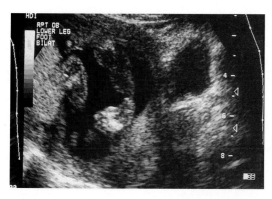

Figure 32-26 Limb anomalies associated with aneuploidy include talipes (clubfoot).

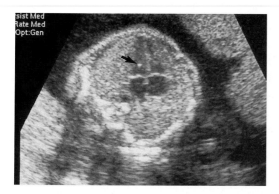

Figure 32-27 An isolated echogenic foci may be insignificant. When identified with other anomalies, aneuploidy should be considered.

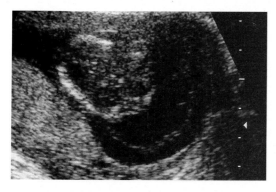

Figure 32-28 A cystic hygroma was revealed in a 14-week pregnancy. Hydrops with pleural effusions and ascites was also evident. Amniocentesis confirmed Turner's syndrome.

mately 1% of conceptions, although most fetuses will spontaneously abort in the first trimester.[12] Only 1 in 5000 will continue to 16 to 20 weeks of gestation.[21]

Physical features of triploidy include heart defects, renal anomalies, omphalocele, and meningomyelocele. Cranial defects associated with triploidy include holoprosencephaly, agenesis of the corpus callosum, hydrocephalus, and Dandy-Walker malformation. Facial anomalies may be present and include low-set ears, **hypertelorism,** cleft lip and palate, and micrognathia. Cryptorchidism, ambiguous genitalia, syndactyly, and talipes may also be observed.

Triploidy is considered a lethal condition, with those surviving the gestational period dying shortly after birth. A mosaic form of triploidy may be compatible with survival, although these infants are affected with mental retardation.

Ultrasound findings. Sonographic features of triploidy include the above findings in addition to severe IUGR and placental changes (hydatidiform degeneration). Oligohydramnios is often present and may hamper adequate visualization of the fetus.

TURNER'S SYNDROME

Turner's syndrome (45,X) is a genetic abnormality marked by the absence of the X or Y chromosome. It is not associated with advanced maternal age. It occurs in every 1 of 5000 to 10,000 births.[23] Patients may present with an elevated MSAFP when a cystic hygroma is present.

Cystic hygroma (32-28) is one of the most pathognomonic findings for this disorder. Other physical features include cardiac anomalies, which are present in 20%, with coarctation of the aorta being the most common.[7] Generalized lymphedema and hydrops may also be present. Renal anomalies such as horseshoe kidney, renal agenesis, hydronephrosis, and hypoplastic kidney may coexist. Short femurs are also associated with Turner syndrome.[1]

Most fetuses with Turner's syndrome will spontaneously abort. The prognosis is especially grave when the fetus presents with a large cystic hygroma and edema or hydrops (Figure 32-29). If the hygroma is isolated, it may regress in utero. The prognosis after birth depends on the severity of associated anomalies. Female infants who survive will have immature sexual development, amenorrhea, short stature, a webbed neck, cubitus valgus (abnormal elbow angle), and a shield chest with widely-spaced nipples. They may also have poor hearing, and hormone replacement is necessary for sexual development. Turner's children usually have normal intelligence.[27]

Ultrasound findings. The ultrasound findings for Turner's syndrome are listed above and may also include oligohydramnios, especially when severe renal anomalies are present.

REVIEW QUESTIONS

1. Describe the technique used for chorionic villus sampling.
2. How would you differentiate sonographically between trisomies 13, 18, and 21?
3. What sonographic findings would you specifically search for in a patient at risk for a Down syndrome fetus?
4. Discuss the difference between an anomaly that is transmitted in an autosomal-recessive fashion and one that is transmitted in an autosomal-dominant fashion.
5. What sonographic findings would most specifically suggest Turner's syndrome, trisomy 18, and trisomy 13?

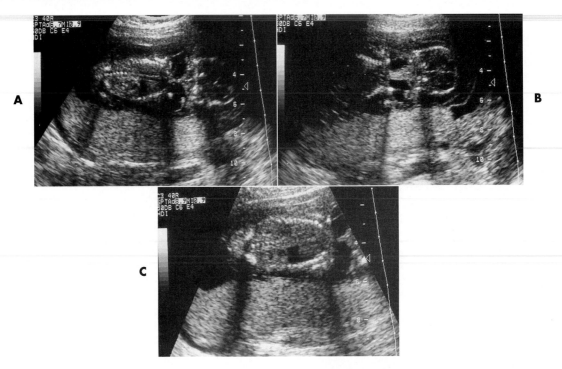

Figure 32-29   Turner's syndrome **A,** Cystic hygroma is noted in the nuchal region. **B,** Hydrops was also evident. Note the significant edema around the fetal head and the pleural effusions **(C).** Turner syndrome with hydrops carries a grave prognosis.

ACKNOWLEDGMENT

I would like to acknowledge the sonographers, Ginny, Maria, and Lucy, in the Maternal Fetal Center at Florida Hospital, Orlando, Florida for continually sharing their interesting cases with me, so that I am able to share a piece of their knowledge. I would also like to thank the perinatologists, Drs. Fuentes and Almalt for allowing me to continue to expand my skills and knowledge under their mentoring. I would also like to thank the sonographers in the Florida Hospital Radiology Ultrasound department who also add to my teaching file. Finally, I would like to recognize Beck Hutchinson, librarian, and the Florida Hospital College of Health Sciences library staff for their expertise in searching for and acquiring the research materials needed for this project.

REFERENCES

1. Benacerraf BR: *Ultrasound of fetal syndromes,* Philadelphia, 1998, Churchill Livingstone.
2. Benacerraf BR, Harlow BL, Frigoletto FD: Hypoplasia of the middle phalanx of the fifth digit: a feature of the second trimester fetus with Down syndrome, *J Ultrasound Med* 9:389, 1990.
3. Bevis DCA: Composition of liquor amnii in haemolytic disease of newborn, *Lancet* 2:443, 1950.
4. Bilardo C: Second trimester ultrasound markers for fetal aneuploidy, *Early Hum Dev* 47(suppl):S31, 1996
5. Callen PW: *Ultrasonography in obstetrics and gynecology,* Philadelphia, 1994, WB Saunders.
6. Elias S, Simpson JL, editors: *Maternal serum screening for fetal genetic disorders,* New York, 1992, Churchill Livingstone.
7. Fleischer AC and others: *Sonography in obstetrics and gynecology: principles & practice,* ed 5, Stamford, Conn, 1996, Appleton & Lange
8. Golbus MS and others: Prenatal genetic diagnosis in 3000 amniocenteses, *N Engl J Med* 300:157, 1979.
9. Haddow JE and others: Prenatal screening for Down's syndrome with use of maternal serum markers, *N Engl J Med* 327:588, 1992.
10. Hytten FE, Lind T: *Diagnostic indices in pregnancy,* Basel, Switzerland, 1973, Giba-Geigy.
11. Itoh H and others: Nuchal-fold thickening in Down syndrome fetuses: transient appearance and spontaneous resolution in the second trimester, *J Perinat Med* 21:139, 1993.
12. Jauniaux E and others: Prenatal diagnosis of triploidy during the second trimester of pregnancy, *Obstet Gynecol* 88:983, 1996.
13. Jeanty P: Prenatal detection of simian crease, *J Ultrasound Med* 9:131, 1990.
14. Jeanty P and others: How to improve your amniocentesis technique, *Am J Obstet Gynecol* 146:593, 1983.
15. Martinez JM and others: Fetal heart rate and nuchal translucency in detecting chromosomal abnormalities other than Down syndrome, *Obstet Gynecol* 92:68, 1998.
16. Milunsky A, Sapirstein VS: Prenatal diagnosis of open neural tube defects using the amniotic fluid acetylcholinesterase assay, *Obstet Gynecol* 59:1, 1982.
17. Nyberg DA, Mahony BS, Pretorius, DH, editors: *Diagnostic ultrasound of fetal anomalies: text and atlas,* St Louis, 1990, Mosby.

18. Pandya PP and others: First-trimester fetal nuchal translucency thickness and risk for trisomies, *Obstet Gynecol* 84:420, 1994.

19. Pandya PP and others: Chromosomal defects and outcome in 1015 fetuses with increased nuchal translucency, *Ultrasound Obstet Gynecol* 5:15, 1995.

20. Reece EA and others: Embryoscopy: a closer look at first-trimester diagnosis and treatment, *Am J Obstet Gynecol* 166:775, 1992.

21. Rijhsinghani A and others: Risk of preeclampsia in second-trimester triploid pregnancies, *Obstet Gynecol* 90:884, 1997.22. Salihu HM, Boos R, Schmidt W: Antenatally detectable markers for the diagnosis of autosomally trisomic fetuses in at-risk pregnancies, *Am J Perinatol* 14:257-261, 1997.

23. Sanders RC and others: *Structural fetal abnormalities: the total picture,* St Louis, 1996, Mosby.

24. Schloo R and others: Distal limb deficiency following CVS? *Am J Genetics* 42:404, 1992.

25. Scrimgeour JB: Amniocentesis: technique and complications. In Emery AEH, editor: *Antenatal diagnosis of genetic disease,* Baltimore, 1973, Williams & Wilkins.

26. Toriello HV: General principles of human genetics, *Clin Commun Disord* 2:1, 1992.

27. United Kingdom Collaborative Study on Alpha-fetoprotein in Relation to Neural Tube Defects: Maternal serum alpha-fetoprotein measurement in antenatal screen for anencephaly and spina bifida in early pregnancy, *Lancet,* 1:1323, 1977.

28. Vintzileos AM and others: The use of second-trimester genetic sonogram in guiding clinical management of patients at increased risk for fetal trisomy 21, *Obstet Gynecol* 87:948, 1996.

29. Wapner FJ, Jackson LG, Davis GH: Chorionic villus sampling: first trimester cytogenetic and biochemical fetal diagnosis, *Female Patient* 10:95, 1985.

30. Williamson R and others: Direct gene analysis of chorionic villi: a possible technique for first trimester antenatal diagnosis of haemoglobinopathies, *Lancet* 2:1125, 1981.

31. Zimmermann R and others: Serum parameters and nuchal translucency in first trimester screening for fetal chromosomal abnormalities, *Br J Obstet Gynaecol* 103:1009, 1996.

CHAPTER 33

Clinical Ethics for Obstetric Sonography

Frank A. Chervenak
Laurence B. McCullough

beneficence - quality or state of being beneficent (doing good)

confidentiality - the nondisclosure of certain information except to another authorized person

ethics - discipline dealing with what is good and bad and with moral duty and obligation

informed consent - consent to surgery by a patient or to participation in a medical experiment by a subject after achieving an understanding of what is involved

respect for autonomy - relation to or concern with self-governing or self-directing freedom and especially moral independence

---

Sonographers, along with their physician colleagues, must be prepared to identify and manage clinical ethical issues that arise in their relationships with their patients.[4,9] In this chapter we provide an overview of clinical ethics and then consider the moral responsibilities of obstetric sonographers regarding four clinical ethical issues: competence to perform obstetric ultrasound and referral to specialists; routine screening; disclosure of results; and confidentiality.

CLINICAL ETHICS

In the history of philosophy, ethics is defined as the disciplined study of morality. Morality concerns right and wrong conduct (what we ought or ought not do) and good and bad character (the kinds of persons we should become and the virtues we should cultivate in doing so). Both aspects of morality are of importance for the clinical ethics of sonography.

In a pluralistic, multicultural society such as the United States, there are many sources of moral beliefs and behavior, including personal experience, the traditions and experiences of families, communities, ethnic and racial groups, and geographic regions; the variety of world religions; and national identity and history, including the laws of the states and of the federal government. These sources of moral beliefs can sometimes come into conflict. Morality should not be confused with ethics, which seeks to articulate clear, consistent, coherent, and clinically applicable accounts of moral conduct and character by providing arguments for what morality *ought* to be.

Two academic disciplines have contributed to the development of ethics as an intellectual discipline. The first, theologic or religious ethics, appeals to particular or general religious commitments. There are several problems with this approach. First, religions disagree both intramurally and extramurally about conduct and character. Second, people of no religious persuasion are excluded from the dialogue. Finally, medical ethics, at least in countries such as the United States, must confront the fact that the health care professions are secular and that the society that they serve is morally pluralistic.[9] Religious ethics provides an inadequate foundation for secular professional ethics in a culturally diverse society.

The second academic discipline involved in ethics is philosophy. To be applicable in a medical context, ethics must transcend moral pluralism by offering an approach with minimal, ideally nonexistent, ties to any substantive prior commitment about moral conduct and character. This is what philosophical ethics attempts to do because it requires only a commitment to the results of rational discourse, in which all substantive commitments about what morality ought to be are open to question. Every such substantive claim requires intellectual justification in the form of a rigorous ethical analysis and argument. Philosophic ethics, therefore, properly serves as the foundation for medical ethics, especially in an international context.[8]

The beginning point for clinical ethics in sonography is an analysis of the ethical obligation that serves as the foundation of the patient-sonographer relationship: the sonographer's obligation to protect and promote the interests of the patient as a member of the obstetric team. This commitment creates the health care professional's moral authority, i.e., ethical justification for the professional's power, which takes the forms of clinical judgment, recommendations, and technical interventions. This relationship derives from the patient-physician relationship because the sonographer's moral authority to care for patients derives from the physician's moral authority as the patient's principal caregiver.

From its recorded beginnings in ancient Greece in about the fifth century BCE, Western medicine has made a distinctive claim to know what is in the clinical interests of the patient. One expression of this claim is *primum non nocere*, which means, "First do no harm." In ethics, this is known as the *ethical principle of nonmaleficence*.[1,9] This ethical principle only partially explains what is in the patient's interests, however, because medicine, and therefore sonography, seeks to benefit patients, not simply avoid harming them. The use of obstetric ultrasound, like other medical interventions, must be justified by the goal of seeking the greater balance of clinical "goods" over "harms," not simply avoiding harm to the patient at all cost. This ethical principle is called *beneficence* and is a more adequate basis for ethics in sonography than is nonmaleficence.[1,9]

The principle of beneficence obligates the obstetric sonographer to seek the greater balance of clinical goods over harms in the care of pregnant patients. Goods and harms are to be defined and balanced from a rigorous clinical perspective.[2,9] The goods that obstetric sonography should seek for patients are preventing early or premature death (not preventing death at all costs); preventing and managing disease, injury, and handicapping conditions; and alleviating unnecessary pain and suffering.[2,9] Pain and suffering are unnecessary and therefore represent clinical harms to be avoided when they do not contribute to seeking the goods of the beneficence-based clinical judgment. Pain is a physiologic phenomenon involving central nervous system processing of tissue damage. Suffering is a psychologic phenomenon involving blocked intentions, plans, and projects. Pain usually causes suffering, and one can suffer without being in pain.[2]

In the twentieth century, first in the United States and more recently in other Western democracies, it has been recognized that patients, including pregnant women, have their own perspective on their interests that should be respected as much as the clinician's perspective on the patient's interests. A patient's perspective on her interests is shaped by wide-ranging and sometimes idiosyncratic values and beliefs.[9] *Autonomy* refers to a person's capacity to formulate, express, and carry out value-based preferences.[1,2] The ethical principle of respect for autonomy obligates the sonographer to acknowledge the integrity of a patient's values and beliefs and of her value-based preferences; to avoid interfering with the expression or implementation of these preferences; and, when necessary, to assist in their expression and implementation. This principle generates the autonomy-based obligations of the sonographer.[9] For example, it is an autonomy-enhancing strategy for a woman to be enabled to insert a vaginal probe herself to make the experience more comfortable and less threatening. Unlike beneficence-based clinical judgment, no specific goods and harms can be defined because these definitions are left to each individual patient. These range widely and include biopsychosocial dimensions of health as well as spiritual, religious, aesthetic, and other personal concerns.

Protecting and promoting the interests of the pregnant woman and the interests of the fetal patient in a pregnancy going to term are the basic goals or purposes of obstetric care.[9] Sonographic examination plays a crucial role in implementing these goals.

Maternal interests are protected and promoted by both autonomy-based and beneficence-based obligations of the sonographer to the pregnant woman. Fetuses are incapable of having their own perspective on their interests because the immaturity of their central nervous system renders them incapable of having the requisite values or beliefs. Thus there can be no autonomy-based obligations to the fetus.[5,9] Fetal interests in sonography are understood exclusively in terms of beneficence. This principle explains the moral (as distinct from legal) status of the fetus as a patient and generates the serious ethical obligations owed by physicians and sonographers to the fetus.[5,9] In the technical language of beneficence the sonographer has beneficence-based obligations to the fetal patient in a pregnancy going to term, to protect and promote fetal interests and those of the child it will become, as these are understood from a rigorous clinical perspective. The clinical goods to be sought for the fetal patient include prevention of premature death, disease, and handicapping conditions and of unnecessary pain and suffering. It is appropriate, therefore, to refer to fetuses as patients, with the exception of previable fetuses that are to be aborted.[9]

The pregnant woman also has beneficence-based obligations to the fetal patient because she is its moral fiduciary when the pregnancy will be taken to term. She is therefore morally expected to protect and promote the fetal patient's interests and those of the child it will become.[9] When a pregnant woman elects to have an abortion, however, these fiduciary obligations do not exist. A sonographer with moral objections to abortion should keep two things in mind: First, the moral judgment and decision of the pregnant woman to end her pregnancy should not be criticized or commented on in any way; her autonomy demands respect in the form of the sonographer and physician being neutral to her judgment and decision. Second, the sonographer is free to follow his or her conscience and to withdraw from further involvement with patients who elect abortion. Physicians should as a matter of office policy respect this important matter of individual conscience on the part of the sonographer.[9]

FOUR MAJOR CLINICAL ETHICAL ISSUES

COMPETENCE AND REFERRAL IN ULTRASOUND EXAMINATION

The ethical obligation to provide competent obstetric ultrasound examinations derives from both beneficence and respect for autonomy. Either principle alone, and certainly both in combination, require sonographers and physicians to provide patients with accurate and reliable clinical information. To meet this ethical obligation, the clinician must address the following ethical considerations.

First, ensuring an appropriate level of competence imposes a rigorous standard of training and continuing education. Two problems result when sonographers do not maintain this baseline level of competence in the techniques and interpretation of ultrasound imaging: (1) They may cause unnecessary harm to the pregnant woman or fetal patient, for example, from mistaken diagnosis of fetal anomalies, thus violating beneficence-based obligations. (2) Incomplete or inaccurate reporting of results by the sonographer to the physician and therefore by the physician to the pregnant woman undermines the informed consent process regarding the management of pregnancy. This constitutes an unacceptable ethical violation of autonomy-based obligations of the sonographer to the pregnant woman. Because physicians rely heavily on them, the

general competence of obstetric sonographers is essential to avoiding these ethically unacceptable consequences for the exercise of the pregnant woman's autonomy.

Second, these obligations have important implications for physicians who employ a sonographer. Such physicians are ethically obligated to adequately supervise the sonographer's clinical work. To do this adequately the physician should know more than the sonographer, especially about the application of sonographic findings to the diagnosis of anomalies. This more advanced fund of clinical and scientific knowledge is essential for the physician to fulfill his or her additional ethical obligation to regularly review the sonographer's work. In addition, physicians should provide the opportunity for continuing education of obstetric sonographers.

In medical care, patients properly rely for their protection on the personal and professional integrity of their clinicians. A crucial aspect of that integrity on the part of physicians is willingness to refer to specialists when the limits of their own knowledge are being approached. Integrity should also be one of the fundamental virtues of sonographers and, thus, a standard for judging professional character. Like other virtues, such as self-sacrifice and compassion, integrity directs sonographers to focus primarily on the patient's interests as a way to blunt mere self-interest.[9] As sonography continues to develop as a profession, it will need to identify, address, and manage in a responsible fashion incentives to mere self-interest on the part of sonographers, especially concerning compensation packages and productivity.

Sonographers who work with specialists who receive patients on referral should be aware of and prepared to manage two clinical ethical challenges. Like all sonographers, they have an ethical obligation to ensure that they maintain their standards of general competence. Sonographers as a group have beneficence-based obligations to the population of pregnant patients receiving ultrasound services. The patient population relies on sonographers' self-regulation as the means to guarantee that these beneficence-based obligations are fulfilled. This ethical concern becomes even more important in the clinically complex and demanding setting of a specialty referral practice.

The second concern for sonographers involves discovering avoidable errors that a colleague has made in previous ultrasound examinations. The specialist may sometimes have the ethical obligation to present findings to a pregnant woman that the referring physician should have been competent to detect but did not, possibly due to faulty technique or interpretation. In such an instance, the sonographer's integrity is an essential safeguard of the patient's autonomy against the self-interest of the specialist, who may wish to avoid potential loss of income that might result from a conflict with the referring physician. The sonographer should not fail to bring to the attention of the referral specialist (not the patient directly) his or her concern about the inadequacies of the referring physician's sonographic technique. If necessary, the sonographer should become an advocate, even a vigorous advocate for disclosure of such information to the pregnant woman. Failure to make such a disclosure undermines professional integrity and therefore the moral authority of health care professionals. When the sonographer disagrees with the clinical judgment of his or her supervising physician, communication about this matter should be professional (not personal) and direct, but not in the presence of the patient.

ROUTINE ULTRASOUND SCREENING OF PREGNANT WOMEN

In many countries, such as Germany, Great Britain, and Scandinavia, routine obstetric ultrasound examination at about 18 weeks of gestation has become the standard of obstetric care. In other countries, including the United States, this is not the case. Debate in the United States about routine ultrasound examination has been conducted almost exclusively in terms of medical judgment, that is, the principle of beneficence applied to both the fetus and the pregnant woman. The RADIUS study, for example, used exclusively beneficence-based outcomes of perinatal morbidity and mortality.[7] Its findings that routine obstetric ultrasound had no effect on these outcomes and therefore would involve unjustified costs, has been strongly challenged.[10] The result of this ongoing debate is residual uncertainty about how to balance the goods and harms of routine obstetric ultrasound examinations.[6]

The clinical ethical issues here focus on the physician's responsibilities under informed consent, an autonomy-based concern. We believe that this debate should therefore be expanded to include reference to the health care professional's autonomy-based obligations regarding the informed consent process. This process includes disclosure of and discussion about what ultrasound examinations can and cannot detect, the level of sophistication of the ultrasound techniques employed, and the incomplete and sometimes uncertain interpretation of ultrasound images.

In the face of medical uncertainty about the clinical goods and harms of routine ultrasound, it is obligatory to inform pregnant patients about that uncertainty and to give them the opportunity to make their own choices about how that uncertainty should be managed. We have argued that prenatal informed consent for sonogram (PICS) should be an indication for the routine use of obstetric ultrasound,[6,9] despite the contested claim that routine ultrasound has no effect on perinatal morbidity and mortality.[7]

The timing of routine ultrasound should be governed, as a rule, by the ethical principle of respect for autonomy because the information obtained is relevant to the woman's decision about whether she will seek an abortion. In pregnancies that will be taken to term, routine ultrasound during the second trimester can enhance a pregnant woman's autonomy. If anomalies are detected and she does not choose abortion, she may begin to prepare herself for the decisions that she will confront later about the management of those anomalies in the intrapartum and postpartum periods. Providing this information early in pregnancy permits a pregnant woman ample time to deal with its psychologic and other sequelae before she must confront such decisions.

DISCLOSURE OF RESULTS OF ULTRASOUND EXAMINATIONS

Significant clinical ethical issues arise about the disclosure of results of ultrasound examinations. First, there should be an adequate informed consent process, as just described. In routine examinations it is also important to inform the woman of the possibility of confronting an anomaly that will lead her to decide whether to terminate the pregnancy or take it to term.[6,9] Sonographers are justified to disclose findings of normal anatomy directly to the pregnant woman. Disclosure of, and discussion about, abnormal findings—if such disclosure and discussion are to respect and to enhance maternal autonomy and avoid unnecessary psychologic harm to the pregnant woman—are the responsibilities of the physician. This is because such discussion should occur in the context of the alternatives available to manage a pregnancy complicated by abnormal ultrasound findings. Sonographers, neither by training nor experience, can claim the clinical competence to engage in such discussions; physicians can and therefore should.

The second clinical ethical issue concerns the phenomenon of apparent bonding of pregnant women to their fetuses as a result of the pregnant woman seeing the ultrasound images.[3] Such bonding can sometimes benefit pregnancies that will be taken to term but can also at other times complicate decisions to terminate a pregnancy. We recommend that these matters, like abnormal findings, be discussed with the pregnant woman.

A third issue is a matter of ongoing debate: the disclosure of the fetus's gender.[9,11] We propose that respect for maternal autonomy dictates responding frankly to requests from the pregnant woman for information about the fetus's gender. The pregnant woman should be made aware of the uncertainties of ultrasound gender identification as part of the disclosure process. The sonographer can use his or her own experience to help the pregnant woman understand those uncertainties.

A fourth clinical ethical issue may, at first, seem a non-issue, (videotaping or photography of "baby pictures"). There is nothing intrinsically wrong with the practice if it is a side product of a legitimate ultrasound examination. In fact, it may help the bonding of the prospective parents to the fetal patient. However, when videotaping or Polaroid photography are performed to generate revenues, this practice trivializes the ultrasound examination and may result in harm because problems that could be diagnosed could be missed.

CONFIDENTIALITY OF FINDINGS

Confidentiality concerns the obligation of care givers to protect clinical information about patients from unauthorized access.[9] The obligation of confidentiality derives from the principles of beneficence—patients will be more forthcoming—and respect for autonomy—the patient's privacy rights are protected. Others, including the pregnant woman's spouse, sex partner, and family, should be understood as third parties to the patient-sonographer relationship. Diagnostic information about a woman's pregnancy is confidential. It can therefore be justifiably disclosed to third parties *only* with the pregnant woman's *explicit permission*. This is because a potentially acceptable condition for releasing confidential information, avoiding grave harm to others, does not apply in this context.[1,9] To avoid awkward situations, sonographers and their supervising physicians should establish policies and procedures that reflect this analysis of the ethics of confidentiality.

The ethics of confidentiality when the pregnant woman is less than the age of 18 years should be the same as when the patient is 18 years of age and older. The law, however, may complicate matters because pregnancy does not emancipate a minor in every jurisdiction and because different jurisdictions give different levels of protection to the privacy of the physician-patient relationship when the patient is under the age of 18 years.

REVIEW QUESTIONS

1. What are the major ethical obligations of obstetric sonographers to their patients?
2. What role do the ethical principles of beneficence and respect for autonomy play in generating these obligations?
3. How should sonographers respond when they have concerns about the adequacy of ultrasound examinations preferred by referring physicians?

REFERENCES

1. Beauchamp TL and others: *Principles of biomedical ethics,* ed 3, New York, 1989, Oxford University Press.
2. Beauchamp TL and others: *Medical ethics: the moral responsibilities of physicians,* Englewood Cliffs, NJ, 1984, Prentice-Hall.
3. Campbell S and others: Ultrasound scanning in pregnancy: the short-term psychological effects of early real time scans, *J Psychosomat Obstet Gynecol* 1:57, 1986.
4. Chervenak FA and others: Ethics in obstetric ultrasound, *J Ultrasound Me*d 8:493, 1989.
5. Chervenak FA and others: Perinatal ethics: a practical analysis of obligations to mother and fetus, *Obstet Gynecol* 66:442, 1985.
6. Chervenak FA and others: Prenatal informed consent for sonogram (PICS): an indication for obstetrical ultrasound, *Am J Obstet Gynecol* 161(4):857, 1989.
7. Ewigman BG and others: Effect of prenatal ultrasound screening on perinatal outcome, *N Engl J Med* 329:483, 1993.
8. McCullough LB: Methodological concerns in bioethics, *J Med Phil* 11:17, 1986.
9. McCullough LB and others: *Ethics in obstetrics and gynecology,* New York, 1994, Oxford University Press.
10. Skupski DW and others: Is routine ultrasound screening for all patients? *Clin Perinat* 21:707, 1994.
11. Warren MA: *Gendercide: the implications of sex selection,* Totowa, NJ, 1985, Rowman and Littlefield.

PART VIII

*F*etal *A*natomy

CHAPTER 34

The Placenta

Sandra L. Hagen-Ansert

KEY TERMS

abruptio placenta - premature detachment of the placenta from the maternal wall

battledore placenta - cord insertion into the margin of the placenta

Braxton-Hicks contractions - spontaneous painless uterine contractions described originally as a sign of pregnancy; they occur from the first trimester to the end of pregnancy

chorionic plate - that part of the chorionic membrane that covers the placenta

chorionic villi - vascular projections from the chorion

circummarginate placenta - chorionic plate of the placenta is smaller than the basal plate, with a flat interface between the fetal membranes and the placenta

circumvallate placenta - chorionic plate of the placenta is smaller than the basal plate; the margin is raised with a rolled edge

decidua basalis - the part of the decidua that unites with the chorion to form the placenta

decidua capsularis - the part of the decidua that surrounds the chorionic sac

ductus venosus - connection that is patent during fetal life from the left portal vein to the systemic veins (inferior vena cava)

ligamentum venosum - transformation of the ductus venosus in fetal life to closure in neonatal life

lower uterine segment (LUS) - lowest segment of the uterus at the junction of the internal os and sacrum

molar pregnancy - also known as gestational trophoblastic disease; abnormal proliferation of trophoblastic cells in the first trimester

placenta accreta - growth of the chorionic villi superficially into the myometrium

placenta increta - growth of the chorionic villi deep into the myometrium

placenta percreta - growth of the chorionic villi through the myometrium.

placenta previa - placenta completely covers the lower uterine segment (internal os)

placental grading - arbitrary method of classifying the maturity of the placenta with a grading scale of 0 to 3

placental migration - the placenta is attached to the uterine wall; as the uterus enlarges the placenta "moves" with it; therefore a low-lying placenta may move out of the uterine segment in the second trimester

succenturiate placenta - one or more accessory lobes connected to the body of the placenta by blood vessels

vasa previa - occurs when the intramembranous vessels course across the cervical os

Wharton's jelly - mucoid connective tissue that surrounds the vessels within the umbilical cord

---

The development of the placenta has always been of interest to anatomists, researchers, obstetricians, and ultrasonographers. Combined studies using transvaginal ultrasonography, hysteroscopy, chorionic villus sampling, and hysterectomy specimens from the first trimester of pregnancy have recently indicated the absence of continuous blood flow in the intervillous space before 12 weeks of gestation.[7]

The major role of the placenta is to permit the exchange of oxygenated maternal blood (rich in oxygen and nutrients) with deoxygenated fetal blood. Maternal vessels coursing posterior to the placenta circulate blood into the placenta, whereas blood from the fetus reaches this point through the umbilical cord.[3] The placenta is effectively studied by antenatal ultrasound. Valuable information regarding placental configuration, location, maturity, pathology, and maturation irregularities may be assessed.

It is recognized that the anatomic components of the placenta are discernible from as early as the 7th to 8th week of gestation. By the end of the first trimester, sonography can determine the location and position of the placenta and identify specific components of the placenta.

EMBRYOGENESIS

The chorion, amnion, yolk sac, and allantois constitute the embryonic or fetal membranes. These membranes develop from the zygote. Implantation of the blastocyst occurs 6 to 7 days after fertilization. Enlargement of trophoblasts helps to anchor the blastocyst to the endometrial lining. The placenta has two components, the fetal portion, developed from the chorion frondosum **(chorionic plate),** and a maternal portion, the **decidua basalis,** formed by the endometrial surface (Figure 34-1).

The transformation of cells into glycogen and lipoid cells characterizes the decidual reaction. This occurs in response to ovarian hormones (estrogen and progesterone). The development of the placenta is seen in the changes in the decidua (Box 34-1).

As the embryo and membranes grow, the **decidua capsularis** is stretched. The **chorionic villi** on the associated part of the chorionic sac gradually atrophy and disappear (smooth chorion or chorion laeve). The chorionic villi related to the decidua basalis increase rapidly in size and complexity (villous chorion or chorion frondosum).

The fetal chorion is the fusion of the trophoblast and extraembryonic mesenchyme. There are two types of trophoblastic cells: the syncytiotrophoblast is the outer layer of multinuclear cells, and the cytotrophoblast is the inner layer of mononuclear cells (Box 34-2).

The major functioning unit of the placenta is the chorionic villus (Figure 34-2). Within the chorionic villus are the intervillous spaces. The maternal blood enters the intervillous spaces. The cotyledons are cobblestone in appearance and composed of several mainstem villi and their branches. They are covered with a thin layer of the decidua basalis.

Before birth, the fetal membranes and placenta perform the following functions and activities: protection, nutrition, respiration, and excretion (Box 34-3). At birth or parturition, they are separated from the fetus and cast from the uterus as the afterbirth.

The maternal placental circulation may be reduced by a variety of conditions that decrease uterine blood flow, such as severe hypotension, renal disease, or placental infarction. Placental defects can cause intrauterine fetal growth restriction (IUGR). The net effect is that there is a reduction between the fetal and maternal blood.

The fetal placenta is anchored to the maternal placenta by the cytotrophoblastic shell and anchoring villi. It provides a large area where materials may be exchanged across the placental membrane and interposed between fetal and maternal circulation. It has been demonstrated that the embryo favors an environment low in oxygen during early development and that oxygen levels in placental tissue are low in the early first trimester.[6]

The placenta is dedicated to the survival of the fetus. Even when exposed to a poor maternal environment (e.g., when the mother is malnourished, diseased, or smokes or takes cocaine, the placenta can often compensate by be-

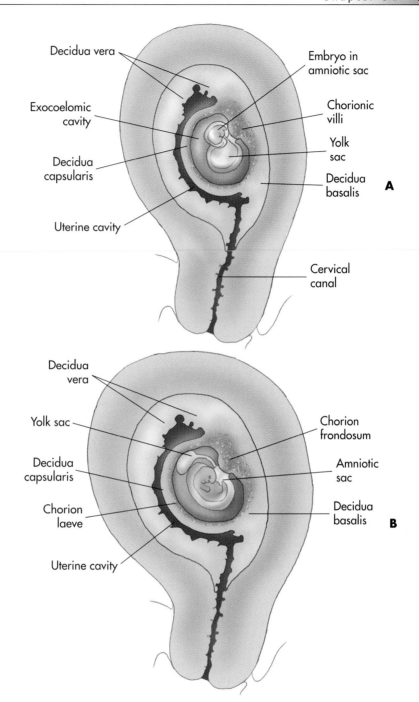

Figure 34-1   A, The placenta has two components, the fetal portion, developed from the chorion frondosum (chorionic plate), and a maternal portion, the decidua basalis, formed by the endometrial surface. **B,** The chorionic villi gradually atrophy and disappear (chorion laeve). The chorionic villi in the decidua basalis increase rapidly in size and complexity.

coming more efficient.[10] Unfortunately, there are limits to the placenta's ability to cope with external stresses. Eventually, if multiple or severe enough, these stresses can lead to placental damage, fetal damage, and even intrauterine demise and pregnancy loss.[10]

Deoxygenated blood leaves the fetus and passes through the umbilical artery to the placenta. As the cord attaches to the placenta, the arteries divide into a number of radically disposed vessels that branch into the chorionic plate before entering the villi. There is normally no gross intermingling of fetal and maternal blood. The placental membrane consists of fetal tissues separating the maternal and fetal blood.

PLACENTAL MEMBRANE

The placental membrane is often called a barrier because there are a few compounds, endogenous and exogenous, that are unable to cross the placental membranes in detectable amounts. The placenta has three main activities: metabolism, endocrine secretion, and transfer. All are essential for maintaining the pregnancy and promoting normal embryonic development. After birth, the placenta, umbilical cord, and associated membranes are expelled from the uterus.

CORDAL ATTACHMENTS

The attachment of the cord is usually near the center of the placenta. Abnormal cordal attachments to the placenta are battledore and velamentous placenta. A **battledore placenta** refers to the insertion of the umbilical cord at the

---

> ### BOX 34-1 DECIDUAL CHANGES
>
> - **Decidua basalis:** The decidual reaction that occurs between the blastocyst and the myometrium
> - **Decidua capsularis:** The decidual reaction occurring over the blastocyst closest to the endometrial cavity
> - **Decidua vera (parietalis):** A reaction changes in the endometrium opposite the site of implantation

---

> ### BOX 34-2 FETAL CHORION
>
> - **Chorion frondosum:** The fetal trophoblastic tissue, that together with the decidua form the area for maternal and fetal circulation
> - **Chorion laeve:** The chorion around the gestational sac on the opposite side of implantation
> - **Chorionic plate:** The fetal surface of the placenta
> - **Basal plate:** The maternal surface of the placenta

---

margin of the placenta (Figure 34-3). It usually has no clinical significance unless the cord is avulsed during delivery. The velamentous placenta refers to a membranous insertion of the cord. In a small number of cases (less than 2%) it may be associated with significant fetal hemorrhage, especially if the membrane carrying the vessels is positioned across the internal os **(vasa previa).**

YOLK SAC

The yolk sac has a role in the transfer of nutrients to the embryo during the 2nd and 3rd weeks while the uteroplacental circulation is developing. By 9 weeks, the yolk sac has diminished to less than 5 mm in diameter. It is connected to the midgut by a narrow yolk stalk, and by 12 weeks the tiny yolk sac lies within the chorionic cavity between the amnion and chorionic sac.

IMPLANTATION OF THE PLACENTA

Normally the placenta will implant on the anterior, fundal, or posterior wall of the uterus. Occasionally the placenta will implant low in the uterus, causing a condition called **placenta previa.**

MEMBRANES

The fetal membranes consist of the chorion, amnion, allantois, and yolk sac. The chorion originates from the trophoblastic cells and remains in contact with the trophoblasts throughout pregnancy. The amnion develops at the 28th menstrual day and is attached to the margins of the embryonic disk. As the embryo grows and folds ventrally, the junction of the amnion is reduced to a small area on the ventral surface of the embryo to form the umbilicus.

Expansion of the amniotic cavity occurs with the production of amniotic fluid. By 16 weeks the amnion fuses

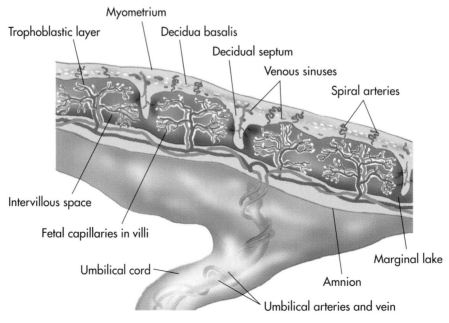

Figure 34-2 The major functioning unit of the placenta is the chorionic villus. The spiral arteries, venous sinuses, and uterine arteries line the periphery of the placenta.

with the chorion and can no longer be seen on ultrasound as two separate membranes. If the separation extends beyond 16 weeks it may be associated with polyhydramnios or prior amniocentesis. Hemorrhage may also have this appearance.

The secondary yolk sac forms after regression of the primary yolk sac at 28 menstrual days on the ventral surface of the embryonic disk. Before 5 menstrual weeks, the amniotic sac and secondary yolk sac have been pressed together with the embryonic disk between. This structure is suspended within another balloon (the chorion cavity) by the connecting stalk. The yolk sac becomes displaced from the embryo and lies between the amnion and the chorion (see Figure 34- 1).

THE AMNIOTIC SAC AND AMNIOTIC FLUID

The amnion forms a sac that contains amniotic fluid. The sac encloses the embryo and forms the epithelial covering of the umbilical cord. Most of the amniotic fluid comes from the maternal blood by diffusion across the amnion from the decidua parietalis and intervillous spaces of the placenta.

In the first trimester the fetus begins to excrete urine into the sac to fill the amniotic cavity. The fetus swallows this fluid, and the cycle continues throughout pregnancy. The amniotic fluid serves as a protective buffer for the embryo and fetus. In addition, the fluid provides room for the fetal movements to occur and assists in regulating fetal body temperature.

THE PLACENTA'S ROLE AS AN ENDOCRINE GLAND

The chronic villi are the functional endocrine units of the placenta. A central core with abundant capillaries is surrounded by an inner layer, cytotrophoblast, and an outer layer, syncytiotrophoblast. The inner layer produces neuropeptides, and the outer layer produces the protein hormones human chorionic gonadotropin (hCG) and human placental lactogen (hPL), along with the sex steroids estrogen and progesterone.

After the 7th week of gestation, most progesterone is produced by the syncytiotrophoblast from maternally derived cholesterol precursors. Progesterone production is exclusively a maternal-placental interaction, with no contribution from the fetus. The production of placental estrogen involves an intricate pathway requiring maternal, placental, and fetal contributions.

The function of the hCG is to maintain the corpus luteum in early pregnancy. It is elevated shortly after conception and peaks at 8 to 10 weeks. The hPL is responsible for the promotion of lipolysis and an antiinsulin action that serves to direct nutrients to the fetus.

THE UMBILICAL CORD

DEVELOPMENT

The umbilical cord forms during the first 5 weeks of gestation. The cord is surrounded by a mucoid connective tissue called **Wharton's jelly.** The intestines grow at a faster

rate than the abdomen and herniate into the proximal umbilical cord at approximately 7 weeks and remain there until approximately 10 weeks. The insertion of the cord into the ventral abdominal wall is an important sonographic anatomic landmark because scrutiny of this area will reveal abdominal wall defects such as omphalocele, gastroschisis, or limb-body wall complex.

The umbilical cord has one large vein and two smaller arteries. One umbilical artery is found in approximately 1% of all singleton births and 7% of twin gestations. It is seen more commonly in diabetic mothers and is associated with low birthweight infants. Congenital malformations, (genitourinary, cardiovascular, facial, and musculoskeletal), are seen in 25% to 50% of infants with one umbilical artery.

ULTRASOUND OF THE UMBILICAL CORD

The vessels of the cord may be followed with real-time ultrasound as they leave the placenta to enter the fetal ab-

---

BOX 34-3   FUNCTION OF THE PLACENTA

RESPIRATION
Oxygen in maternal blood diffuses across the placental membrane into fetal blood by diffusion. Carbon dioxide passes in the opposite direction. The placenta acts as "fetal lungs."

NUTRITION
Water, inorganic salts, carbohydrates, fats, proteins, and vitamins pass from maternal blood through the placental membrane into fetal blood.

EXCRETION
Waste products cross membrane from fetal blood and enter maternal blood. Excreted by mother's kidneys.

PROTECTION
Some microorganisms cross placental border.

STORAGE
Carbohydrates, proteins, calcium, and iron are stored in placenta and released into fetal circulation.

HORMONAL PRODUCTION
Produced by syncytiotrophoblast of placenta: human chorionic gonadotropin, estrogens, progesterone.

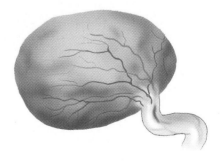

Figure 34-3   A battledore placenta refers to the insertion of the umbilical cord at the margin of the placenta.

domen and travel toward the liver and iliac arteries (Figure 34-4). From the left portal vein, the umbilical blood flows either through the **ductus venosus** to the systemic veins (inferior vena cava or hepatic veins) by passing the liver or through the right portal sinus to the right portal vein. The ductus venosus forms the conduit between the portal system and the systemic veins.

Sonographically, the ductus venous appears as a thin intrahepatic channel with echogenic walls. It lies in the groove between the left lobe and the caudate lobe. The ductus venosus is patent during fetal life until shortly after birth, when transformation of the ductus into the **ligamentum venosum** occurs (beginning in the 2nd week after birth).

The umbilical arteries may be followed caudal from the cord insertion, in their normal path adjacent to the fetal bladder to the iliac arteries. On ultrasound, the sonographer may look at the cord in a transverse plane to see the large umbilical vein and two smaller arteries. Another approach to image the umbilical arteries is to image the fetal bladder in a transverse or coronal plane. The umbilical arteries will run along the lateral margins of the fetal bladder and are well seen with color flow Doppler. In the postpartum stage, the umbilical arteries become the superior vesical arteries.

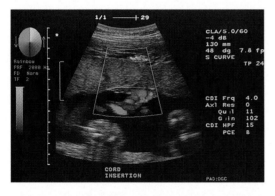

Figure 34-4 Color Doppler may demonstrate the umbilical cord as it exits the placenta.

SONOGRAPHIC EVALUATION OF THE NORMAL PLACENTA

Two surfaces of the placenta merit special attention because they are important in assessing normal placental anatomy, evaluating placental abruption, and grading the placenta.

The fetal surface of the placenta (portion of the placenta nearest the amniotic cavity) is represented by the echogenic chorionic plate that courses along the placental tissue and is found at the junction with the amniotic fluid. This linear density is further enhanced by the strong interface of the amnion covering the chorionic plate (Figure 34-5).

The second surface is the basal plate or maternal portion of the placenta, which lies at the junction of the myometrium and the substance of the placenta (see Figure 34-5). Maternal blood vessels from the endometrium (endometrial veins) run behind the basal plate and are often confused with placental abruption.[14] This represents the normal vascularity of this region. The endometrial veins are more apparent when the placenta is located in the fundus or posteriorly within the uterine cavity.

The substance of the placenta assumes a relatively homogenous pebble-gray appearance during the first part of pregnancy and is easily recognized with its characteristically smooth borders. The thickness of the placenta varies with gestational age, with a minimum diameter of 15 mm in fetuses greater than 23 weeks.[8] The size of the placenta rarely exceeds 50 mm in the normal fetus (Figure 34-6). Enlarged placentas are most often associated with Rh sensitization, diabetes of pregnancy, or congenital anomalies. The sonographer must maintain a perpendicular measurement of the placental width in relation to the myometrial wall when evaluating the width of the placenta. **Braxton-Hicks contractions** (normal contractions of pregnancy) should not be confused for placental pathology.

Several sonolucent areas within the placenta may confuse the sonographer unfamiliar with the wide range of placental variants. Cystic structures representing large fetal

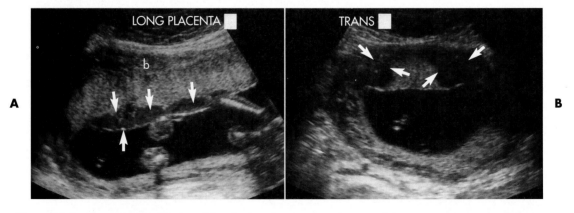

Figure 34-5 **A,** Longitudinal image of the placenta demonstrates the smooth homogeneous texture of the organ. Areas of echolucencies *(arrows)* are shown along the inner margin of the chorionic plate *(arrow)*. The basal surface *(b).* of the placenta is well seen along the myometrial surface of the uterus **B,** Transverse image of the placenta as it lies along the anterior uterine wall. Echolucencies are seen representing the intervillous lakes *(arrows)*.

vessels are commonly observed coursing behind the chorionic plate and between the amnion and chorion layers (Figure 34-7). Real-time observation of blood flow or color Doppler (Figure 34-8) helps to differentiate these vessels.[5] Deposits of fibrin may also be found in the intervillous space posterior to the chorionic plate, and blood flow will not be seen in fibrinous areas.[8,11]

Echo-spared regions may also be seen within the placental substance in the center of the placental lobes (cotyledons), which have been referred to as placental lakes.[8,14] Blood flow should be identified within these areas. Placental veins may also be seen within the mass of the placenta.

PLACENTAL POSITION

The position of the placenta is readily apparent on most obstetric ultrasound studies. The placenta may be located within the fundus of the uterus, along the anterior or posterior uterine walls (Figure 34-9), or laterally, or it may be dangerously implanted over or near the cervix, (placenta previa) (Figure 34-10).

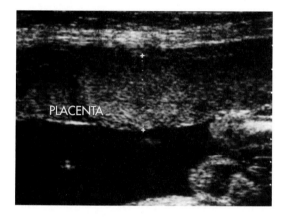

Figure 34-6   The thickness of the placenta measures over 7 cm in this Rh-sensitized pregnancy. Calipers should be placed perpendicular to the placental borders.

Occasionally the placenta originates in the fundus of the uterus and proceeds along the anterior wall (fundal anterior placenta) or along the posterior uterine wall (fundal posterior placenta). In early pregnancy the chorion frondosum (primitive placenta) appears to completely surround the chorionic cavity (circumferential placenta).

The sonographer should always describe the position of the placenta. The placenta should be scanned longitudinally to see whether it extends into the lower segment. If it does, a transverse scan should be obtained to determine whether the placenta is located centrally or whether it lies to one side of the cervix. Oblique scans may be necessary to visualize the relationship of the placenta to the cervix.

For the sonographer to visualize the internal os of the cervix, the patient should have a full bladder. In this way the relationship of the placenta to the internal os can be visualized (Figure 34-11). In theory this works well. In practice, it is not always easy for the sonographer to view the internal os with the patient's bladder full. If a patient is actively bleeding or in active labor, the sonographer may not have time to wait for the patient to fill her bladder. If the fetal head is low in the pelvis, diagnosis of a posterior placenta previa may be difficult because the fetal skull bones block transmission of the ultrasound at a critical point. If the fetal head can be elevated out of the pelvis, it may be possible to distinguish between a posterior low-lying position and a posterior previa position. Other methods to demonstrate the os include tilting the patient in a slight Trendelenburg position (head lower than body) to relieve pressure of the uterus on the **lower uterine segment** or using the transvaginal or transperineal approach.

An overfilled bladder may push the internal os up, making it appear higher than it actually is. This may give the false impression of a previa. Emptying the bladder reduces the pressure on the lower uterine segment and allows the cervix to assume a more normal position. The placenta may in fact not be a previa at all.

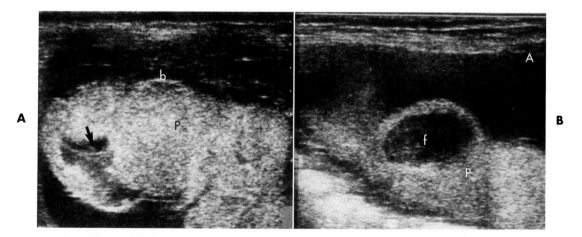

Figure 34-7   **A,** Subchorionic cystic area of the placenta at 29 weeks of gestation. Blood flow was obvious under real time imaging *(arrow). b,* Basal plate; *p,* placenta. **B,** Subchorionic cystic area at 24 weeks of gestation, with internal echoes, representative of blood flow *(f).* Color Doppler imaging may aid in detecting areas of blood flow. *A,* Amniotic fluid; *p,* placenta.

Describing the location of the placenta has clinical importance. A previa noted on a scan alerts the obstetrician that no pelvic examination should be performed on the patient. A finger inadvertently pushed through an unknown previa can result in an amount of bleeding that frightens not only the patient but the physician. If a placenta is noted to be a low-lying presentation early in pregnancy, the placenta location can be followed with consecutive scans to see whether this location persists.

When the placenta appears to lie on both anterior or posterior uterine walls, check for a laterally positioned placenta. When the placenta does not appear to communicate, a **succenturiate placenta** should be considered. This is a condition in which there are additional placental lobes joined to the main placenta by blood vessels. There is a risk that these connecting blood vessels may rupture or that an extra lobe may be inadvertently left in the uterus after delivery; therefore the clinician should be notified of this condition.[8]

The concept that the placenta changes its position within the uterine cavity has been termed *migration*, imply-

ing that the placenta actually moves and relocates.[9] It may be that the placenta actually does not move but that the position appears changed because of the physiologic changes occurring around it (i.e., enlargement of the uterus and development of the lower uterine segment).

Although the majority of placentas that are considered previas in the second trimester convert to fundal or low-lying placentas by the third trimester, there are exceptions. If the placenta is a complete previa in the second trimester, it is unlikely to change its position drastically. In all likelihood when the third trimester arrives, it will remain a complete previa.

PLACENTAL GRADING
The textural characteristics of the developing placenta have been described.[2] The changes in the maturing placenta have been commonly referred to as **placental grading.** It is known that the maturation of the placenta does not occur at the same rate or to the same degree in all pregnancies. Maternal disease states (e.g., diabetes, hypertension, Rh disease) may affect the maturation process.

Grading the placenta involves the evaluation of the basal plate, placental substance, and chorionic plate (Figure 34-12). The grading classification is as follows[2]:

- **GRADE 0:** Represents the earliest placental grade, with a smooth, well-defined chorionic plate, homogeneous placental tissue, and regular basal plate (without echogenic densities). This is the typical grade of a placenta less than 28 weeks of gestation (Figure 34-13, *A*).
- **GRADE 1:** Characteristic undulation (indentation) of the chorionic plate with spotlike densities dispersed throughout the placental tissue (calcium deposits) and with a regular basal plate (Figure 34-13, *B*).
- **GRADE 2:** Indentations of the chorionic plate with linear commalike densities extending from the chorionic plate into the placental substance but not reaching the

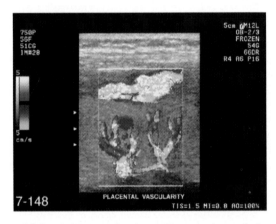

Figure 34-8 Color Doppler shows the normal vascularity of the marginal lakes, capillaries, and basal area of the placenta.

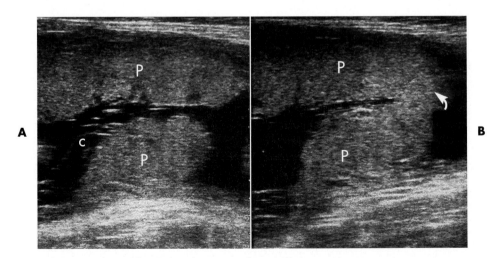

Figure 34-9 A, Placenta *(P)* appears to be located on both anterior and posterior uterine walls. *C,* Umbilical cord. **B,** By scanning laterally, the placenta is seen to communicate *(arrow),* representing a lateral placenta rather than a succenturiate lobed placenta.

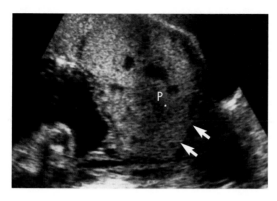

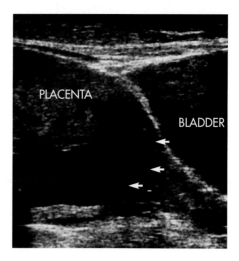

Figure 34-10 Placenta previa. *Arrows* point to the placenta *(p)* implanted over the cervical os.

Figure 34-11 Ultrasound clearly shows the internal os of the cervix *(arrows)*. The placenta is implanted away from the os.

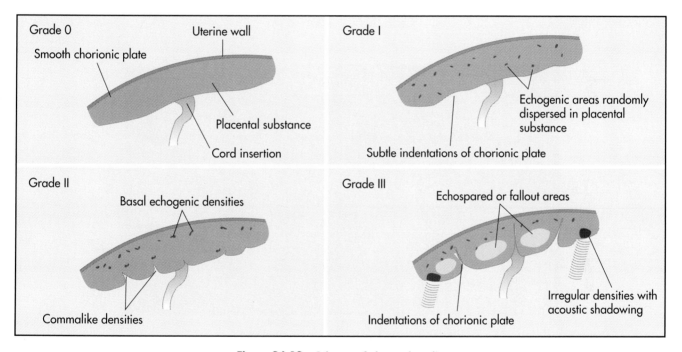

Figure 34-12 Schema of placental grading.

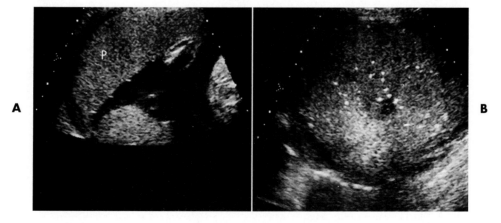

Figure 34-13 **A,** Fundal, anterior, grade 0 placenta at 20 weeks of gestation. Note the smooth homogeneous echo pattern characteristic of this early grade. There are no calcifications within the placenta *(p)* or along the basal plate. **B,** Fundal, grade 1 placenta at 39 weeks of gestation, showing the characteristic echogenic densities within the placental substance.

basal plate. Along the basal plate, linear echogenic densities are noted (Figure 34-14, *A*).

- **GRADE 3:** Highest grade of the placenta. The comma-like densities reach the basal plate as the placental septae are deposited with calcium, which surrounds the placental lobes (cotyledons), resulting in complete circles of calcium. Echo-spared areas may be found in the center, with highly echogenic basal echoes that may produce acoustic shadowing (Figures 34-14, *B*, and 34-15).

When two grades are present the placental grade should be assigned to the highest grade. Only 15% to 20% of placentas reach grade 3 status at term.[2] Premature aging of the placenta (grade 3 placenta before 34 weeks) may indicate an impending complication, such as intrauterine growth restriction or preeclampsia, whereas it is common to see immature placenta in patients with gestational diabetes or Rh incompatibility.[5]

EVALUATION OF THE PLACENTA AFTER DELIVERY

The normal term placenta has several characteristics at delivery. It measures about 15 to 20 cm in diameter, is discoid in shape, weighs about 600 g, and measures less than 4 cm in thickness. The clinician ascertains that the placenta has been delivered intact to avoid complications of postpartum hemorrhage or infection. Membranes of the amnion and chorion are inspected for color and consistency, with attention to meconium staining or signs of infection. The length of the umbilical cord is noted (and measured in the pathology laboratory). Short cords of less than 30 cm may result in traction during labor and delivery, leading to avulsion of the cord, abruption, or inversion of the uterus. Long cords are more likely to prolapse, become twisted around the fetus, or tie in true knots.

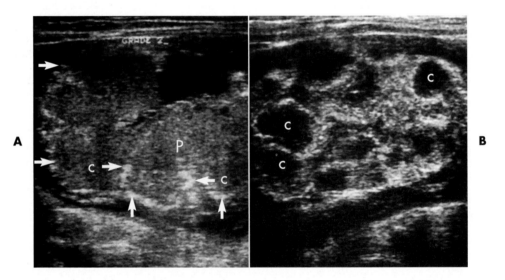

Figure 34-14 **A,** Fundal, grade 2 placenta at 33 weeks of gestation showing calcifications lining up along the basal plate *(arrows)* and within the placenta *(p)*. *c,* Cotyledons. **B,** Fundal, grade 3 placenta at 42 weeks of gestation showing calcifications encasing several cotyledons *(c)*.

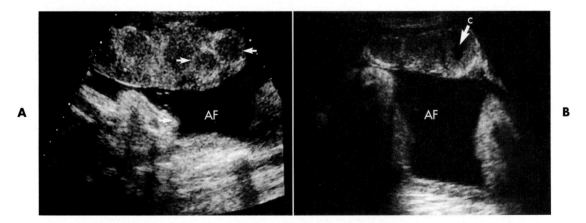

Figure 34-15 **A,** Ringlike calcifications consistent with a grade 3 placenta observed at the lateral aspect of the placenta. *AF,* Amniotic fluid. **B,** A grade 3 placenta noted with the center of the cotyledon *(c)* outlined. *AF,* Amniotic fluid.

PLACENTOMEGALY

Placentomegaly is an enlarged placenta weighing more than 600 g. On ultrasound examination the placenta thickness measures more than 5 cm. Maternal diabetes and Rh incompatibility are primary causes for placentomegaly (Box 34-4).

ABNORMALITIES OF THE PLACENTA

The major pathologic processes seen in the placenta that can adversely affect pregnancy outcome include intrauterine bacterial infections, decreased blood flow to the placenta from the mother, and immunologic attack of the placenta by the mother's immune system.[10] Intrauterine infections (most commonly the result of migration of vaginal bacteria through the cervix into the uterine cavity) can lead to severe fetal hypoxia as a result of villous edema (fluid build up within the placenta itself).[10] Both chronic and acute decreases in blood flow to the placenta can cause severe fetal damage and even death.

As well as supplying the fetus with nutrition, the placenta is a barrier between the mother and fetus, protecting the fetus from immune rejection by the mother, a pathologic process that can lead to intrauterine growth restriction or even demise.[10] In addition to these major pathologic categories, many other insults, such as placental separation, cord accidents, trauma, and viral and parasitic infections, can adversely affect pregnancy outcome by affecting the function of the placenta (Table 34-1).[10]

FIBRIN DEPOSITION

Fibrin is a protein derived from fibrinogen. It is found throughout the placenta, but is most pronounced in the floor of the placenta (in the septa) and increases continuously throughout pregnancy. Fibrin deposits on the villi may increase their mechanical stability; the deposits may be the result of eddies in the turbulent flow—more flow equals increased fibrin deposits. Fibrin may also be attributed to the regulatiom of intervillous circulation.

Ultrasound findings. On ultrasound examination, this fibrin deposition (subchorionic) appears as hypoechoic area beneath the chorionic plate of the placenta (see Figure 34-13, *B*). Differential diagnosis of fibrin deposition includes a venous lake or a subchorionic hematoma. A venous lake shows increased flow with color flow Doppler. It may be difficult to distinguish fibrin deposits from a hematoma on ultrasound.

PLACENTA PREVIA

The placenta normally implants in the body of the uterus; however, in 1 of 200 pregnancies the placenta implants over or near to the internal os of the cervix.[12] This condition is called placenta previa.

The placenta may be considered (1) a complete or total previa, (2) a partial previa, (3) a marginal previa, or (4) low-lying (Figure 34-16). With complete previa the cervical internal os is completely covered by placental tissue; this occurrence has been found in 20% of patients with previa. The majority of patients present with some form of previa. A partial previa only partially covers the internal os. A marginal previa does not cover the os, but its edge comes

---

BOX 34-4	PLACENTA SIZE

PLACENTOMEGALY
Maternal diabetes
Maternal anemia
α-Thalassemia
Rh sensitivity
Fetomaternal hemorrhage
Chronic intrauterine infections
Twin-twin transfusion syndrome
Congenital neoplasms
Fetal malformations

SMALL PLACENTA
Intrauterine growth restriction
Intrauterine infection
Chromosomal abnormality

TABLE 34-1   LESIONS OF THE PLACENTA

Lesion Significance	Incidence Etiology	Clinical Findings
Intervillous thrombosis	36%: Bleeding from fetal vessels	Fetal-maternal hemorrhage
Massive perivillous fibrin deposition	22%: Pooling and stasis of blood in intervillous space	None
Infarct	25%: Thrombosis of maternal vessel or retroplacental bleed and associated condition	Depends on extent
Subchorionic fibrin	20%: Pooling and stasis of blood in subchorionic space	None
Hydatidiform change	<1%: Complete mole	Predisposes to choriocarcinoma
	<1%: Partial mole	Associated with symptoms of preeclampsia
Chorioangioma	1%: Vascular malformation	Usually none, depends on size

to the margin of the os. Although a low-lying placenta is implanted in the lower uterine segment, its edge does not reach the internal os.

A pregnancy complicated by placenta previa is at high risk because of the risk of life-threatening hemorrhage. As the pregnancy progresses into the third trimester, two very important changes occur. First, the lower uterine segment is developing, that is, thinning and elongating in preparation for labor. As the lower uterine segment develops, the placental attachment to the lower uterine wall may be disrupted, resulting in bleeding. Second, the cervix softens and some dilation can occur before the onset of labor. Cervical dilation may also disrupt the attachment of a placenta located over or near the cervical os.

Earlier in gestation, "complete previa" may be noted in about 5% of second-trimester pregnancies, with 90% resolving by term as the placenta migrates with the growth of the uterus. Asymptomatic partial previas are seen in as many as 45% of second-trimester pregnancies, with over 95% resolving before delivery.

Three factors are associated with placenta previa: advanced maternal age, multiparity, and prior cesarean section or uterine surgery.[1] Complications of placenta previa include premature delivery, life-threatening maternal hemorrhage, increased risk of **placenta accreta,** increased risk of postpartum hemorrhage, and IUGR.

Clinically the patient may present with painless, bright, red vaginal bleeding in the third trimester. About 25% of patients will present with bleeding in the first 30 weeks. As many as 20% are associated with uterine premature contractions. Abnormal lie (either transverse or breech) is associated with placenta previa.

When a patient presents with third-trimester bleeding, diagnosis is imperative because the treatment will be different based on the clinical diagnosis. If the clinical diagnosis is placental abruption, the obstetrician will deliver the fetus or it may die. If the diagnosis is placenta previa, the fetus is preterm, and the mother is not bleeding heavily, the clinical management may be conservative, with transfusion and close observation until the point where the fetus is mature or the pregnancy must be terminated because of bleeding.

When the time for delivery arrives, if the placenta completely covers the os, the fetus will have to be delivered by cesarean section. If the placenta only partially covers the os, it is possible that the fetus may deliver vaginally. The pressure of the fetus as it passes through the cervix and birth canal may compress the part of the placenta that has been disrupted and stop the bleeding (Box 34-5).

Ultrasound findings. The sonographer must be cautious in examining the lower uterine segment in relation to the location of the placenta. The maternal urinary bladder may be used as a landmark to identify the location of the internal cervical os (see Figure 34-11). The sonographer should be cautious of misinterpreting a low-lying placenta covering the internal os secondary to an overdistended bladder. The patient should be asked to empty her bladder, and the lower uterine segment should be rescanned to see the lower segment of the placenta in relation to the os.

Although ultrasound allows easy localization of the placenta, the diagnosis of previa is difficult at times. Early in pregnancy, while the uterus is small, the relative endometrial surface covered by the placenta is large.[9] As the pregnancy progresses, however, the amount of endometrial surface the placenta covers decreases. Therefore placentas can appear as previas early in pregnancy and may be marginal. As the lower uterine segment develops, however, and the placenta decreases relative to the uterus in size, there may be an increase in distance between the lower edge of the placenta and the internal os (Figure 34-17). The relationship of the placenta changes as pregnancy progresses, and a large number of low-lying placentas become fundal placentas by term.

Focal uterine contractions may also be misleading and a pitfall in diagnosing previa. The lower uterine segment should be scanned early in the ultrasound examination. If a contraction occurs, the sonographer may go on with the normal examination and reexamine the lower uterine segment in 20 minutes.

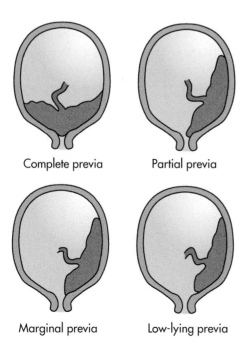

Complete previa   Partial previa

Marginal previa   Low-lying previa

Figure 34-16 Types of placenta previa.

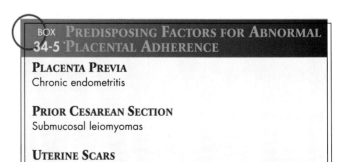

BOX
34-5 **PREDISPOSING FACTORS FOR ABNORMAL PLACENTAL ADHERENCE**

PLACENTA PREVIA
Chronic endometritis

PRIOR CESAREAN SECTION
Submucosal leiomyomas

UTERINE SCARS
Intrauterine synechiae

If the fetus is vertex and in the last trimester of pregnancy, the sonographer should examine the fetal head in relationship to the posterior wall of the uterus and the mother's sacrum. A distance of more than 1.5 cm indicates there will not be enough room for the placenta to be between the fetal head and posterior uterine wall.

The transperineal approach is also useful in evaluating the lower uterine segment when the definition of the placenta needs to be clarified. The transvaginal transducer is ideal for this approach.[4] (The transducer should be prepared as for a transvaginal examination, with a protective covering). The transducer is placed along the maternal labia to demonstrate the maternal bladder, the internal os (directed in a vertical orientation), the lower uterine segment, the fetal head, and the placenta (if previa). Longitudinal and transverse scans are carefully made to delineate the relation of the placenta to the cervical os.

ACCRETA, INCRETA, PERCRETA

Placenta accreta is the abnormal adherence of part or all of the placenta with partial or complete absence of the decidua basalis. Chorionic villi grow into the myometrium, and the placental villi are anchored to muscle fibers rather than to the intervening decidual cells. Placenta accreta occurs in approximately 1 in 2500 deliveries.[11]

Placenta increta is further extension of the placenta through the myometrium. **Placenta percreta** is penetration of the uterine serosa. These conditions result from the underdeveloped decidualization of the endometrium.

The risk of placenta accreta increases in patients with placenta previa.[11] Without prior uterine surgery, the risk of accreta at the time of delivery with placenta previa is about 5%, increasing to 25% if there has been one previous cesarean section and to as high as 45% when there have been two or more previous uterine surgeries (Table 34-2).

Ultrasound findings. The sonographer should evaluate the placenta previa to look for the absence of hypoechoic subplacenta venous channels and myometrium beneath the placenta. In placenta percreta the placental vessels extend within the urinary bladder wall. The perineal scanning approach may help the sonographer further define the lower uterine segment and the vascularity of the placenta in relationship to the maternal bladder.

SUCCENTURIATE PLACENTA

The succenturiate placenta is the presence of one or more accessory lobes connected to the body of the placenta by blood vessels (Figure 34-18). The incidence occurs in 3% to 6% of pregnancies.

Normally, the placenta is oval with a shape that varies somewhat depending on its site of implantation and areas of atrophy. When the placenta develops a secondary lobe or several other smaller lobes, these are called succenturiate lobes. These lobes have a tendency to develop infarcts and necrosis (50% of deliveries). They may create a "placenta previa" or be retained in utero after delivery.

The retention of the succenturiate lobe at delivery may result in postpartum hemorrhage and infection. Rarely, rupture of the connecting vessels may occur during delivery, causing fetal hemorrhage and demise.

Ultrasound findings. The sonographer should look for a discrete lobe that has "placenta texture" but is separate from the main body of the placenta. With color flow Doppler, vascular bands are seen connecting the lobes. The succenturiate placenta varies in appearance; it may be as large as the main lobe of the placenta and appear as two placentas. In 33% of bilobed placentas, the umbilical cord is attached to the main lobe of the placenta.

CIRCUMVALLATE PLACENTA

A **circumvallate placenta** is the attachment of the placental membranes to the fetal surface of the placenta rather than to the placental margin (Figure 34-19). This abnormality occurs in 1% to 2% of pregnancies. It results in placental villi around the border of the placenta that are not covered by the chorionic plate. A circumvallate placenta is diagnosed when the placental margin is folded, thickened, or elevated with underlying fibrin and hemorrhage.[12] It is associated with premature rupture of

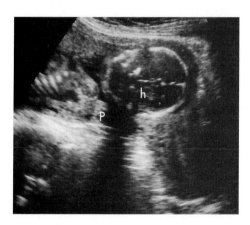

Figure 34-17 A lower uterine segment in the longitudinal plane shows the placental tissue *(p)* lying between the maternal sacrum and the fetal head *(h)*.

Type Bleeding	Invasion of Chorionic Villi Has Occurred	Blood Loss
Placenta accreta	Superficially into myometrium	Mild
Placenta increta	Deep into myometrium	Moderate
Placenta pecreta	Through the myometrium	Severe

TABLE 34-2 PLACENTA ACCRETA, PLACENTA INCRETA, AND PLACENTA PECRETA

Data from http://telpath2.med.utah.edu/WebPath/PLACHTML/PLACO70.html

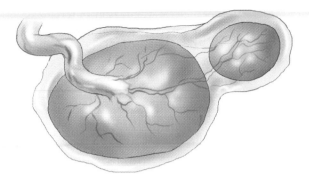

Figure 34-18 A succenturiate placenta is the presence of one or more accessory lobes connected to the body of the placenta by blood vessels.

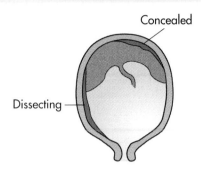

Figure 34-20 Types of placental abruption.

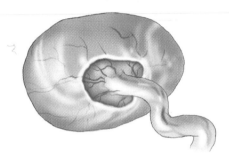

Figure 34-19 A circumvallate placenta is the attachment of the placental membranes to the fetal surface of the placenta rather than to the placental margin.

the membranes, premature labor, hemorrhage, and placental abruption.[7]

CIRCUMMARGINATE PLACENTA

This condition is diagnosed when the placental margin is not deformed. It is found in 20% of placentas. Prematurity has been found as a complication.

Ultrasound findings. Ultrasound findings are nonspecific because the placental shape is not distorted.

PLACENTAL ABRUPTION

Placental abruption is a premature placental detachment and occurs in 1 in 120 pregnancies. Bleeding in the decidua basalis occurs with separation (Figure 34-20). The mortality rate ranges from 20% to 60% and accounts for 15% to 25% of perinatal deaths. Clinically the patient may present with any of the following signs: preterm labor, vaginal bleeding, abdominal pain, fetal distress or demise, and uterine irritability. **Abruptio placenta** may be further classified as retroplacental or marginal.

Maternal hypertension is seen in 50% of severe abruptions and is considered a risk factor. Hypertension is chronic in half of these cases; in the other half it is pregnancy-induced. Other risk factors for abruption include a previous history of abruption, perinatal death, short umbilical cord, premature delivery, fibroids, trauma, placenta previa, and cocaine and other drugs. The recurrence of pla-

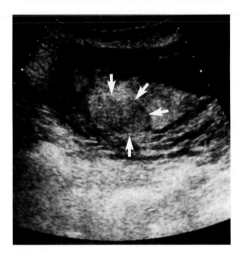

Figure 34-21 Transverse image of a retroplacental abruption. The texture of the placenta is inhomogeneous *(arrows).*

cental abruption ranges from 5% to 16% in subsequent pregnancies.

RETROPLACENTAL ABRUPTION

Retroplacental abruption results from the rupture of spiral arteries and is a "high-pressure" bleed. It is associated with hypertension and vascular disease. If the blood remains retroplacental, the patient has no visible bleeding (Figure 34-21).

MARGINAL ABRUPTION

Marginal abruption results from tears of the marginal veins and represents a "low-pressure" bleed. It is associated with cigarette smoking. The hemorrhage dissects beneath the placental membranes and is associated with little placental detachment. A subchorionic hemorrhage accumulates at the site separate from the placenta.

Ultrasound findings. Upon examination of the placenta, the sonographer will notice an abnormality in the texture and size of the placenta. If a hemorrhage is present, the echogenicity depends on the age of the hemorrhage; the acute bleed is hyperechoic to isoechoic, and the chronic bleed is more hypoechoic. The bleed may be retro-

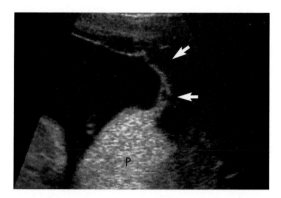

Figure 34-22   Ultrasound showing an abruption. *Arrows* point to the echolucent collection of blood lateral to the edge of the placenta. *p*, Placenta.

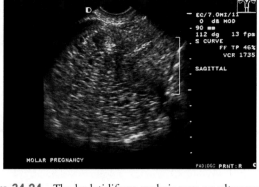

Figure 34-24   The hydatidiform mole is seen on ultrasound as multiple tiny vesicles throughout the uterine cavity.

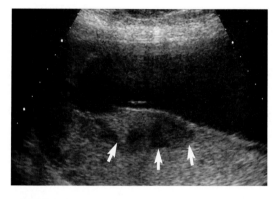

Figure 34-23   Thrombus within the intervillous spaces occurs in one third of the pregnancies. The inhomogeneity of the placenta is seen with sonolucent areas within the texture of the placenta *(arrows)*.

placental or subchorionic. Careful analysis should be made from the normal villus attachment of the placenta to the uterine wall to detect an abnormal collection of blood secondary to hemorrhage (Figure 34-22).

INTERVILLOUS THROMBOSIS

The presence of thrombus within the intervillous spaces occurs in one third of pregnancies. It results from intraplacental hemorrhage caused by breaks in the villous capillaries. Usually there is little risk to the fetus, although the condition is associated with Rh sensitivity and elevated alpha-fetoprotein levels from a fetal-maternal hemorrhage.

Ultrasound findings. On ultrasound examination, sonolucent lucencies are seen within the homogeneous texture of the placenta. These lucencies increase with advanced gestational age and indicate maturity of the placenta (Figure 34-23).

PLACENTA INFARCTS

Infarcts are common, found in 25% of pregnancies, and are usually small with no clinical significance. Large infarcts may reflect underlying maternal vascular disease.

PLACENTAL TUMORS

GESTATIONAL TROPHOBLASTIC DISEASE

Gestational trophoblastic disease is commonly known as **molar pregnancy** and is found in 1 in 1200 pregnancies. There are three groups of molar pregnancy: complete mole (may develop into choriocarcinoma), partial or incomplete mole, and coexistent mole and fetus. Clinical symptoms include extreme nausea and vomiting (from elevated levels of hCG), vaginal bleeding, uterine size larger than dates, and preeclampsia. In this group, 15% to 25% will develop malignant gestational trophoblastic disease (choriocarcinoma).

Ultrasound findings. The sonogram shows uterine size larger than dates, no identifiable fetal parts, and an inhomogeneous texture of the placenta that represents the multiple vesicular changes throughout the placenta (Figure 34-24). Bilateral theca luetin cysts are seen in the ovaries secondary to the hyperstimulation of the elevated hCG.

A partial mole carries little malignant potential. It is associated with an abnormal fetus or fetal tissue. On ultrasound examination a reduced amount of amniotic fluid is noted without defined fetal parts. The placenta is thick with multiple intraplacental cystic spaces.

A coexistant mole and fetus is very rare; the mole may result from a hydatidiform degeneration of twin fetuses. This condition is more likely when two placentas are present. The abnormal placenta is hyperechoic with multiple small cysts. The coexisting fetus is live with a normal placenta.

CHORIOANGIOMA

Second to trophoblastic disease, chorioangioma is the most common "tumor" of the placenta, occurring in 1% of pregnancies. The tumor is usually small and consists of a benign proliferation of fetal vessels; the majority are capillary hemangiomas that arise beneath the chorionic plate (Figure 34-25).[15] Complications include polyhydramnios, fetal hydrops, fetal cardiomegaly, IUGR, and fetal demise. The ma-

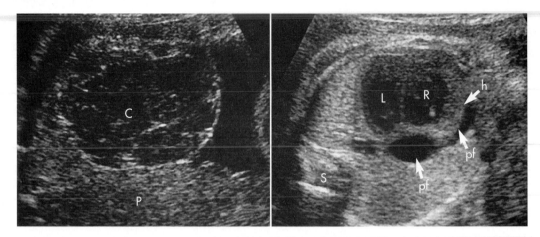

Figure 34-25 Chorioangioma *(C)* of the placenta of a fetus on the left side with dilation and hypertrophy *(h)* of the right cardiac ventricle *(R)* shown on the right side. Pleural fluid *(pf)* is shown. *L,* Left ventricle; *p,* placenta; *S,* spine.

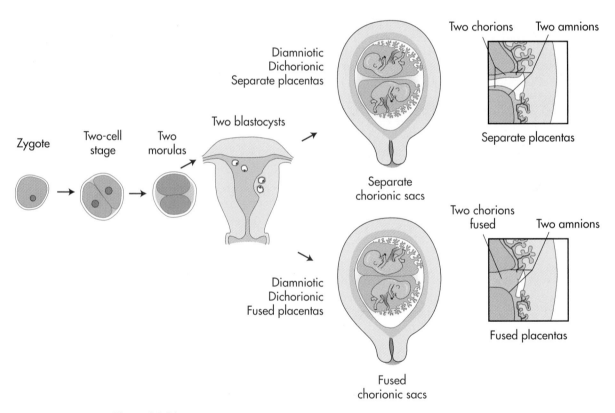

Figure 34-26 Possible dichorionicity and diamnionicity of monozygotic twins.

ternal serum alpha-fetoprotein may be elevated. Premature labor is another complication of large chorioangiomas and is thought to be related to polyhydramnios.[15]

Ultrasound findings. Ultrasound examination shows a circumscribed solid or complex mass that protrudes from the fetal surface of the placenta. It may be located near the umbilical cord site. The sonographer should look for polyhydramnios and fetal hydrops.

THE PLACENTA IN MULTIPLE GESTATION

Monozygotic twins are associated with all three types of membranes: dichorionic/diamniotic (di/di), monochorionic/diamniotic (mo/di), or monochorionic/monoamniotic (mo/mo), depending on when during gestation the twinning event occurred (Figure 34-26). If the membranes

BOX
34-6

MULTIPLE GESTATION PREGNANCIES AND PLACENTAS

Dizygotic (fraternal twins)
Derived from two zygotes
Diamniotic/dichorionic/two placentas
Occurs during first 4 days of gestation

Monozygotic (identical twins)
Dervied from one zygote
Monochorionic/diamniotic/one placenta
Occurs during 1st week of gestation
Monochorionic/monoamniotic/one placenta
Occurs during 2nd week of gestation

RISKS INVOLVED
Monochorionic
Placental vascular anastomosis
Monoamniotic
Entanglement of umbilical cord

are di/di, the pregnancy is probably dizygotic (97% chance), with only a 3% chance it is a monozygotic pregnancy. If the membranes are mo/di or mo/mo, they are from a monozygotic pregnancy.

Ultrasound findings. The sonographer should be able to carefully scan the uterus to determine the site and number of the placentas to differentiate the type of multiple gestation present. Refer to Chapter 31 for further discussion of multiple gestations (Box 34-6).

REVIEW QUESTIONS

1. Describe the composition of the fetal membranes.
2. Where is the chorionic plate located?
3. What is the major functioning unit of the placenta?
4. Where is the decidua basalis found?
5. Name the functions of the placenta.
6. What is a velamentous placenta?
7. When should the amnion fuse with the chorion?
8. What is the significance of a single umbilical artery?
9. Name the primary causes for placentomegaly.
10. Name the complications and sonographic findings of placenta previa.
11. What is placenta accreta?
12. Discuss the difference between a circumvallate, succenturiate, circummarginate, and battledore placenta.
13. What type of placental bleed is most dangerous to the fetus?

REFERENCES

1. Ananth CV, Smulian JC, Vintzileos AM: The association of placenta previa with history of cesarean delivery and abortion: a metaanalysis, *Am J Obstet Gynecol* 177:1071, 1997.
2. Grannum PT, Berkowitz, RD, Hobbins JC: The ultrasonic changes in the maturing placenta and their relation to fetal pulmonic maturity, *Am J Obstet Gynecol* 133:915, 1979.
3. Guyton AC: Pregnancy and lactation. In Guyton AC, editor: *Textbook of medical physiology*, Philadelphia, 1981, WB Saunders.
4. Hertzberg BS and others: Diagnosis of placenta previa during the third trimester: role of transperineal sonography, *Am J Radiol* 159:83, 1992.
5. Hobbins JC, Winsberg F, Berkowitz RL: The placenta. In Hobbins JC, Winsberg F, and Berkowitz RL, editors: *Ultrasonography in obstetrics and gynecology*, ed 2, Baltimore, 1983, Williams & Wilkins.
6. Jaffe R, Jauniaux E, Hustin J: Maternal circulation in the first-trimester human placenta: myth or reality? *Am J Obstet Gynecol* 176:695, 1997.
7. Jauniaux E, Campbell S: Ultrasonographic assessment of placental abnormalities, *Am J Obstet Gynecol* 163:1650, 1990.
8. Jeanty P, Romero R: *Obstetrical ultrasound*, New York, 1984, McGraw-Hill.
9. King DL: Placental migration demonstrated by ultrasonography, *Radiology* 109:167, 1973.
10. Kliman HJ: Behind every healthy baby is a healthy placenta, http://info.med.yale.edu/obgyn/kliman/Placenta/behind.html, accessed 1998.
11. Miller DA, Chollet JA, Goodwin TM: Clinical risk factors for placenta previa-placenta accreta, *Am J Obstet Gynecol* 177:210, 1997.
12. Pritchard JA, MacDonald PC: Obstetric hemorrhage. In *Williams' obstetrics*, ed 16, New York, 1980, Appleton Century-Crofts.
13. Sistrom CL, Ferguson JE: Abnormal membranes in obstetrical ultrasound: incidence and significance of amniotic sheets and circumvallate placenta, *Ultrasound Obstet Gynecol* 3:249, 1993.
14. Spirit BA, Gordon, LP, Kagan EH: Sonography of the placenta. In Sanders RC, James AE, editors: *The principles and practice of ultrasonography in obstetrics and gynecology*, ed 3, Norwalk, Conn, 1985, Appleton-Century-Crofts.
15. Spirt BA and others: Antenatal diagnosis of chorioangioma of the placenta, *Am J Radiol* 135:1273, 1980.

BIBLIOGRAPHY

Ball RH, Buchmeier, SE, Longnecker M: Clinical significance of sonographically detected uterine synechiae in pregnant patients, *J Ultrasound Med* 16:465, 1997.

Barton, SM: Placental abruption. In Frederickson H, Wilkins-Haug L, editors: *Ob-gyn secrets*, St Louis, 1991, Mosby.

Benirschke K, Kaufmann P: *Pathology of the human placenta*, ed 2, New York, 1990, Springer-Verlag.

Callen P: *Ultrasonography in obstetrics & gynecology*, ed 3, Philadelphia, 1994, WB Saunders.

Fox H: *Pathology of the placenta*, Philadelphia, 1978, WB Saunders.

Jurkovic D and others: Transvaginal color Doppler assessment of the uteroplacental circulation in early pregnancy, *Obstet Gynecol* 77:365, 1991.

Klaisle D: The placenta. In Frederickson H, Wilkins-Haug L, editors: *Ob-gyn secrets*, St Louis, 1991, Mosby.

Nyberg D, Mahony B, Pretorius D: *Diagnostic ultrasound of fetal anomalies*, St Louis, 1990, Mosby.

Trierweiler MW: Abnormal placentation. In Frederickson H, Wilkins-Haug L, editors: *Ob-gyn secrets*, ed, St Louis, 1991, Mosby.

CHAPTER 35

The Umbilical Cord

Sandra L. Hagen-Ansert

KEY TERMS

allantoic duct - elongated duct that contributes to the development of the umbilical cord and placenta during the first trimester

battledore placenta - marginal or eccentric insertion of the umbilical cord into the placenta

false knots of the umbilical cord - occurs when blood vessels are longer than the cord; they fold on themselves and produce nodulations on the surface of the cord

gastroschisis - anomaly in which part of the bowel remains outside the abdominal wall without a membrane

hemangioma of the cord - vascular tumor within the umbilical cord

membranous or velamentous insertion of the cord - cord inserts into the membranes before it enters the placenta

nuchal cord - occurs when the cord is wrapped around the fetal neck

omphalocele - failure of the bowel, stomach, liver to return to the abdominal cavity; completely covered by a peritoneal-amniotic membrane

omphalomesenteric cyst - cystic lesion of the umbilical cord

single umbilical artery - high association of congenital anomalies with single umbilical artery

superior vesical arteries - after birth the umbilical arteries become the superior vesical arteries

true knots of the umbilical cord - may be formed when a loop of cord is slipped over the fetal head or shoulders during deliver

umbilical herniation - failure of the anterior abdominal wall to close completely at the level of the umbilicus

vasa previa - occurs when the umbilical cord vessels cross the internal os of the cervix

Wharton's jelly - myxomatous connective tissue that surrounds the umbilical vessels and varies in size

yolk stalk - umbilical duct connecting the yolk sac with the embryo

DEVELOPMENT AND NORMAL ANATOMY OF THE UMBILICAL CORD

The umbilical cord is the essential link for oxygen and important nutrients between the fetus, the placenta, and the mother. The amnion covers the cord and blends with the fetal skin at the umbilicus. The vascular connections within the cord serve a reverse function in the fetus; the vein carries oxygenated blood to the fetus while the arteries bring venous blood back to the placenta.

The amniotic membrane covers the fetal surface of the placenta and the multiple vessels that branch from the umbilical vein and arteries. The cord should normally insert into the center of the placenta.

DEVELOPMENT

The umbilical cord forms during the first 5 weeks of gestation (7 menstrual weeks) as a fusion of the omphalomesenteric (yolk stalk) and allantoic ducts.[5] The umbilical cord acquires its epithelial lining as a result of the enlargement of the amniotic cavity and the result of envelopment of the cord by amniotic membrane. The intestines grow at a faster rate than the abdomen and herniate into the proximal umbilical cord at approximately 7 weeks and remain there until approximately 10 weeks.[6] The insertion of the umbilical cord into the ventral abdominal wall is an important sonographic anatomic landmark because scrutiny of this area will reveal abdominal wall defects such as omphalocele, gastroschisis, or limb-body wall complex.

ANATOMY

The umbilical cord is covered by the amniotic membrane. The cord includes two umbilical arteries and one umbilical vein (Figure 35-1) and is surrounded by a homogeneous substance called Wharton's jelly. Wharton's jelly is a myxomatous connective tissue that varies in size and may be imaged with high-frequency ultrasound transducers. The diameter of the cord usually measures 1 to 2 cm

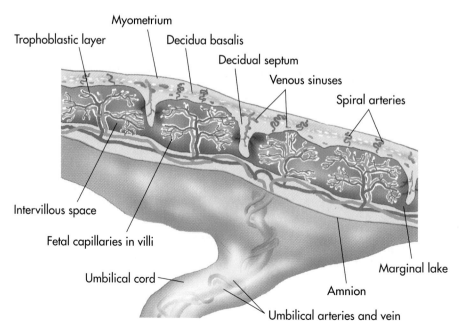

Figure 35-1 Organization of the mature placenta.

(variations in cord diameter are usually attributed to Wharton's jelly). The normal length of the cord is 40 to 60 cm; it is difficult to assess the length reliably with ultrasound.

The umbilical artery arises from the fetal internal iliac vessels, courses alongside the fetal bladder and exits the

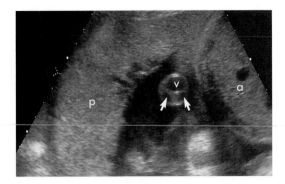

Figure 35-2 Transverse view of the normal three-vessel cord. The umbilical vein *(v)* is the largest vessel, with two smaller arteries *(arrows)* spiraling around the vein. *a,* Abdomen; *p,* placenta.

umbilicus to form part of the umbilical cord. The left umbilical vein enters the umbilicus and joins the left portal vein as it courses through the liver.[1] The right umbilical vein usually regresses at 6 weeks gestation and is not seen by ultrasound. Persistence of the right umbilical vein is rare and may be related to an involution of the left umbilical vein. If it persists, the right umbilical vein enters the right lobe of the liver to join the right portal vein. At least 50% of these cases have other fetal anomalies.

ULTRASOUND OF THE UMBILICAL CORD

The umbilical cord has one large vein and two smaller arteries (Figure 35-2). The umbilical vein transports oxygenated blood from the placenta, and the paired umbilical arteries return deoxygenated blood from the fetus to the placenta for purification. The umbilical cord is identified at the cord insertion into the placenta and at the junction of the cord into the fetal umbilicus. The arteries spiral with the larger umbilical vein (Figure 35-3), which is surrounded by Wharton's jelly (Figure 35-4). Absent cord twists may be associated with decreased fetal movement and a poor pregnancy outcome.[3]

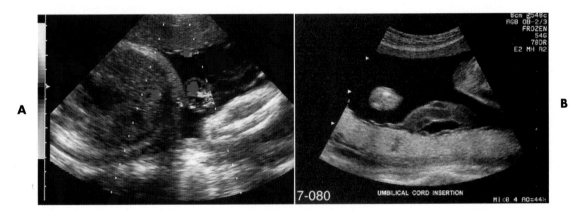

Figure 35-3 **A,** Normal insertion of the umbilical cord shown with color Doppler as it inserts into the fetal abdomen. **B,** The umbilical cord may be seen as it exits the placental surface.

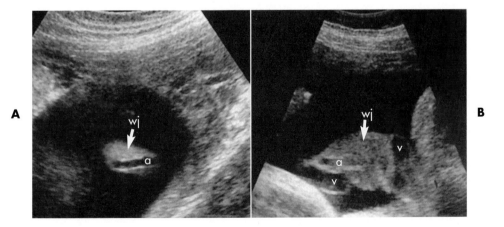

Figure 35-4 **A,** Wharton's jelly *(wj)* observed in a 30-week fetus. One of the umbilical arteries *(a)* is in view. **B,** Wharton's jelly *(wj)* is present adjacent to one of the umbilical arteries *(a)* and the single umbilical vein *(v)* is observed in a 35-week fetus. Wharton's jelly is an important structure to recognize when performing cordocentesis procedures in which the needle is directed into the cord vessels.

The umbilical vein diameter increases throughout gestation, reaching a maximum diameter of 0.9 cm by 30 weeks of gestation. The umbilical cord has been found to be significantly larger in fetuses of mothers with gestational diabetes than in the normal population; the increase in width is attributed mainly to an increase in Wharton jelly content.[9]

The three vessels of the cord may be followed with real-time ultrasound as they enter the abdomen and travel toward the liver and iliac arteries (Figure 35-5). From the left portal vein, the umbilical blood flows either through the *ductus venosus* to the systemic veins (inferior vena cava or hepatics) by passing the liver or through the right portal sinus to the right portal vein.[1] The ductus venosus forms the conduit between the portal system and the systemic veins.

Sonographically the ductus venosus appears as a thin intrahepatic channel with echogenic walls. It lies in the groove between the left lobe and the caudate lobe. The ductus venosus is patent during fetal life until shortly after birth, when transformation of the ductus into the *ligamentum venosum* occurs (beginning in the second week after birth).

The umbilical arteries may be followed caudally from the cord insertion, in their normal path adjacent to the fetal bladder to the iliac arteries. On ultrasound, the sonographer may look at the cord in a transverse plane to see the one large umbilical vein and two smaller umbilical arteries. Another sonographic approach to see the arteries is to look lateral to the fetal bladder in a transverse or coronal plane. The umbilical arteries run along the lateral margin of the fetal bladder and are well imaged with color flow Doppler. In the postpartum stage, the umbilical arteries become the **superior vesical arteries.**

ABNORMAL UMBILICAL CORD (LENGTH AND WIDTH)

Although the umbilical cord varies in length and width, researchers have found specific problems associated with a cord that varies from normal dimensions. The normal length of the cord measures 40 to 60 cm and is difficult to assess reliably with ultrasound (Figure 35-6).

A short umbilical cord measures less than 35 cm in length. This condition is associated with or predisposed to the following:

- Oligohydramnios
- Restricted space (as in multiple gestations)
- Intrinsic fetal anomaly
- Tethering of the fetus by an amniotic band
- Inadequate fetal descent
- Cord compression
- Fetal distress

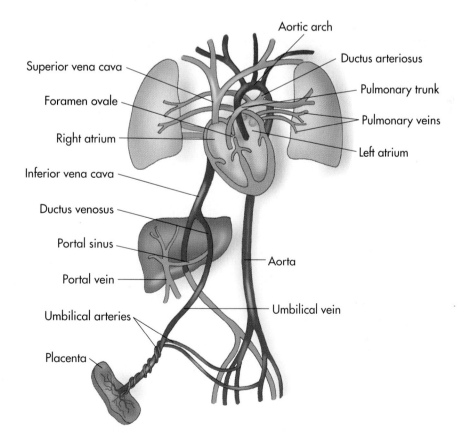

Figure 35-5 The umbilical vein leaves the placenta to deliver nutrients to the fetus. From the left portal vein the umbilical blood flows either through the ductus venosus to the inferior vena cava or hepatics or through the right portal sinus to the right portal vein. The iliac arteries drain into the umbilical arteries.

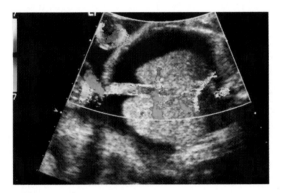

Figure 35-6 **A,** The umbilical cord is shown in a sagittal plane in a 33-week fetus, outlining the cord borders *(b),* the umbilical vein *(v),* and the arteries *(arrows).* The spirals of the cord vessels and Wharton's jelly are outlined. Abnormal cord twists may indicate a higher risk for stillbirth. **B,** Cross-sections of the umbilical cord. *Arrows,* Umbilical arteries; *v,* umbilical vein.

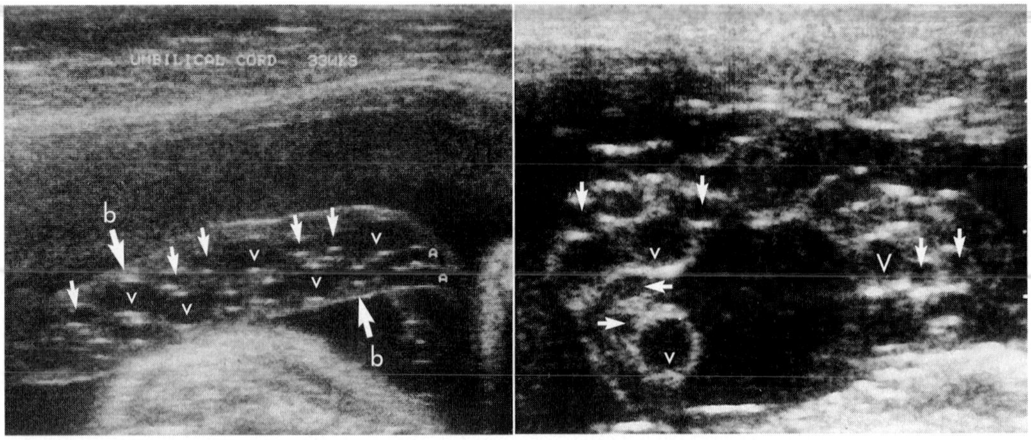

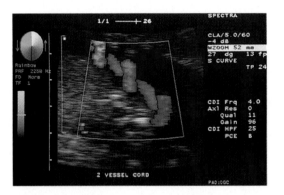

Figure 35-7 As the cord is held vertically, vessels along the anterior surface spiral downward from high left to low right, angled like the left side of the letter *V,* indicate a left helix.

Figure 35-9 This hydropic fetus showed decreased movement over 24 hours. The cord is shown without its usual twisting and coiling, indicating decreased fetal movement.

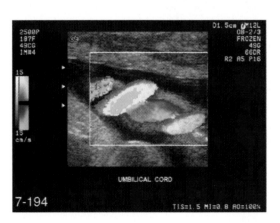

Figure 35-8 This two-vessel cord has a right twist; the fetus had multiple congenital anomalies.

Coiling of the umbilical cord is normal and is related to fetal activity. The normal cord may coil as many as 40 times, usually to the left. The helical twisting of the cord can be easily determined by gross pathologic inspection.[3] With the cord held vertically, vessels along the anterior surface that spiral downward from high left to low right, angled like the left side of the letter V, indicate a left helix (Figure 35-7). The incidence of a "left" twist of the cord is found in 7:1 pregnancies. The significance of this is that a fetus with a "right" twist in the cord has a higher incidence of fetal anomalies than with a "left" twist (Figure 35-8).

The absence of cord twisting is an indirect sign of decreased fetal movement (Figure 35-9). This event occurs in a small (4.3%) number of deliveries; however, it may lead to increased mortality and morbidity. Other obstetric problems seen with a short umbilical cord include preterm delivery, decreased heart rate during delivery, meconium staining secondary to fetal distress, and fetal anomalies. If the cord is completely atretic, the fetus is attached directly to the placenta at the umbilicus and an omphalocele is always present.

It has been theorized that the length of the umbilical cord is determined partly by the amount of amniotic fluid present in the first and second trimesters, as well as fetal mobility. Therefore, the presence of oligohydramnios, am-

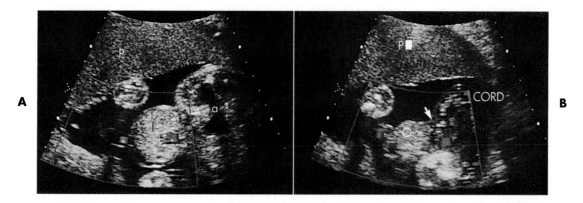

Figure 35-10   A, Image of a liver-filled omphalocele in a 26-week fetus showing hepatic vessel flow within the herniated liver. *a,* Abdomen; *P,* placenta. **B,** In the same fetus, color enhancement aids in the confirmation of the cord vessels entering the base of the omphalocele *(O, arrow); P,* placenta. No other anomalies were found and the karyotype was normal.

niotic bands, or limitation of fetal movement for any reason may impede umbilical cord growth.

A long umbilical cord measures greater than 80 cm and may be associated with or predisposed to the following:

- Polyhydramnios
- Nuchal cord (occurs in 25% of deliveries)
- True cord knots (occurs in 0.5% of deliveries); may be difficult to distinguish from "false" cord knot or redundancy of cord–true knots cause vascular compromise and fetal demise
- Umbilical cord compression, cord presentation, and prolapse of the cord leads to fetal distress
- Umbilical cord stricture or torsion resulting from excessive fetal motion

The diameter of the umbilical cord has been measured from 2.6 to 6.0 cm. Variations in cord diameter are usually attributed to diffuse accumulation of Wharton's jelly. This condition has been associated with maternal diabetes, edema secondary to fetal hydrops, Rh incompatibility, and fetal demise.

UMBILICAL CORD MASSES

Umbilical cord masses are not very common in the fetus. Many of the "masses" seen on ultrasound may be attributed to focal accumulation of Wharton's jelly and may be isolated or associated with an omphalocele or cyst. A cystic mass in the cord is usually omphalomesenteric or allantoic in origin. These are generally small (less than 2 cm), tend to be near the fetal end of the cord, and resolve by the second trimester. Cysts that persist beyond the first trimester usually are associated with other fetal anomalies and aneuploidy.

Other masses associated with the umbilical cord include:

- Omphalocele (cord runs through the middle of this mass as it protrudes from the umbilicus)
- Gastroschisis (cord usually found to the right of this mass)
- Umbilical herniation
- Teratoma of the umbilical cord
- Aneurysm of the cord

- Varix of the cord (may be intraabdominal)
- Hematoma of the cord (usually iatrogenic–cordocentesis or amniocentesis)
- True knot of the cord
- Angioma of the cord (well-circumscribed echogenic mass that may cause increased cardiac failure and hydrops–alphafetoprotein level is increased; associated with a cyst caused by transudation of fluid from a hemangioma)
- Thrombosis of cord secondary to compression or kinking, focal cord mass, true cord knots, velamentous cord insertion, cord entanglement in monoamniotic twins (commonly seen with fetal demise)

OMPHALOCELE

Omphalocele occurs 1:5000 births and results from failure of the intestines to return to the abdomen. The hernia may consist of a single loop of bowel or it may contain most of the intestines (Figure 35-10). The covering of the hernia sac is epithelium from the umbilical cord.

GASTROSCHISIS

Gastroschisis is usually a right paraumbilical defect involving all layers of the abdominal wall, usually measuring 2 to 4 cm. The small bowel always eviscerates through the defect (Figure 35-11). The loops of bowel are never covered by a membrane; thus they are directly exposed to amniotic fluid and elevated alpha-fetoprotein levels. Other organs that may eviscerate are large bowel, stomach, a portion of the gastrointestinal system and, rarely, liver.

UMBILICAL HERNIATION

Umbilical herniation occurs when the intestines return normally to the abdominal cavity and then herniate either prenatally or postnatally through an inadequately closed umbilicus (Figure 35-12).

OMPHALOMESENTERIC CYST

Omphalomesenteric cyst is a cystic lesion of the umbilical caused by persistence and dilation of a segment of the

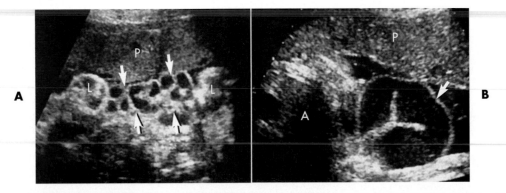

Figure 35-11   A, Gastroschisis showing herniated bowel *(arrows)* in the amniotic cavity. Cesarean section was performed at 36 weeks of gestation because of a nonreactive nonstress test with variable decelerations and absent breathing. A small-for-gestational age infant with a left-side gastroschisis was delivered. *L,* Limbs; *P,* placenta. **B,** Isolated bowel segment *(arrow)* observed in another fetus with gastroschisis at 29 weeks of gestation. Bowel dilation (29 mm) and obstruction (meconium ileus) are shown. Note the haustral markings within the obstructed bowel. *A,* Abdomen; *P,* placenta.

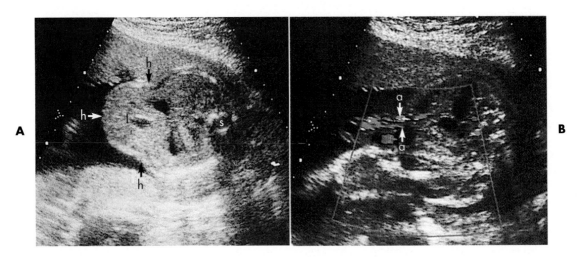

Figure 35-12   A, Umbilical hernia *(h, arrows)* observed in a fetus with Carpenter syndrome (acrocephalopoly-syndactyly). *l,* Liver; *s,* spine. **B,** In the same fetus, at the cord insertion level using color imaging, the umbilical arteries are observed entering the abdomen *(a)* in a normal location. This excludes the diagnosis of omphalo-

omphalomesenteric duct lined by epithelium of gastrointestinal origin. During the third week of early development, the omphalomesenteric duct joins the embryonic gut and the yolk sac. This is closed by the 16th week of gestation; however, in some cases small vestigial remnants of duct may be found in normal umbilical cords (Figure 35-13). The omphalomesenteric cyst is found closer to the fetal cord insertion and may vary in size (up to 6cm). This condition affects females over males with a ratio of 5:3. In addition, there may be an associated condition of Meckel's diverticulum.

HEMANGIOMA OF THE CORD

A **hemangioma of the cord** arises from the transthelial cells of the vessels of the umbilical cord. Pathologically, this angiomatous nodule is surrounded by edema and myxomatous degeneration of Wharton's jelly. The sites of origin are the main vessels of the umbilical cord, and it may involve more than one vessel. This condition is rare;

however, when found near the placental end of the cord the size varies from small to large (to 15 cm). The fetus may develop nonimmune hydrops.

HEMATOMA OF THE CORD

Trauma to the umbilical vessels may occasionally cause extravasation of blood into Wharton's jelly. This occurs usually near the fetal insertion of the cord. The umbilical vein is most frequently involved. If the blood clot is new, the mass is hyperechoic on ultrasound; if the clot is old, the mass is hypoechoic and septated. Complications have been reported as high as 47% to 52% fetal mortality.

THROMBOSIS OF THE UMBILICAL VESSELS

Thrombosis of the umbilical vessels is occlusion of one or more vessels of the umbilical cord; primarily it occurs in the umbilical vein. The incidence is higher in infants of diabetic mothers (1:82) than in nondiabetic mothers

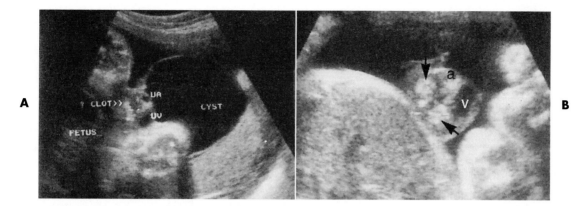

Figure 35-13   A, Omphalomesenteric cyst observed in a 34-week fetus. Clot formation was found within one artery. A single umbilical artery *(UA)* was viewed in proximal sections of the cord close to the cyst, and three vessels were noted distally. *UV,* Umbilical vein. **B,** In the same fetus, clot is observed *(arrows).* At birth, a 10-cm, serous-filled cyst consistent with omphalomesenteric cyst was confirmed. The cyst weighed 1 lb.

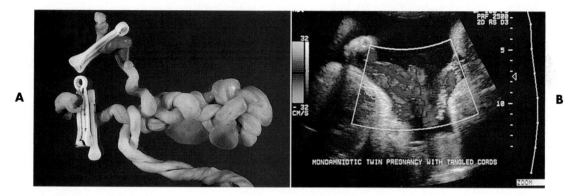

Figure 35-14   A, Pathologic specimen of a umbilical cord with multiple knots. **B,** Ultrasound image of a mono-amniotic twin pregnancy showing multiple knots and tangles within the cord. Doppler flow showed decreased velocity in the blood flow.

(2:3918). Thrombosis may be primary or secondary to torsion, knotting, looping, compressions, or hematoma. The sonographer should look for aneurysmal dilation of the cord and the presence of fetal hydrops. Other maternal factors are phlebitis and arteritis. The prognosis is poor in the fetus with umbilical vein thrombosis.

UMBILICAL CORD KNOTS

TRUE KNOTS OF THE CORD

True knots of the umbilical cord have been associated with long cords, polyhydramnios, intrauterine growth restriction, and monoamniotic twins. The knots may be single or multiple, with increased incidence of congenital anomalies (Figure 35-14). The mortality rate is 8% to 11%. In these cases there is a flattening or dissipation of Wharton jelly and venous congestion distal to the knot, as well as vascular thrombi within the cord.

The knot may be formed when a loop of cord is slipped over the infant's head or shoulders during delivery. Usually the umbilical vessels are protected by Wharton's jelly

and are not constricted enough to cause fetal anoxia in this condition.

Color Doppler is useful to record absence of blood flow within the umbilical cord. When Doppler is used to image a false knot, flow is not completely constricted but may appear to show constriction secondary to fetal activity and tension on the cord as the fetus moves.

FALSE KNOTS OF THE CORD

False knots of the umbilical cord are seen when the blood vessels are longer than the cord. Often they are folded on themselves and produce nodulations on the surface of the cord (Figure 35-15).

NUCHAL CORD

Nuchal cord is the most common cord entanglement in the fetus. Multiple coils around the fetal neck have been reported (Figure 35-16).[4] A single loop of cord has been seen in over 20% of deliveries; two loops have been found in 2.5%. Trouble begins as the fetus descends into the birth canal during delivery and the coils tighten to suffi-

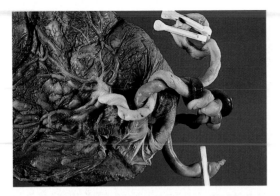

Figure 35-15 Pathologic specimen of a double placenta with a false knot.

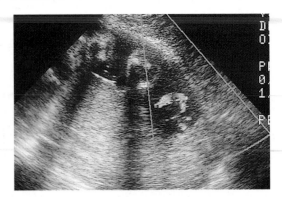

Figure 35-17 Color Doppler shows the marginal insertion of the cord into the edge of the placenta instead of into the middle of the placenta.

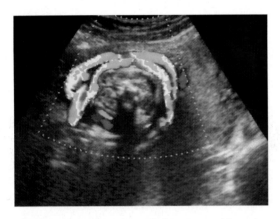

Figure 35-16 Nuchal cord is well demonstrated by color Doppler as it wraps multiple times around the fetal neck.

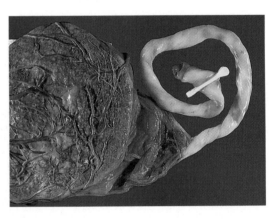

Figure 35-18 Pathologic specimen of the membranous insertion of the cord into the membranes of the placenta.

ciently reduce the flow of blood through the cord. Fetal heart deceleration, meconium-stained amniotic fluid, and babies requiring resuscitation are seen more frequently when there is a cord entanglement.

UMBILICAL CORD INSERTION ABNORMALITIES

MARGINAL INSERTION OF THE CORD (BATTLEDORE PLACENTA)

The differential proliferation of placenta villi may result in eccentric insertion of the umbilical cord into the placenta. The cord implants into the edge of the placenta **(battledore placenta)** instead of into the middle of the placenta (Figure 35-17). This is significant when the cord is inserted near the internal os, because labor may cause the cord to prolapse or be compressed during contractions. The marginal insertion occurs in 2% to 10% of singleton births, 20% of twins, and 18% of pregnancies with a single umbilical artery.

MEMBRANEOUS OR VELAMENTOUS INSERTION OF THE CORD

Membranous or **velamentous insertion of the cord** occurs when the cord inserts into the membranes before it enters the placenta rather than inserting directly into the

placenta (Figure 35-18). This condition occurs in 1% of singleton births, 12% of twins, and 9% of pregnancies with a single umbilical artery. There is an increased risk of thrombosis, cord rupture during delivery, or vasa previa.

One theory states that velamentous insertion occurs when most of the placental tissue grows laterally, leaving the initially centrally located cord in an area that becomes atretic. Another theory shows a defect in the implantation of the cord that occurs in the site of the trophoblast in front of the decidua capsularis instead of the area of trophoblast that forms the placental mass. The implantation occurs in the chorion laeve where the umbilical vessels lie on the membranous surface.

Velamentous umbilical cord insertion is associated with higher risk of low birth weight, small for gestational age, preterm delivery, low Apgar scores, and abnormal intrapartum fetal heart rate pattern.

Associated anomalies occur in under 10% of pregnancies with velamentous insertion of the cord. These anomalies include esophageal atresia, obstructive uropathies, congenital hip dislocation, spina bifida, ventricular septal defect, and cleft palate. There has been reported an increased risk for intrauterine growth restriction and premature birth.

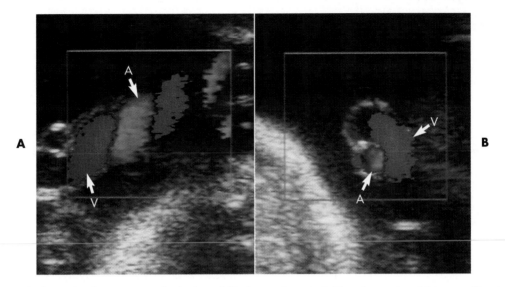

Figure 35-19   Color-flow imaging of a single umbilical artery in sagittal **(A)** and transverse **(B)** images. The single umbilical artery *(a, blue)* and umbilical vein *(v, red)* are shown. The fetus had posterior urethral valve syndrome.

VASA PREVIA AND PROLAPSE OF THE CORD

Prolapse of the umbilical cord occurs when the cord lies below the presenting part. This condition may exist whenever the presenting part does not fit closely and fails to fill the pelvic inlet; further risk is incurred if the membranes rupture early. Compression of the cord reduces or cuts off the blood supply to the fetus and may result in fetal demise. Abnormal fetal presentation occurs in nearly half of the prolapse cord cases. A slightly higher risk is incurred when the fetus is in a transverse or breech presentation.

Vasa previa is defined as the presence of umbilical cord vessels crossing the internal os of the cervix. The mortality may be high, ranging from 60% to 70% for vaginal delivery and is caused from rupture of the vessels and fetal exsanguination. Color Doppler is the best method of detection in the ultrasound examination. Vasa previa may be due to many factors: velamentous insertion of the cord, succenturiate lobe of the placenta, or low-lying placenta with marginal insertion of the cord near the internal os.

CORD PRESENTATION AND PROLAPSE

Cord presentation and prolapse of the umbilical cord through the cervix into the vagina occurs in 0.5% of deliveries. An occult prolapse occurs when the cord lies alongside the presenting part. The perinatal mortality rate of 25% to 60% is due to cord compression during vaginal delivery. Conditions predisposing to cord presentation and prolapse are as follows:

- Abnormal fetal presentation
- Nonengagement of the fetus because of prematurity
- Long umbilical cord
- Abnormal bony pelvic inlet
- Leiomyomas

- Polyhydramnios
- Vasa previa
- Velamentous insertion of the cord
- Marginal insertion of the cord in a low-lying placenta
- Incompetent cervix with premature rupture of the membranes

PREMATURITY

Two factors contribute to failure of the fetus to fill the pelvic inlet cavity: small presenting part, and increased frequency of abnormal presentations in premature labor. Fetal mortality is high in the premature population secondary to birth trauma and anoxia.

MULTIPLE PREGNANCY

Multiple pregnancy factors include failure of adequate adaptation of the presenting part to the pelvis, higher incidence of abnormal presentation, polyhydramnios, and premature rupture of the membranes of the second twin when it is unengaged.

OBSTETRIC PROCEDURES

One third of cord prolapse problems are produced during obstetric procedures:

- Artificial rupture of membranes
- Disengaging the head
- Flexion of an extended head
- Version and extraction

SINGLE UMBILICAL ARTERY

A **single umbilical artery** occurs in 0.2% to 1% of singleton births and 3.5% of twin pregnancies; it is more frequent in miscarriages and autopsy series (Figures 35-19 and 35-20). Reports have found single umbilical artery in 18% of pregnancies with marginal insertion of the cord and in 9% of membranous insertion of the cord. The probable cause is atrophy of one of the um-

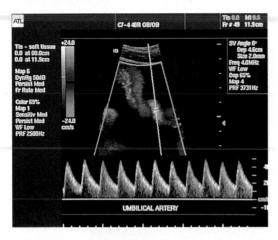

Figure 35-20 Color Doppler shows normal umbilical artery flow in a fetus with a two-vessel cord.

bilical arteries in the early development stage. The left umbilical artery is absent a slightly higher percentage of time than the right.

Single umbilical artery has been associated with the following:

- Congenital anomalies in 20% to 50% of cases
- Increased incidence of intrauterine growth restriction (small placenta)
- Increased perinatal mortality
- Increase incidence of chromosomal abnormalities (trisomies 18, 13, and 21, Turner's syndrome, and triploidy)

Infants with single umbilical arteries have associated anomalies that affect other organ system, such as the following[2]:

- Musculoskeletal 23%
- Genitourinary 20%
- Cardiovascular 19%
- Gastrointestinal 10%
- Central nervous systems 8%

Multiple studies have investigated normal measurements of the vessels within the umbilical cord. A three-vessel cord showing artery to artery difference of more than 50% was defined as hypoplastic umbilical artery. A study of 100 pregnancies found that between 20 and 36 gestational weeks all pregnancies with a single umbilical artery had a transverse umbilical artery diameter of greater than 4 mm and all pregnancies with two umbilical arteries had a transverse umbilical arterial diameter of less than 4 mm.[7] In another study the diameter of the umbilical artery was greater than 50% of that of the umbilical vein in the fetus with a single umbilical artery.[8]

The sonographic detection of a single umbilical artery should prompt the investigation of further fetal anomalies. The incidence of associated anomalies has been reported to range from 25% to 50%. The major anomalies have included cardiac defects, skeletal abnormalities, abdominal wall defects, diaphragmatic hernia, holoprosencephaly, and hydrocephalus.

Variations in the number of umbilical arteries have also been reported. More than three vessels in the cord have been documented in conjoined twins.

REVIEW QUESTIONS

1. When does the umbilical cord form?
2. The intestines are seen to herniate into umbilical cord on ultrasound between what periods in development?
3. What covers the umbilical cord?
4. The two umbilical arteries arise from which vessels?
5. With what conditions might a short umbilical cord be associated?
6. If an enlarged cord diameter was seen on a follow-up sonogram after cordocentesis, what would be the most likely cause of this mass?
8. Describe a marginal insertion of the cord.
9. Define vasa previa.
10. The absence of cord twisting is an indirect sign of what condition?
11. Describe the difference between a true knot and false knot of the umbilical cord.
12. What is the risk of a velamentous insertion of the cord?
13. List the conditions that may predispose to cord presentation and prolapse.
14. Describe the significance of finding a single umbilical artery.

REFERENCES

1. Callen P: *Ultrasonography in obstetrics & gynecology,* ed 3, Philadelphia, 1994, WB Saunders.
2. Dudiak CM and others: Sonography of the umbilical cord, *Radiographics* 15:1035, 1995.
3. Finberg HJ: Avoiding ambiguity in the sonographic determination of the direction of umbilical cord twists, *J Ultrasound Med* 11:185, 1992.
4. Heinonen S and others: Perinatal diagnostic evaluation of velamentous umbilical cord insertion, *Obstet Gynecol* 87:112, 1996.
5. Moore KL: *Before we are born: basic embryology and birth defects,* ed 3, Philadelphia, 1989, WB Saunders.
6. Moore KL: *Essentials of human embryology,* Toronto, 1988, BC Decker.
7. Persutte WH, Lenke RR: Transverse umbilical arterial diameter: technique for the prenatal diagnosis of single umbilical artery, *J Ultrasound Med* 13:763, 1994.
8. Sepulveda W and others: Umbilical vein to artery ratio in fetuses with single umbilical artery, *Ultrasound Obstet Gynecol* 8:5, 1996.
9. Weissman A and others: Sonographic measurements of the umbilical cord in pregnancies complicated by gestational diabetes, *J Ultrasound Med* 16:691, 1997.

BIBLIOGRAPHY

Bornemeier S and others: Sonographic evaluation of the two vessel umbilical cord: a comparison between umbilical arteries adjacent to the bladder and cross-sections of the umbilical cord, *J Diag Med Sonogr* 12:260,1996,

Chow JS and others: Frequency and nature of structural anomalies in fetuses with single umbilical arteries, *J Ultrasound Med* 17:765,1998.

Ellis JW: Disorders of the placenta, umbilical cord, and amniotic fluid. In Ellis JW, Beckmann CRB, editors: *A clinical manual of obstetrics,* Norwalk, Conn, 1983, Appleton-Century Crofts.

Fitzgerald MJT and others: *Human embryology,* Philadelphia, 1994, Bailliere Tindall.

Nyberg DA and others: *Diagnostic ultrasound of fetal anomalies,* St Louis, 1990, Mosby.

Oxorn H: *Human labor & birth,* ed 5, New York, 1986, Appleton Century Crofts.

Petrikovsky B and others: Prenatal diagnosis and clinical significance of hypoplastic umbilical artery, *Prenatal Diagn* 16:938, 1996.

Romero R and others: *Prenatal diagnosis of congenital anomalies,* Norwalk, Conn, 1988, Appleton & Lange.

Sauerbrei EE and others: *A practical guide to ultrasound in obstetrics and gynecology,* ed 2, Philadelphia, 1998, Lippincott Raven.

CHAPTER 36

Amniotic Fluid and Membranes:
Polyhydramnios and Oligohydramnios

Sandra L. Hagen-Ansert

OBJECTIVES

- Describe how amniotic fluid is derived
- Detail the production of amniotic fluid
- List the functions of amniotic fluid
- Describe how to assess amniotic fluid volume by three methods
- Recognize abnormal volumes of amniotic fluid
- Differentiate amniotic band syndrome from amniotic sheets

DERIVATION AND CHARACTERISTICS OF AMNIOTIC FLUID
ASSESSMENT OF ABNORMAL AMNIOTIC FLUID VOLUME
ABNORMAL VOLUMES OF AMNIOTIC FLUID
AMNIOTIC BAND SYNDROME
AMNIOTIC SHEETS AND SYNECHIAE

REVIEW QUESTIONS

KEY TERMS

amniotic bands - multiple fibrous strands of amnion that develop in utero that may entangle fetal parts to cause amputations or malformations of the fetus

amniotic cavity - forms early in gestation and surrounds the embryo; amniotic fluid fills the cavity to protect the embryo and fetus

amniotic fluid - produced by the umbilical cord and membranes, the fetal lung, skin, and kidney

amniotic fluid index - the uterus is divided into four quadrants; each "quadrant" is evaluated with the transducer perpendicular to the table in the deepest vertical pocket without fetal parts; the four quadrants are added together to determine the amniotic fluid index

chorion frondosum - the portion of the chorion that develops into the fetal portion of the placenta

maximum or deep vertical pocket - another method (used more often in multiple-gestation pregnancy) to determine the amount of amniotic fluid; pocket less than 2 cm may indicate oligohydramnios; greater than 8 cm indicates polyhydramnios

oligohydramnios - too little amniotic fluid; associated with intrauterine growth restriction, renal anomalies, premature rupture of membranes, postdate pregnancy, and other factors

placental insufficiency - produces redistribution of fetal blood flow away from the kidneys and toward the brain to counterattack the hypoxia

polyhydramnios - too much amniotic fluid; associated with central nervous system disorder, gastrointestinal anomalies, fetal hydrops, skeletal anomalies, renal disorders, and other factors

subjective assessment of fluid - sonographer surveys uterine cavity to determine visual assessment of amniotic fluid present.

uterine synechiae - scars within the uterus secondary to previous gynecologic surgery.

Amniotic fluid plays a vital role in fetal growth and serves several important functions during intrauterine life. **Amniotic fluid** allows the fetus to move freely within the amniotic cavity while maintaining intrauterine temperature and protecting the developing fetus from injury. Abnormalities of the fluid may interfere with the normal fetal development and cause structural abnormalities or may represent an indirect sign of an underlying anomaly, such as neural tube defect or gastrointestinal disorder.

This chapter focuses on the production and echogenicity of amniotic fluid, assessment and disorders of amniotic fluid volume, and the use of amniotic fluid volume in the diagnosis of fetal disorders.

DERIVATION AND CHARACTERISTICS OF AMNIOTIC FLUID

The **amniotic cavity** forms early in fetal life and is filled with amniotic fluid that completely surrounds and protects the embryo and, later, fetus. The amnion can be visualized in most pregnancies before the 12th week (Figure 36-1). It appears as a thin membrane separating the amniotic cavity, which contains the fetus, from the extraembryonic coelom and the secondary yolk sac (Figure 36-2).[7]

Amniotic fluid is produced by the umbilical cord and membranes, lungs, skin, and kidneys.[11] The mechanisms of amniotic fluid production and consumption, as well as the composition and volume of amniotic fluid, depend on gestational age.[4] Early in gestation the major source of amniotic fluid is the amniotic membrane, a thin membrane lined by a single layer of epithelial cells. During this stage of development, water crosses the membrane freely, and the production of amniotic fluid is accomplished by active transport of electrolytes and other solutes by the amnion, with passive diffusion of water following in response to osmotic pressure changes.[4]

As the fetus and placenta mature, amniotic fluid production and consumption change to include movement of fluid across the chorion frondosum and fetal skin, fetal urine output and fetal swallowing and gastrointestinal absorption. The **chorion frondosum,** the portion of the chorion that develops into the fetal portion of the placenta, is a site where water is exchanged freely between fetal blood and amniotic fluid across the amnion. Fetal skin is also permeable to water and some solutes, to permit a direct exchange between the fetus and amniotic fluid until keratinization occurs at 24 to 26 weeks.

Fetal production of urine and the ability to swallow begin between 8 and 11 weeks of gestation and become the major pathways for amniotic fluid production and consumption after this time period. The fetus swallows amniotic fluid, which is absorbed by the digestive tract. The fetus also produces urine, which is passed into the surrounding amniotic fluid. Fetal urination into the amniotic sac accounts for nearly the total volume of amniotic

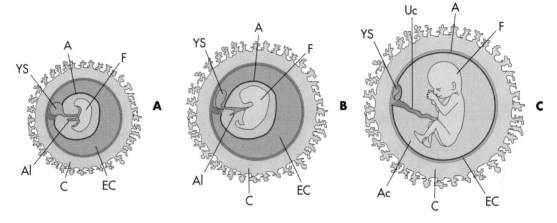

Figure 36-1 A, Four-week gestation. The amnion is formed from cells found on the interior of the developing cell mass that is to become the fetus and placenta. *F,* Fetus; *YS,* yolk sac; *C,* chorion; *Al,* allantois; *A,* amnion; *EC,* extraembryonic coelom. **B,** Six-week gestation. **C,** Eight-week gestation. *Ac,* Amniotic cavity; *Uc,* Umbilical cord.

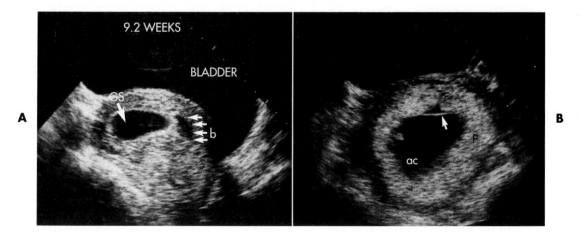

Figure 36-2 A, Sagittal scan through the uterine fundus demonstrating a normal-appearing gestational sac *(GS)* at 9.2 weeks with evidence of an implantation bleeding site *(b) (arrows).* **B,** Transverse scan demonstrating the amnion *(arrow)* dividing the amniotic cavity *(ac)* and chorionic cavity. *P,* Placenta.

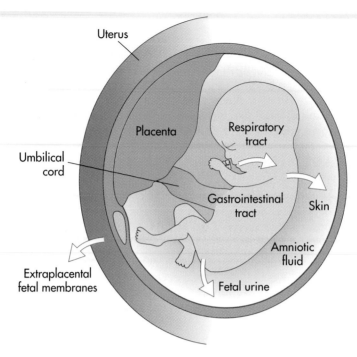

Figure 36-3 Schematic drawing of amniotic fluid formation.

fluid by the second half of pregnancy, so the quantity of fluid is directly related to kidney function.[6] A fetus with malformed kidneys or renal agenesis produces little or no amniotic fluid.

The amount of amniotic fluid is regulated not only by the production of fluid, but also by removal of the fluid by swallowing, by fluid exchange within the lungs, and by the membranes and cord (Figure 36-3). Normal lung development depends critically on the exchange of amniotic fluid within the lungs. Inadequate lung development may occur when severe oligohydramnios is present, placing the fetus at high risk for developing small or hypoplastic lungs.

Amniotic fluid has the following six functions:

1. Acts as a cushion to protect the fetus
2. Allows embryonic and fetal movements
3. Prevents adherence of the amnion to the embryo
4. Allows symmetric growth
5. Maintains a constant temperature
6. Acts as a reservoir to fetal metabolites before their excretion by the maternal system

The volume of amniotic fluid increases during the first two trimesters, with the average increment per week of 25 ml from the 11th to the 15th week and 50 ml from the 15th to 28th week of gestation.[17] In the last trimester the mean amniotic fluid volume does not change significantly.[17] The sonographer must be aware of the relative differences in amniotic fluid volume throughout pregnancy. During the second and early third trimester of pregnancy, amniotic fluid appears to surround the fetus and should be readily apparent (Figure 36-4). From 20 to 30 weeks of gestation, amniotic fluid may appear somewhat generous, although this typically represents a normal amniotic fluid variant (Figure 36-5). By the end of pregnancy, amniotic fluid is scanty, and isolated fluid pockets may be the only visible areas of fluid.

Subjective observation of amniotic fluid volumes throughout pregnancy helps the sonographer determine the norm and extremes of amniotic fluid. The amniotic fluid index aids in estimating the amount of amniotic fluid present in the uterine cavity. The amount of fluid volume correlates with fetal and placental weight. The small-for-age fetus has decreased amniotic fluid; the large-for-age fetus has increased volume of fluid.

Amniotic fluid generally appears echo-free, although occasionally fluid particles (particulate matter) may be seen (see Figure 36-4). Vernix caseosa (fatty material found on fetal skin and in amniotic fluid late in pregnancy) may be seen within the amniotic fluid.

In accordance with the guidelines for obstetric scanning, every obstetric examination should include a thorough evaluation of amniotic fluid volume. When extremes in amniotic fluid volume (hydramnios or oligohydramnios) are found, targeted studies for the exclusion of fetal anomalies are recommended.

ASSESSMENT OF ABNORMAL AMNIOTIC FLUID VOLUME

There are several ways to assess the amount of amniotic fluid throughout the pregnancy. This assessment becomes important in the second and third trimesters to help determine fetal well-being. Fluid may be classified as normal, polyhydramnios, or oligohydramnios. There are several methods to achieve this measurement, including subjective assessment, four-quadrant assessment, or measurement of the single deepest pocket of fluid.

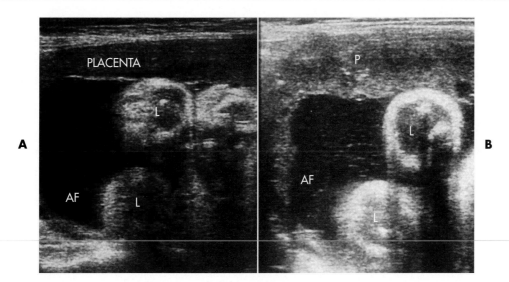

Figure 36-4 A, Amniotic fluid *(AF)* in the uterine fundus revealing an echo-free fluid appearance. *L,* limbs. **B,** At 38 weeks of gestation, the amniotic fluid is mixed with particulate matter or vernix. *P,* Placenta.

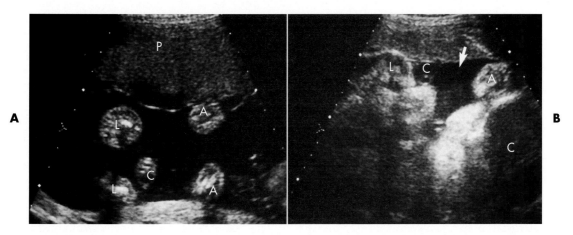

Figure 36-5 A, Amniotic fluid in a 20-week pregnancy outlining the legs *(L)* and arms *(A).* This is a typical appearance of the abundance of amniotic fluid during this period of pregnancy. *C,* Umbilical cord; *P,* placenta. **B,** Amniotic fluid *(arrow)* in a 35-week pregnancy demonstrating an amniotic fluid pocket *(arrow)* surrounded by fetal parts and the placenta. The amount of amniotic fluid compared with the fetus and placenta is less at this stage of pregnancy. *A,* Arms; *C,* cranium; *L,* legs.

Subjective Assessment. Subjective assessment is performed as the sonographer initially scans "through" the entire uterus to determine the *visual eye-ball* assessment of the fluid present, the lie of the fetus, and the position of the placenta (Figure 36-6). When amniotic fluid is assessed subjectively, decreased amniotic fluid is identified by an overall sense of crowding of the fetus and obvious lack of amniotic fluid and/or inability to identify any significant pockets of fluid in any sector of the uterus.[17] Excessive fluid is defined subjectively when there is an obvious excess of fluid and when a transverse ultrasound done at various levels of the uterine cavity identifies a fluid pocket in which one can comfortably place a cross-section of the fetal trunk.[17]

This subjective assessment is more successful in the hands of experienced sonographers than in the beginner's assessment. A more definitive determination of amniotic fluid volume is with the four-quadrant method.

Four-Quadrant Assessment. A method has been developed for evaluating and quantifying amniotic fluid volume at different intervals during a pregnancy.[13] The uterine cavity is divided into four equal quadrants by two imaginary lines perpendicular to each other (Figure 36-7). The largest vertical pocket of amniotic fluid, excluding fetal limbs or umbilical cord loops, is measured. The sum of the four quadrants is called the **amniotic fluid index (AFI).** Normal values have been calculated for each gestational age (plus or minus 2 standard deviations). Normal is 8 to 22 cm; decreased is less than 5 cm; and increased is greater than 22 cm (Figure 36-8).

The sonographer must be careful to hold the transducer perpendicular to the table (not the curved skin surface) when determining these pockets of fluid. Also, care must be taken not to include the thickness of the maternal uterine wall in the measurement. As the gain is increased

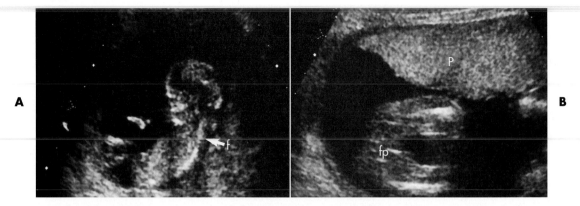

Figure 36-6 **A,** Amniotic fluid around a 13-week fetus in a sitting position. Note the hand in front of the fetal chest. Amniotic fluid appears in black. *f,* Fetus. **B,** Amniotic fluid around an 18-week fetus. The fetus appears to be surrounded by amniotic fluid (black areas). *P,* Placenta; *fp,* fetal pelvis.

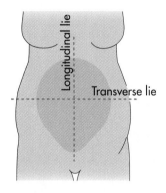

Figure 36-7 The amniotic cavity is divided into quadrants by two imaginary lines perpendicular to each other. The largest pocket of fluid is measured in each quadrant.

slightly, the uterine wall may be determined. Also, the use of color helps the sonographer separate the umbilical cord loops from areas within the pockets of fluid. The transducer should be moved until the cord loops and/or fetal limbs are not within the pocket.

Single Pocket Assessment. Clinicians have described other criteria to define the presence of abnormal fluid volumes (Figure 36-9). The **maximum vertical pocket** (fluid should measure greater than 1 cm rule) assessment of amniotic fluid is done by identifying the largest pocket of amniotic fluid (Figure 36-10). The depth of the pocket is measured at right angles to the uterine contour and placed into three categories: (1) less than 2 cm, indicating oligohydramnios; (2) 2 to 8 cm, indicating normal amniotic fluid; and (3) greater than 8 cm, indicating polyhydramnios.[16]

The Effect of Maternal Hydration. A study was performed to see if maternal hydration would increase the AFI in women with low AFIs.[9] The control group was instructed to drink their normal amount of fluid; the hydration group was instructed to drink 2 L of water in addition to their usual amount of fluid 2 to 4 hours before the posttreatment AFI was determined. The mean posttreatment AFI was significantly greater in the hydration group. The findings sug-

gested that maternal oral hydration increased the amniotic fluid volume in women with decreased fluid levels.

The Preferred Method. Of all the three techniques used to assess amniotic fluid volumes, the AFI is the only technique that is both valid and reproducible.[16] The AFI is very helpful in a busy laboratory where multiple sonographers evaluate patients and there may be varying opinions of what normal, decreased, or increased amniotic fluid looks like.

Amniotic fluid volume should be one component of a composite of fetal assessment techniques, including measurements such as fetal abdominal trunk circumferences, Doppler flow studies, and other fetal biophysical activities.[27]

ABNORMAL VOLUMES OF AMNIOTIC FLUID
Abnormal volumes of amniotic fluid may suggest that the fetus has a congenital anomaly. Amniotic fluid volume may be assessed subjectively, or the AFI may be helpful in detecting abnormally increased **(polyhydramnios)** (Box 36-1) or decreased amniotic fluid volumes **(oligohydramnios)** (Box 36-2).

Polyhydramnios. Polyhydramnios is a common finding in pregnancy. Several large studies have reported the incidence to be 0.20% to 1.6%.[6] These studies also indicate that polyhydramnios is associated with increased perinatal mortality and morbidity and maternal complications.

By clinical definition, polyhydramnios is an excessive amount of fluid. The uterine size is larger than expected for gestational dates. Often the patient will come for an ultrasound with the remark, "rule out multiple gestation, molar pregnancy, or size greater than dates."

If polyhydramnios occurs before the 24th week, it is considered acute. Chronic polyhydramnios is usually first diagnosed in the third trimester. Acute polyhydramnios is more serious, because perinatal death is the usual outcome secondary to premature delivery of the fetus.[5]

Other conditions associated with increased amniotic fluid volume include maternal diabetes mellitus, fetal macrosomia, and Rh isoimmunization. Diabetes mellitus is associated with an increased frequency of hydramnios

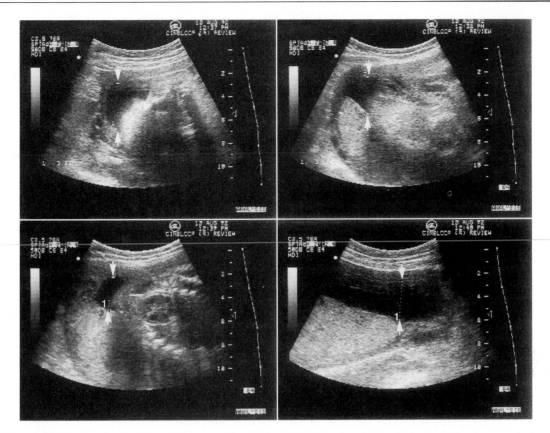

Figure 36-8 The four-quadrant technique of amniotic fluid assessment. This technique produces an amniotic fluid index (AFI). The uterus is divided into four equal parts, and the largest vertical pocket of amniotic fluid in each quadrant is measured, excluding fetal limbs or umbilical cord. The sum of the four quadrants is the AFI, which equals 14.2 cm at 31 weeks. This is within normal limits.

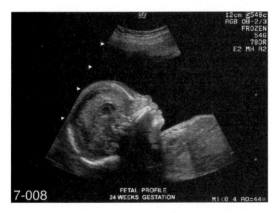

Figure 36-9 Longitudinal view of the fetal profile at 24 weeks of gestation. The amniotic fluid enables the facial detail to be well imaged. A single vertical pocket is measured perpendicular to the floor.

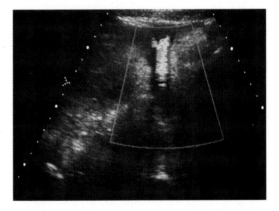

Figure 36-10 The sonographer must use color Doppler to make sure the umbilical cord is not in the way when making a single vertical measurement.

and represents the most common maternal cause of elevated amniotic fluid volume, especially when poorly controlled.[5]

Increased amniotic fluid volume produces uterine stretching and enlargement that may lead to preterm labor as well as various other maternal symptoms. In addition, the acute onset of hydramnios may be painful, compress other organs or vascular structures, cause hydronephrosis of the kidneys, or produce shortness of breath from compression of the organs on the diaphragm.[5]

Once polyhydramnios has been diagnosed, the prognosis for pregnancy is guarded. There is an increased perinatal mortality and morbidity as well as an increased maternal morbidity and mortality.[6] The mother has an increased risk of developing pregnancy-induced hypertension, preterm labor, or postpartum hemorrhage.

Etiology of polyhydramnios. The amniotic fluid compartment is in a dynamic equilibrium with the fetal and maternal compartments. In polyhydramnios the equilibrium shifts so that the net transfer of water is into the amniotic space (Figure 36-11).[5] Many factors are involved in the regulation of amniotic fluid volume (e.g., swallowing, urination, uterine-placental blood flow, fetal respiratory movements, fetal membrane physiology).

One study found that the time of onset of polyhydramnios was helpful in predicting outcome and suggesting the type of fetal anomaly likely to be present.[2] Of neonates who were normal at birth but who had developed severe polyhydramnios, 93% had done so after 30 weeks of gestation. Primary central nervous system abnormalities were diagnosed at or before 30 weeks of gestation in all cases. In neonates with primary gastrointestinal abnormalities, polyhydramnios was diagnosed after 30 weeks of gestational age in 83% of the patients.

Polyhydramnios is often associated with central nervous system disorders, which causes depressed swallowing. With gastrointestinal abnormalities, often a blockage (atresia) of the esophagus, stomach, duodenum, and small bowel results in ineffective swallowing. Fetal hydrops, skeletal anomalies, and some renal disorders (usually uni-

---

BOX 36-1 CONGENITAL ANOMALIES ASSOCIATED WITH POLYHYDRAMNIOS

GASTROINTESTINAL SYSTEM
Esophageal atresia and/or tracheoesophageal fistula
Duodenal atresia
Jejunoileal atresia
Gastroschisis
Omphalocele
Diaphragmatic hernia
Meckel's diverticulum
Congenital megacolon
Meconium peritonitis
Annular pancreas
Pancreatic cyst

HEAD AND NECK
Cystic hygroma
Goiter
Cleft palate
Epignathus

RESPIRATORY SYSTEM
Cystic adenomatoid malformation
Congenital hydrothorax
Extralobar sequestration
Primary pulmonary hypoplasia
Congenital pulmonary lymphangiectasia
Pulmonary cyst
Asphyxiating thoracic dystrophy

CARDIOVASCULAR SYSTEM
Arrhythmias
Coarctation of the aorta
Myxomas and hemangiomas
Ectopia cordis
Cardiac tumors
Heart anomalies with hydrops

CENTRAL NERVOUS SYSTEM
Anencephaly
Hydrocephaly
Microcephaly
Iniencephaly
Hydranencephaly
Holoprosencephaly
Encephalocele
Spina bifida
Dandy-Walker malformation

GENITOURINARY SYSTEM
Ureteropelvic junction obstruction
Posterior urethral valves
Urethral stenosis
Multicystic kidney disease
Large ovarian cyst
Mesoblastic nephroma
Bartter syndrome
Megacystis microcolon hypoperistalsis syndrome

SKELETAL SYSTEM
Thanatophoric dwarf
Campomelic dwarf
Osteogenesis imperfecta
Heterozygous achondroplasia
Arthrogryposis multiplex
Klippel-Feil syndrome
Nager acrofacial dysostosis
Achondrogenesis

CONGENITAL INFECTIONS
Cytomegalovirus
Toxoplasmosis
Listeriosis
Congenital hepatitis

MISCELLANEOUS
Sacrococcygeal teratoma
Cranial teratoma
Cervical teratoma
Congenital sarcoma
Placental chorioangioma
Cavernous hemangioma
Metastatic neuroblastoma
Myotonic dystrophy
Fetal acetaminophen toxicity
Retroperitoneal fibrosis
Multisystem anomalies
Pena-Shokeir syndrome
Cutaneous vascular hemarthrosis
Twin reversed arterial perfusion sequence/acardiac anomaly

From Nyberg DA, Mahony BS, Pretorius DH: *Diagnostic ultrasound of fetal anomalies: text and atlas,* St Louis, 1990, Mosby.

lateral) may be associated with hydramnios. Many congenital anomalies are found in association with hydramnios (see Box 36-1).

Ultrasound findings. Sonographic signs of polyhydramnios are as follows[13]:

- Appearance of a freely floating fetus within the amniotic cavity
- Accentuated fetal anatomy as increased amniotic fluid improves image resolution
- Freely moving fetus
- AFI equal to or greater than 20 cm

Oligohydramnios. Oligohydramnios is an overall reduction in the amount of amniotic fluid. The incidence of oligohydramnios is estimated to be between 0.5% to 5.5% of all pregnancies, depending on the population tested and the criteria used for diagnosis.[12] Criteria for oligohydramnios are based on subjective experience and estimations of the AFI . Oligohydramnios may be defined as an AFI of less than 5 cm. A gray zone for decreased fluid ranges from 5 to 9 cm when a four-quadrant approach is used.[13]

The association between intrauterine growth restriction (IUGR) and decreased amniotic fluid (oligohydramnios) is well recognized. There is a four-fold increased risk of growth delay when oligohydramnios is present.[12] Doppler evaluation of the growth-restricted fetus shows abnormal umbilical flow in patients with oligohydramnios.

Second-trimester oligohydramnios is associated with a poor prognosis, especially if maternal serum alpha-fetoprotein level is concurrently elevated.[12] Oligohydramnios has also been associated with fetal renal anomalies, rupture of the intrauterine membranes, and the postdate pregnancy (Figure 36-12). Congenital anomalies and chromosomal abnormalities are also associated with oligohydramnios.

Oligohydramnios may cause fetal deformations such as clubbing of the hands or feet, pulmonary hypoplasia, hip displacement, and phenotypical features of Potter's sequence.[8] Oligohydramnios may be observed as a consequence of first-trimester chorionic villus sampling. Poor scanning resolution is common in pregnancies complicated by oligohydramnios, and limited anatomy surveys are expected.

Placental insufficiency may cause IUGR associated with oligohydramnios. The placental insufficiency produces a redistribution of fetal blood flow away from the kidneys and toward the brain to counterattack the hypoxia. This results in decreased urine output, which decreases fluid volume.

Causes of oligohydramnios are outlined in Box 36-2. Renal disease or other clinical pregnancy problems may lead to diminished amounts of amniotic fluid (see Figures 36-13 and 36-14). Premature rupture of the membranes may occur during the second trimester, so correlation with obstetric history is imperative. Nonanomalous conditions, such as IUGR and postdate pregnancy (beyond 42 weeks), are also causes of oligohydramnios.

Ultrasound findings. If the intrauterine membranes are not ruptured and oligohydramnios is present before 28 weeks of gestation, careful evaluation of the fetal renal system should be made by the sonographer to rule out renal

---

BOX 36-2   CAUSES OF OLIGOHYDRAMNIOS

NONANOMALOUS CONDITIONS
Intrauterine growth restriction
Premature rupture of membranes
Postdate pregnancy (42 weeks)
Chorionic villus sampling

FETAL ANOMALOUS CONDITIONS
Infantile polycystic kidney disease
Renal agenesis
Posterior urethral valve syndrome
Dysplastic kidneys
Chromosomal abnormalities

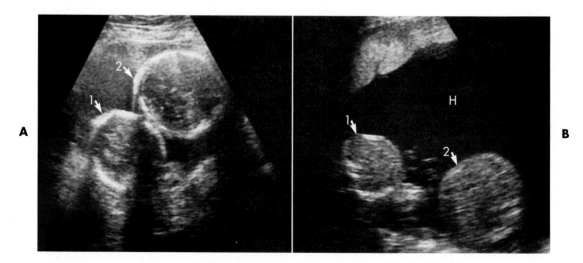

Figure 36-11   Ultrasound demonstrating the discordant growth of twins in the case of a twin-to-twin transfusion syndrome. **A,** The difference in the size of the heads of the twins *(1, 2)*. **B,** The difference in the size of the abdominal circumferences *(1, 2)*. *H,* Hydramnios.

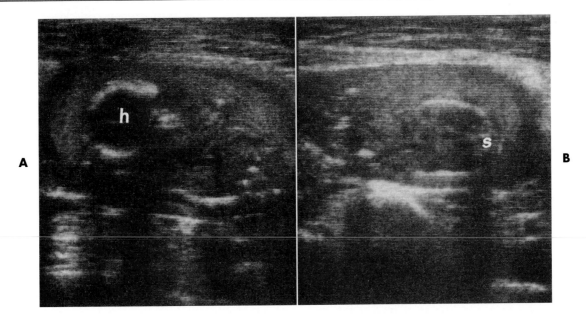

Figure 36-12 Premature rupture of membranes at 16 weeks of gestation with marked oligohydramnios. *h,* Head; *s,* spine.

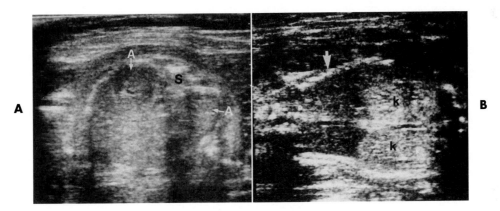

Figure 36-13 **A,** Renal agenesis in a 29-week fetus showing enlarged adrenal glands *(A)* occupying the renal spaces. Oligohydramnios and an absent bladder confirmed the diagnosis. *S,* Spine. **B,** Infantile polycystic kidney disease shown with enlarged and dense kidneys *(k)*. Note the enhanced transmission of sound through the kidneys because of the dilated cystic tubules. Oligohydramnios and absent bladder were coexisting findings.

agenesis, infantile polycystic disease, or posterior urethral valve syndrome. If the oligohydramnios is severe in a fetus with posterior urethral valves, the prognosis is not good. Identification of the renal area may be difficult to assess in the presence of severe oligohydramnios, and the use of color Doppler to demarcate the renal arteries may be helpful for the sonographer to determine if the kidneys are present or not.

In the presence of oligohydramnios, care should be taken when evaluating the fetal growth parameters, because the fetal head and abdomen can be compressed when the fluid level is low. Because the fetus lacks the surrounding fluid protecting it, the circumferences can actually be changed by transducer pressure on the maternal abdomen. This pressure, in turn, may alter the estimated fetal weight by erroneous measurements. On the other hand, prolonged severe oligohydramnios may

cause fetal anomalies secondary to pressure on the fetus by the uterine wall. Such anomalies include pulmonary hypoplasia, abnormal facial features, and abnormal limb development.

When oligohydramnios is suspected, the sonographer should also examine the second-trimester fetus with transvaginal sonography to define fetal anatomy in efforts to detect the anomaly causing the oligohydramnios.

Cord compression by the fetus is another potential cause for fetal asphyxia leading to oligohydramnios. Often the sonographer may see signs of mild cord compression throughout the routine scan, with cardiac decompensation or changes in Doppler flow patterns. Slight rotations of the mother during the examination may stimulate the fetus to roll away from the cord, restoring blood flow. If this cord compression becomes a chronic problem, fetal well-being may be affected.

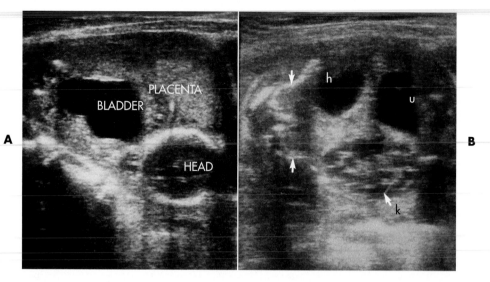

Figure 36-14 A, Posterior urethral valve syndrome in a 17-week fetus showing abnormally distended bladder with a keyhole urethra. Note the significant lack of amniotic fluid. **B,** In the same fetus at 21 weeks of gestation a small thoracic cavity *(arrows),* hydronephrosis *(h),* hydroureter *(u),* and enlargement and mild hydronephrosis of the contralateral kidney *(k)* are noted.

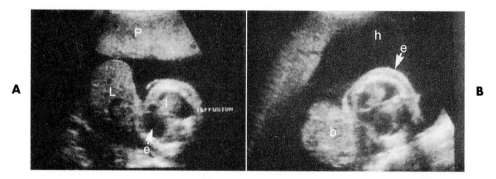

Figure 36-15 A and **B,** Gastroschisis with secondary amniotic bands shown in a 28-week fetus. Eviscerated liver *(L)* and bowel *(b)* are documented. Bilateral pleural effusions *(arrows)* and soft-tissue edema *(e)* in **B** are apparent. Note the hydramnios *(h). l,* Lung; *P,* placenta.

AMNIOTIC BAND SYNDROME

The **amniotic band syndrome** is a common, nonrecurrent cause of various fetal malformations involving the limbs, craniofacial region, and trunk.[10] Various congenital malformation syndromes are supposed to be caused by compression of the fetus by "amniotic bands," which results in developmental abnormalities or fetal death.[7] Amniotic band syndrome may represent a milder form of limb-body wall complex and may be predicted by amniotic bands (fibrous tissue strands) that entangle or amputate fetal parts (Figures 36-15 to 36-17).[14] Facial clefts, asymmetric encephaloceles, constriction or amputation defects of the extremities, and clubfoot deformities are common findings.

The site where the amniotic band cuts across the fetus is evident after birth. The most widely accepted theory for the formation of amniotic bands is that rupture of the amnion leads to subsequent entanglement of various embryonic or fetal parts by fibrous mesodermic bands that emanate from the chorionic side of the amnion.[16] Entrapment of fetal parts by the bands may cause lymphedema, amputations,

or slash defects in nonembryologic distributions. The amnion, which is contiguous with the fetal skin at the umbilicus, is thought to protect the fetus from contact with the chorion.[16] When disruption of the amnion occurs, the fetus may adhere to and fuse with the chorion, with subsequent maldevelopment of the subjacent fetal tissue.

This theory suggests that when gastroschisis results in exteriorization of the liver, the amniotic band syndrome should be strongly considered.[10] One study demonstrated two fetuses with a lateral (instead of midline) encephalocele associated with the amniotic band syndrome. Amputations caused by amniotic bands were found to usually be asymmetric. When syndactylism was seen, the origin was distal in patients with amniotic band syndrome.

Ultrasound findings. The sonographer may observe these bands as the real-time obstetric study is performed to observe where the band is attached to the uterine wall and what, if any, constriction is placed on the fetus. Careful observation with real-time scanning will allow the sonographer to observe if the fetus is free from the band or if

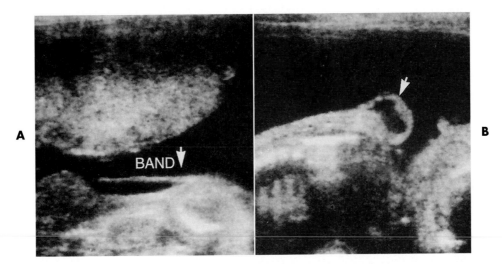

Figure 36-16 In the fetus depicted in Figure 36-15, multiple amniotic bands (**A,** *band*) were found adhering to the abdomen, with attachment to the shoulder (**B,** *arrow*). Normal chromosomes were found by amniocentesis. Amniotic fluid alpha-fetoprotein was extremely elevated (175 MOM) with positive acetylcholinesterase. The fetus was delivered at 28 weeks of gestation because of worsening hydrops. No resuscitative measures were undertaken. Autopsy findings revealed a right paraumbilical gastroschisis with eventration of the liver and intestine. Intestinal malrotation and small bowel obstruction were found. Moderate fetal hydrops with bilateral pleural effusions and pulmonary hypoplasia were noted. An amniotic band or peritoneal band extended from the liver to the thumb. The defect was consistent with a gastroschisis occurring early in embryogenesis because of the intestinal malrotation with secondary amniotic band rupture.

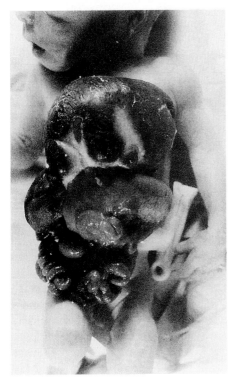

Figure 36-17 Photograph of neonate depicted in Figs. 36-15 and 36-16 with gastroschisis and secondary amniotic band rupture.

movement is restricted. Uterine sheets (synechiae) should not be confused with amniotic bands.

AMNIOTIC SHEETS AND SYNECHIAE

Amniotic sheets are believed to be caused by uterine scars, or **synechiae,** from previous instrumentation of the uterus (usually curettage), cesarean section, or episodes of endometritis.[15] When a pregnancy begins to grow in the uterine cavity, the expanding membranes encounter the scar and wrap around it. The flat portion of the sheet consists of apposed layers of chorion and amnion. The free edge of the sheet is defined by the course of the synechia itself, which may produce a bulbous appearance.[15]

Amniotic sheets arise because of redundant amnionchorion, which may in turn be related to bleeding and subchorionic hemorrhages.[1,3]

Ultrasound findings. Sonographic findings in six patients with amniotic sheets showed a fine echo-dense line in the uterine cavity separated from the uterine wall by an echolucent space.[3] In half of these patients the membrane completely surrounded the fetus. In the others the membrane was freely mobile in the amniotic cavity. Amniotic sheets do not place the fetus at risk for destructive structural malformations.[1]

Amniotic sheets are present in 0.6% of patients having screening obstetric ultrasound examinations.[15] Care should be taken to separate the diagnosis of amniotic sheets from amniotic bands or circumvallate placenta. In the circumvallate placenta the chorion and attached amnion form a raised ridge of tissue at the junction of the chorion and the basal plate.[15] Beyond this ridge the normal vessels on the

fetal surface are absent; after delivery these redundant membranes are described as being adherent to the fetal surface rather than projecting from it.

Both circumvallate placenta and amniotic sheets appear as a thick membrane projecting into the amniotic fluid. Circumvallate placental membranes originate from the edge of the fetal surface of the placenta, while amniotic sheets attach to the uterine wall itself.[15]

REVIEW QUESTIONS

1. Why is the production of amniotic fluid critical to fetal development?
2. Name the six functions of amniotic fluid.
3. What happens to the volume of amniotic fluid as the pregnancy progresses?
4. Describe how to perform the subjective assessment of amniotic fluid.
5. What is the four-quadrant assessment?
6. Describe the single pocket assessment for amniotic fluid.
7. Which assessment method is the most reliable?
8. What is the definition of polyhydramnios?
9. With what abnormal conditions is polyhydramnios associated?
10. Describe how to assess if the fetus has oligohydramnios.
11. What abnormal conditions may be associated with oligohydramnios?
12. What is amniotic band syndrome?
13. Differentiate between amniotic sheets and amniotic band syndrome.

REFERENCES

1. Ball, RH, Buchmeier, SE, Longnecker, M: Clinical significance of sonographically detected uterine synechiae in pregnant patients, *J Ultrasound Med* 16:465, 1997.
2. Barkin SZ and others: Severe polyhydramnios: incidence of anomalies, *Am J Radiol* 148:155-159, 1987.
3. Burrows PE and others: Intrauterine membranes: sonographic findings and clinical significance, *J Clin Ultrasound* 10:1, 1982.
4. Callen PW: *Ultrasonography in obstetrics and gynecology*, Philadelphia, 1994, WB Saunders.
5. Cardwell MS: Polyhydramnios: a review, *Obstet Gynecol Surv* 42:612, 1987.
6. Fleischer AC and others, editors: *The principles and practice of ultrasonography in obstetrics and gynecology*, ed 4, Norwalk, Conn, 1991, Appleton & Lange.
7. Jeanty P and others: Ultrasonic demonstration of the amnion, *J Ultrasound Med* 1:243, 1982.
8. Jeanty P, Romero R: Is there a normal amount of amniotic fluid? In Jeanty P, Romero R, editors: *Obstetrical ultrasound*, New York, 1984, McGraw-Hill.
9. Kilpatrick SJ and others: Maternal hydration increases amniotic fluid index, *Obstet Gynecol* 78: 1098, 1991.
10. Mahony BS and others: The amniotic band syndrome: antenatal sonographic diagnosis and potential pitfalls, *Obstet Gynecol* 152:63, 1985.
11. Nyberg DA, Mahony BS, Pretorius DH, editors: *Diagnostic ultrasound of fetal anomalies: text and atlas*, St. Louis, 1990, Mosby.
12. Peipert JF, Donnenfeld AE: Oligohydramnios: a review, *Obstet Gynecol Surv* 46:325, 1991.
13. Phelan JP and others: Amniotic fluid volume assessment with the four-quadrant technique at 36-42 weeks' gestation, *J Reprod Med* 32:540, 1987.
14. Seeds JW, Cefalo RC, Herbert WN: Amniotic band syndrome, *Am J Obstet Gynecol* 144:243, 1982.
15. Sistrom CL, Ferguson, JE: Abnormal membranes in obstetrical ultrasound: incidence and significance of amniotic sheets and circumvallate placenta, *Ultrasound Obstet Gynecol* 3:249, 1993.
16. Torpin R: *Fetal malformations caused by amnion rupture during gestation*, Springfield, Ill, 1968, Charles C Thomas.
17. Williams, K: Amniotic fluid assessment, *Obstet Gynecol Surv* 48:795, 1993.

BIBLIOGRAPHY

Elias S, Simpson JL, editors: *Maternal serum screening for fetal genetic disorders*, New York, 1992, Churchill Livingstone.

Jeanty P, Romero R, editors: *Obstetrical ultrasound*, New York, 1984, McGraw-Hill.

Jeffrey MF: The role of ultrasound in chorionic villus sampling: a review, *J Diagn Med Sonogr* 3:135, 1986.

Miller ME and others: Compression-related defects from early amnion rupture: evidence for mechanical teratogenesis, *J Pediatr* 98:292, 1981.

Milunsky A, Sapirstein VS: Prenatal diagnosis of open neural tube defects using the amniotic fluid acetylcholinesterase assay, *Obstet Gynecol* 59:1, 1982.

Moore KL, editor: *The developing human: clinically oriented embryology*, ed 4, Philadelphia, 1988, WB Saunders.

Potter EL: Bilateral absence of ureters and kidneys: a report of 50 cases, *Obstet Gynecol* 25:3, 1965.

Romero R and others: The diagnosis of congenital renal anomalies with ultrasound. II. Infantile polycystic kidney disease, *Am J Obstet Gynecol* 150:259, 1984.

Romero R and others: *Prenatal diagnosis of congenital anomalies*, Norwalk, Conn, 1988, Appleton & Lange.

Scrimgeour JB: Amniocentesis: technique and complications. In Emery AEH, editor: *Antenatal diagnosis of genetic disease*, Baltimore, 1973, Williams & Wilkins.

CHAPTER 37

Fetal Head and Neural Tube Defects

Charlotte G. Henningsen

KEY TERMS

acrania - condition associated with anencephaly in which there is complete or partial absence of the cranial bones

alobar holoprosencephaly - most severe form of holoprosencephaly characterized by a single common ventricle and malformed brain; orbital anomalies range from fused orbits to hypotelorism, with frequent nasal anomalies and clefting of the lip and palate

anencephaly - neural tube defect characterized by the lack of development of the cerebral and cerebellar hemispheres and cranial vault; this abnormality is incompatible with life

anomaly - an abnormality or congenital malformation

cebocephaly - form of holoprosencephaly characterized by a common ventricle, hypotelorism, and a nose with a single nostril

cyclopia - severe form of holoprosencephaly characterized by a common ventricle, fusion of the orbits with one or two eyes present, and a proboscis (maldeveloped cylindrical nose)

cystic hygroma - an increase in size of the jugular lymphatic sacs because of abnormal development

holoprosencephaly - a range of abnormalities from abnormal cleavage of the forebrain

hydranencephaly - congenital absence of the cerebral hemispheres because of an occlusion of the carotid arteries; midbrain structures are present, and fluid replaces cerebral tissue

hydrocephalus - ventriculomegaly in the neonate; abnormal accumulation of cerebrospinal fluid within the cerebral ventricles, resulting in compression and frequently destruction of brain tissue

macrocephaly - enlargement of the fetal cranium as a result of ventriculomegaly

meningocele - open spinal defect characterized by protrusion of the spinal meninges

meningomyelocele - open spinal defect characterized by protrusion of meninges and spinal cord through the defect, usually within a meningeal sac

spina bifida - neural tube defect of the spine in which the dorsal vertebrae (vertebral arches) fail to fuse together, allowing the protrusion of meninges and/or spinal cord through the defect; two types exist: spina bifida occulta (skin-covered defect of the spine without protrusion of meninges or cord) and spina bifida cystica (open spinal defect marked by sac containing protruding meninges and/or cord)

spina bifida occulta - closed defect of the spine without protrusion of meninges or spinal cord; alpha-fetoprotein analysis will not detect these lesions

ventriculomegaly - abnormal accumulation of cerebrospinal fluid within the cerebral ventricles resulting in dilation of the ventricles; compression of developing brain tissue and brain damage may result; commonly associated with additional fetal anomalies

EMBRYOLOGY

The central nervous system (CNS) arises from the ectodermal neural plate at around 18 gestational days. The cephalic neural plate develops into the forebrain, and the caudal end forms the spinal cord. The midbrain and hindbrain then form and the neural plate begins to fold. The cranial and caudal neuropores represent unfused regions of the neural tube that will close between 24 and 26 gestational days. The forebrain will continue to develop into the prosencephalon, the midbrain will become the mesencephalon, and the hindbrain will form the rhombencephalon.[4]

At the end of the 3rd week the cephalic end of the neural tube will bend into the shape of a C (cephalic flexure), with the area of the mesencephalon having a very prominent bend. The brain then folds back on itself, and by the beginning of the 5th week another prominent bend, the cervical flexure, appears between the hindbrain and the spinal cord. The brain that originally was composed of three parts has now further divided into five parts. The prosencephalon divides into the telencephalon, which becomes the cerebral hemispheres, and diencephalon, which eventually develops into the epithalamus, thalamus, hypothalamus, and infundibulum. The rhombencephalon also subdivides into the metencephalon, which ultimately becomes the cerebellum and pons, and the myelencephalon, which transforms into the medulla. The fundamental organization of the brain is represented in these five divisions that persist into adult life.[4]

The primitive spinal cord divides into two regions. The alar plate region matures into the sensory region of the cord, and the basal plate region develops into the motor region of the cord. These regions further subdivide into specialized functions. Initially, the spinal cord and vertebral column extend the length of the body. After the first trimester, the posterior portion of the body grows beyond the vertebral column and spinal cord, and the growth of the spinal cord lags behind that of the vertebral column. At birth the spinal cord terminates at the level of the third lumbar vertebra, although by adulthood the cord will end at the level of the second lumbar vertebra.[4]

Neural function begins at 6 weeks of gestation and commences with primitive reflex movements at the level of the face and neck. By 12 weeks of gestation, sensitivity has spread across the surface of the body except at the back and top of the head. The fetus begins to have defined periods of activity and inactivity at the end of the fourth month. Between the fourth and fifth months the fetus can grip objects and is capable of weak respiratory movements. At 6 months of gestation the fetus displays the sucking reflex, and by about 28 weeks there have been significant changes in brain wave patterns.[4]

Many of the congenital malformations of the CNS result from incomplete closure of the neural tube. A wide range of defects may affect the spine and/or brain. The remainder of this chapter presents anomalies of the CNS.

Identification and diagnosis of anomalies of the fetal head and spine can be a complex task. Some of the distinguishing characteristics that help define a specific anomaly are listed in Table 37-1.

ANENCEPHALY

Anencephaly is the most common neural tube defect, with an overall incidence of approximately 1 in 1200 pregnancies.[2] The incidence varies with geographic location; there is a much higher prevalence in the United Kingdom than in the United States. The incidence also varies with gender, having a female prevalence of 4 to 1 over males.[2] There is also a significant recurrence risk of 2% to 3% for subsequent pregnancies for a woman with a history of a prior pregnancy with an open neural tube defect.[21]

Anencephaly, which means absence of the brain, is caused by failure of closure of the neural tube at the cranial end.[2] The result is absence of the cranial vault, complete or partial absence of the forebrain, which may partially develop and then degenerate, and the presence of the brainstem, midbrain, skull base, and facial structures. The remnant brain is covered by a thick membrane called *angiomatous stroma* or *cerebrovasculosa*.

Anencephaly is a lethal disorder, with up to 50% of cases resulting in fetal demise. The remainder die at birth or shortly thereafter.[21] Because of the severity of this disorder, early diagnosis is preferred. Prenatal diagnosis is often made with ultrasound following referral for increased maternal serum alpha-fetoprotein levels, which are extremely high with this defect because of the absent skull and exposed tissue.

The etiology of neural tube defects including anencephaly are numerous. Anencephaly may result from a syndrome such as Meckel-Gruber or a chromosomal ab-

TABLE 37-1	DIFFERENTIAL CONSIDERATIONS FOR CENTRAL NERVOUS SYSTEM ANOMALIES		
Anomaly	**Ultrasound Findings**	**Differential Considerations**	**Distinguishing Characteristics**
Anencephaly	Absence of brain and cranial vault	Microcephaly	No calvarium above orbits
	Froglike appearance	Acrania	
	Cerebrovasculosa	Cephalocele	
Anomaly	**Ultrasound Findings**	**Differential Considerations**	**Distinguishing Characteristics**
Cephalocele	Extracranial mass	Cystic hygroma	Defect in skull
	Bony defect in calvarium		
Anomaly	**Ultrasound Findings**	**Differential Considerations**	**Distinguishing Characteristics**
Dandy-Walker malformation	Posterior fossa cyst	Arachnoid cyst	Cerebellar hemispheres will be splayed
	Splaying of cerebellar hemispheres	Cerebellar hypoplasia	
Anomaly	**Ultrasound Findings**	**Differential Considerations**	**Distinguishing Characteristics**
Vein of Galen aneurysm	Midline cystic structure	Arachnoid cyst	Doppler flow in the cystic space
	Turbulent Doppler flow	Porencephalic cyst	
Anomaly	**Ultrasound Findings**	**Differential Considerations**	**Distinguishing Characteristics**
Porencephalic cyst	Cyst within brain parenchyma	Arachnoid cyst	No mass effect
	No mass effect		Cyst communicating with ventricle
	Communication with ventricle		
Anomaly	**Ultrasound Findings**	**Differential Considerations**	**Distinguishing Characteristics**
Hydranencephaly	Absence of brain tissue	Hydrocephaly	Lack of intact falx
	Fluid-filled brain	Holoprosencephaly	No rim of brain tissue
	Absent or partially absent falx		

normality such as trisomy 13. There is an increased risk in patients with diabetes mellitus, including patients whose disorders are well controlled. Environmental and dietary factors may also increase the prevalence of neural tube defects, including hyperthermia, folate and vitamin deficiencies, and teratogenic levels of zinc. Other teratogens associated with neural tube defects include valproic acid, methotrexate, and aminopterin.[21] Another cause of neural tube defects is amniotic band syndrome, which may manifest with clefting defects.

Ultrasound findings. Anencephaly may be detected with ultrasound as early as 10 to 14 weeks of gestation, although the only sonographic feature may be acrania. The crown-rump length may be normal because the degeneration of the fetal brain is progressive, leading to a reduction in the crown-rump length with advancing gestation.[13] Second-trimester identification of anencephaly is more obvious, with absent cerebral hemispheres evident, as well as absence of the skull.

Sonographic features of anencephaly include the following:

- Absence of the brain and cranial vault (Figure 37-1)
- Rudimentary brain tissue characterized as the cerebrovasculosa (Figures 37-2 and 37-3)
- Bulging fetal orbits, giving the fetus a froglike appearance

Other sonographic findings associated with anencephaly include polyhydramnios, which is seen in 40% to 50% of cases but may not be present until after 26 weeks of gestation,[2] although oligohydramnios may occasionally be identified. Coexisting spina bifida and/or craniorachischisis may be identified in up to 50% of fetuses with anencephaly.[2] Additional anomalies include cleft lip and palate, hydronephrosis, diaphragmatic hernia, cardiac defects, omphalocele, gastrointestinal defects, and talipes.

When severe, microcephaly may be confused with anencephaly, although the presence of the cranium should aid in a definitive diagnosis. Other defects that may mimic anencephaly include acrania (brain is abnormal but present), cephalocele (brain herniation), and amniotic band syndrome (usually asymmetric cranial defects).

ACRANIA

Acrania is a lethal anomaly that manifests as absence of the cranial bones with the presence of complete, although abnormal, development of the cerebral hemispheres. This anomaly occurs at the beginning of the 4th gestational week when the mesenchymal tissue fails to migrate and does not allow bone formation over the cerebral tissue.[24] The prevalence of acrania is rare, with only a few cases re-

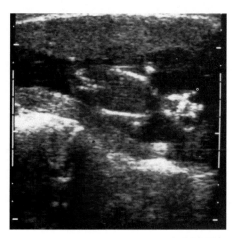

Figure 37-1 A 15-week anencephalic fetus. Note the froglike appearance.

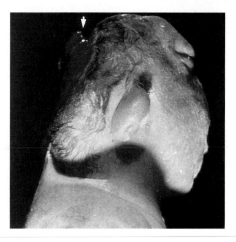

Figure 37-2 Postmortem photograph of anencephaly. The *arrow* points to the rudimentary brain (cerebrovasculosa).

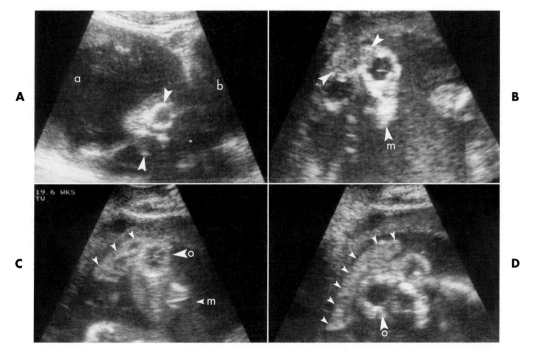

Figure 37-3 **A,** Transabdominal view of fetal cranium at 19.5 weeks of gestation demonstrating only the orbits *(arrows)*. Anencephaly was suspected because of the inability to image the bony skull above the level of the orbits. *a,* Amniotic fluid; *b,* maternal bladder. **B,** In the same fetus, transvaginal coronal imaging more clearly outlines only facial features, confirming the diagnosis of anencephaly. The protruding orbits and absent frontal and parietal bones *(arrows)* are shown. *m,* Mandible. **C,** In the same fetus a side view demonstrates rudimentary brain tissue (cerebrovasculosa) *(arrows)* herniating from the base of the skull. *m,* Mouth *o,* orbit. **D,** In the same fetus a coronal view outlines the herniated brain tissue *(arrows)* extending from the skull above the orbits *(o).*

ported in the literature.[12] In addition, acrania usually progresses to anencephaly as the brain slowly degenerates as a result of exposure to amniotic fluid. Why some cases of acrania do not progress to anencephaly is unknown.[12]

Acrania may be confused with anencephaly, although the presence of significant brain tissue and the lack of a froglike appearance should establish the diagnosis. Other disorders that may mimic acrania include hypophosphatasia and osteogenesis imperfecta, both of which result in hypomineralization of the cranium. The identification of additional findings such as long bone fractures should help to distinguish these disorders from acrania.

Ultrasound findings. Sonographic features of acrania include the following:

- The presence of brain tissue without the presence of a calvarium (Figure 37-4)
- Disorganization of brain tissue
- Prominent sulcal markings (Figsures 37-5 to 37-7)

Acrania may be associated with other anomalies, including spinal defects, cleft lip and palate, talipes, cardiac defects, and omphalocele. Acrania has also been associated with amniotic band syndrome (see Figure 37-4, *B*).

CEPHALOCELE

A cephalocele is a neural tube defect in which the meninges alone or meninges and brain herniate through a defect in the calvarium. *Encephalocele* is the term used to describe herniation of the meninges and brain through the defect; *cranial meningocele* describes the herniation of only meninges (Figure 37-8). Cephaloceles occur at a rate of 1 in 2000 live births.[21]

Cephaloceles involve the occipital bone (Figure 37-9) and are located in the midline in 75% of cases, although they may also involve the parietal and frontal regions.[13]

The prognosis for the infant with a cephalocele varies based on the size, location, and involvement of other brain structures. The presence of brain in the defect, micro-cephaly, and other anomalies worsens the prognosis. An isolated cranial meningocele may have a normal outcome.[18]

Ultrasound findings. The sonographic appearance of a cephalocele largely depends on the location, size, and involvement of brain structures.

Sonographic features of cephaloceles include the following:

- An extracranial mass (Figure 37-10), which may be fluid filled (cranial meningocele) or contain solid components (encephalocele)
- A bony defect in the skull
- Ventriculomegaly, which is more commonly identified with an encephalocele

Another sonographic finding associated with cephaloceles is polyhydramnios. Coexisting anomalies include microcephaly, agenesis of the corpus callosum, facial clefts, spina bifida, cardiac anomalies, and genital anomalies. Chromosomal anomalies and syndromes have been identified with cephaloceles, including trisomy 13 and Meckel-

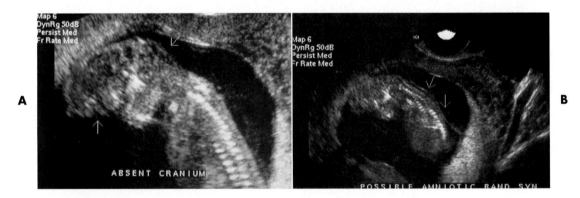

Figure 37-4 Acrania. Patient presented with an elevated maternal serum alpha-fetoprotein. Note the amnion *(arrows)* along the back of the fetus. Amniotic band syndrome was the probable cause.

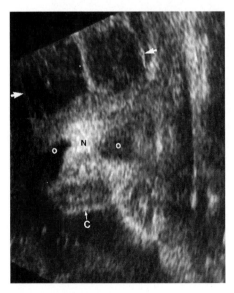

Figure 37-5 Coronal facial view showing absence of the parietal bones *(arrows)*, with highly visible brain tissue *(arrows)* representing acrania or exencephaly. *c*, Chin; *n*, nose; *o*, orbits.

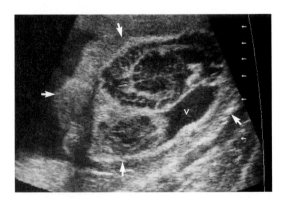

Figure 37-6 In the fetus shown in Figure 37-5 a transverse view shows the disorganized and freely floating brain tissue *(arrows)*. The brain anatomy is enhanced because of the absent skull bones. Note the herniated ventricle *(v)* and sulcal markings.

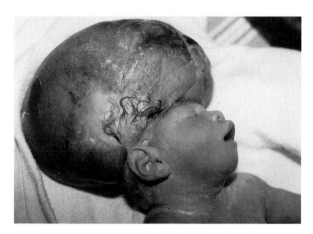

Figure 37-7   Same neonate shown in Figures 37-5 and 37-6, with acrania shortly after birth. The infant died within a few hours.

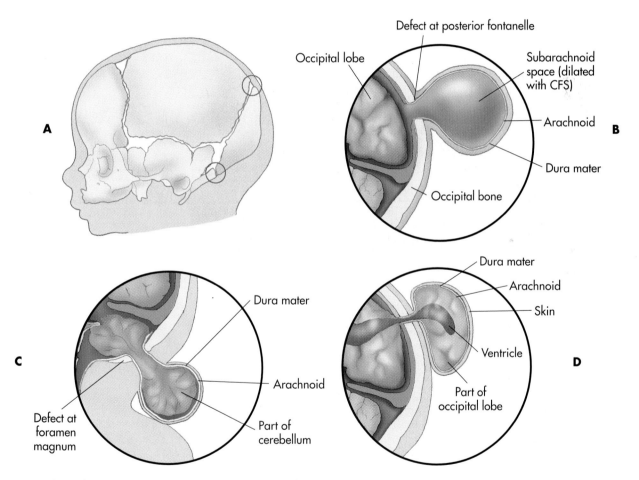

Figure 37-8   Schematic drawings illustrating cranium bifidum (bony defect in the cranium) and the various types of herniation of the brain and/or meninges. **A,** Sketch of the head of a newborn infant with a large protrusion from the occipital region of the skull. The upper circle indicates a cranial defect at the posterior fontanelle, and the lower circle indicates a cranial defect near the foramen magnum. **B,** Meningocele consisting of a protrusion of the cranial meninges that is filled with cerebrospinal fluid. **C,** Meningoencephalocele consisting of a protrusion of part of the cerebellum that is covered by meninges and skin. **D,** Meningohydroencephalocele consisting of a protrusion of part of the occipital lobe that contains part of the posterior horn of a lateral ventricle.

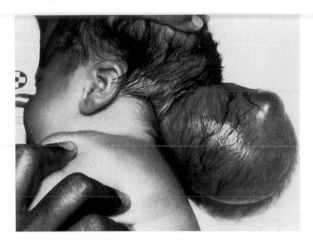

Figure 37-9 Neonate with a posterior occipital encephalocele.

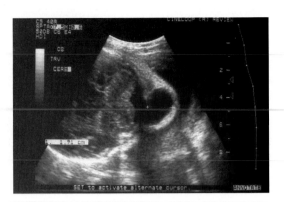

Figure 37-10 Cranial meningocele. The sac protruding from the cranium is fluid-filled.

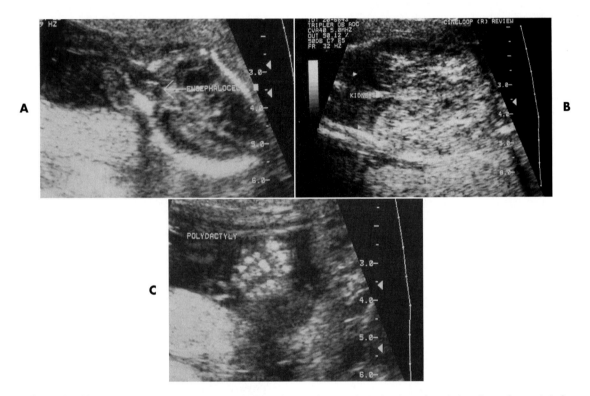

Figure 37-11 Encephalocele as part of Meckel-Gruber syndrome. **A,** Brain tissue herniating from the occipital region. **B,** Large echogenic kidneys consistent with autosomal recessive polycystic kidney disease (ARPKD). **C,** Polydactyly was noted on the hands.

Gruber syndrome, which is an autosomal-recessive disorder characterized by encephalocele, polydactyly, and polycystic kidneys (Figure 37-11). Other syndromes linked with cephalocele include Chemke, cryptophthalmos, Knobloch, dyssegmental dysplasia, von Voss, Roberts', and Walker-Warburg.[21] Cephaloceles located off midline are usually the result of amniotic band syndrome and may be further distinguished by associated limb anomalies and abdominal wall defects.

Cephaloceles may be confused with cystic hygromas, although they lack a cranial defect. Anencephaly may be difficult to distinguish from encephaloceles of significant size, and the presence of the cranial vault with encephalocele should establish the diagnosis. Frontal encephaloceles may be difficult to distinguish from a facial teratoma.[13]

SPINA BIFIDA

Spina bifida encompasses a wide range of vertebral defects that result from failure of neural tube closure. Through this defect the meninges and neural elements may protrude. The defect may occur anywhere along the vertebral

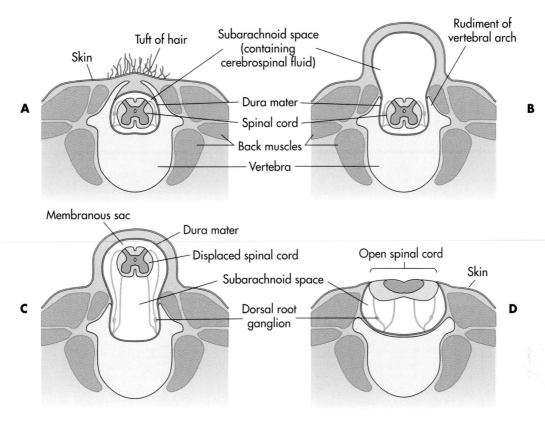

Figure 37-12 Diagrammatic sketches illustrating various types of spina bifida and the commonly associated malformations of the nervous system. **A,** Spina bifida occulta. About 10% of people have this vertebral defect in L5 and/or S1. It usually causes no back problems. **B,** Spina bifida with meningocele. **C,** Spina bifida with meningomyelocele. **D,** Spina bifida with myeloschisis. The types illustrated in **B** to **D** are often referred to collectively as *spina bifida cystica* because of the cystic sac that is associated with them.

column but most commonly occurs along the lumbar and sacral regions. This is the second most common open neural tube defect.[14]

The term *spina bifida* means that there is a cleft or opening in the spine (Figure 37-12). When covered with skin or hair, it is referred to as spina bifida occulta, an anomaly that is associated with a normal spinal cord and nerves and normal neurologic development. Spina bifida occulta is extremely difficult to detect in the fetus. Because the defect is covered by skin, the maternal serum alpha-fetoprotein level will be normal.

When the defect involves only protrusion of the meninges, it is termed a *meningocele*. More commonly the meninges and neural elements protrude through the defect and are termed a *meningomyelocele*. If the defect is very large and severe, it is termed *rachischisis*.

Spina bifida is also associated with varying degrees of neurologic impairment, which may include minor anesthesia, paraparesis, or death.[13] Fetuses with myelomeningoceles often present with the cranial defects associated with the Arnold-Chiari (type II) malformation, which is identified in 90% of patients. The Arnold-Chiari II malformation presents invariably with hydrocephalus because of the cerebellar vermis, which becomes displaced into the cervi-

cal canal. This changes the shape of the cerebellum, giving it a "banana" appearance, and leads to obliteration of the cisterna magna. In addition, caudal displacement of the cranial structures causes scalloping of the frontal bones of the skull, making the fetal head resemble a lemon.[3]

Management of a fetus with spina bifida usually includes serial ultrasound examinations to monitor progression and extent of ventriculomegaly and to follow fetal growth. Fetuses may be delivered early for ventricular shunting, usually by cesarean section to preserve as much motor function as possible.

The prognosis for an infant with spina bifida varies greatly according to the type, size, and location of the defect.[8] Rachischisis is invariably lethal, and higher lesions tend to have a worse prognosis. When intervention is desired, surgical closure of the defect is performed to preserve existing neurologic function. In addition to management of the actual defect, attention to any hydrocephalus, urinary tract anomalies or dysfunction, and orthopedic issues may be part of the long-term care for this child.[21]

Ultrasound findings. Sonographic examination of the fetal spine should include a methodical survey of the spine in the sagittal and transverse planes. The normal fetal spine should demonstrate the posterior ossification centers com-

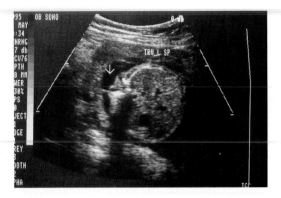

Figure 37-13 Meningomyelocele with the spinal splaying appearing as a V.

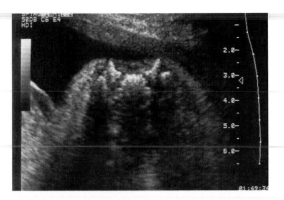

Figure 37-15 Spina bifida with a U-shaped configuration and an open cleft in the skin.

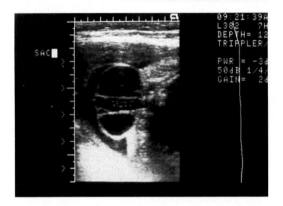

Figure 37-14 Meningomyelocele identified in a fetus with mild ventriculomegaly. Note the neural elements protruding into the sac.

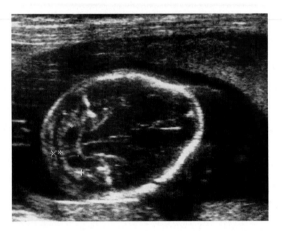

Figure 37-16 Abnormally shaped cerebellum "banana sign" *(calipers; +)* in a 21-week fetus with a lumbosacral meningomyelocele. Note the lemon-shaped frontal bones consistent with frontal bossing.

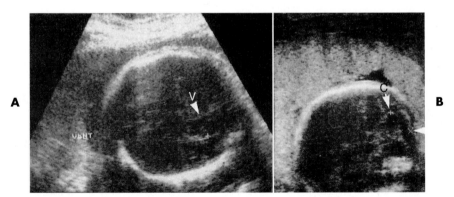

Figure 37-17 **A,** In the fetus shown in Figure 37-19, *B,* views of the brain demonstrate ventriculomegaly with the ventricles *(V; + caliper)* measuring 14 mm in diameter; after birth ventriculoperitoneal shunting was found unnecessary. **B,** A normal-appearing cerebellum *(C; + calipers)* and cisterna magna *(arrowhead; x calipers).*

pleting a spinal circle. The survey of the fetal spine may be impeded when the spine in down, when the fetus is in the breech position, when oligohydramnios is present, and when maternal obesity precludes adequate visualization.

Sonographic features of spina bifida include the following:

• Splaying of the posterior ossification centers with a V or U configuration (Figure 37-13)

• Protusion of a saclike structure that may be anechoic (meningocele) or contain neural elements (myelomeningocele) (Figure 37-14)

• A cleft in the skin (Figure 37-15)

After a spinal defect has been identified, the level and extent of the defect, the presence or absence of neural elements contained in the protruding sac, and associated intracranial findings should be documented.

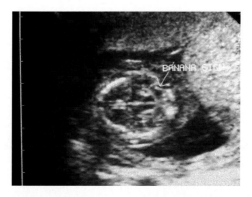

Figure 37-18 Cerebellum is pulled inferiorly, giving it a rounded, banana shape.

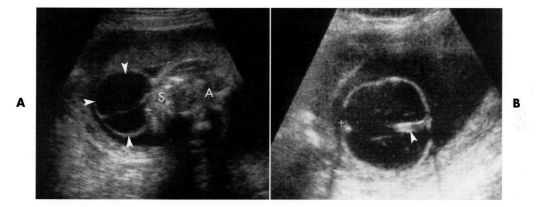

Figure 37-19 **A,** Lumbosacral meningomyelocele *(arrows)* shown in a 21-week fetus, detected on a basic fetal scan. *A,* Abdomen; *S,* spine. **B,** Lumbosacral meningomyelocele measuring 6 cm *(calipers)* observed in a 33-week fetus during a basic fetal scan. Note the spinal elements *(arrow)* within the meningomyelocele sac. Additional anomalies included clubbing of the feet and inward rotation of the legs. Ventriculomegaly was present, but effacement of the cisterna magna was not apparent (see Figure 37-17).

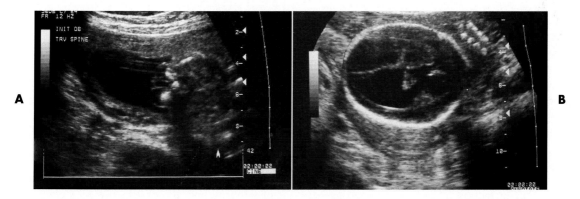

Figure 37-20 **A,** A fetus of 24.6 weeks of gestation with a meningomyelocele. Neural elements were identified in the sac. **B,** A significant amount of ventricular dilation was identified with in the fetal head.

The associated sonographic cranial findings include the following:

- Flattening of the frontal bones, giving the head a "lemon" shape (Figures 37-16 and 37-17)
- Obliteration of the cisterna magna
- Inferior displacement of the cerebellar vermis, giving the cerebellum a rounded, "banana" shape (Figures 37-17 and 37-18)
- Ventriculomegaly (Figures 37-19 and 37-20)

The "lemon sign" is not specific for spina bifida, and similar head shapes have been described with other CNS malformations, such as encephalocele, and non-CNS malformations, such as thanatophoric dysplasia. This appearance may also be indistinguishable from the "strawberry sign" described in association with trisomy 18.

Other sonographic findings associated with spina bifida include talipes, cephaloceles, cleft lip and palate, hypo-

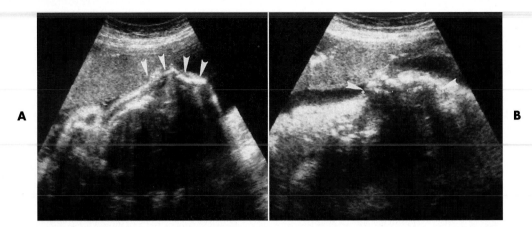

Figure 37-21 **A,** Thoracic meningomyelocele demonstrated with significant disruption of the bony elements *(arrows).* **B,** In the same fetus, another view demonstrating the spinal defect. Coexisting anomalies included significant ventriculomegaly of 27 mm, unilateral renal agenesis, and single umbilical artery.

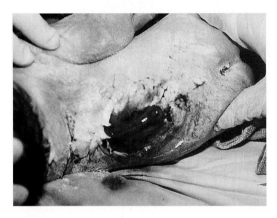

Figure 37-22 Neonate shown in Figure 37-21, demonstrating large thoracic meningomyelocele.

telorism, heart defects, and genitourinary anomalies (Figures 37-21 and 37-22). Spina bifida has also been associated with multiple syndromes and chromosomal anomalies, including trisomy 18. Fetuses exposed to teratogens such as valproic acid (Figure 37-23), methotrexate, and aminopterin are also at greater risk for developing spina bifida. Maternal diabetes, hyperthermia, and folic acid deficiency have also been associated with spina bifida.[21]

DANDY-WALKER MALFORMATION

Dandy-Walker malformation (DWM) is a defect that may have varying degrees of severity. It manifests with agenesis or hypoplasia of the cellebellar vermis with resulting dilation on the fourth ventricle. The occurrence rate is 1 in 25,000 to 35,000.[21]

DWM is thought to occur before the 6th or 7th gestational week as the result of abnormal embryogenesis of the roof of the fourth ventricle. In its milder form, it is referred to as the Dandy-Walker variant. DWM causes 4% of cases of hydrocephalus, which is commonly identified in conjunction with this anomaly.[21]

DWM is associated with other intracranial anomalies about 50% of the time.[21] These include agenesis of the

corpus callosum, aqueductal stenosis, microcephaly, macrocephaly, encephalocele, gyral malformations, and lipomas. Chromosomal anomalies that may be associated with DWM include trisomies 13, 18, and 21. DWM has been associated with several syndromes, including Meckel-Gruber syndrome, Walker-Warburg syndrome, and Aicardi syndrome, and has been linked with congenital infections.[18]

The prognosis for DWM depends on the presence or absence of associated anomalies. Mortality depends highly on other anomalies. Many infants with isolated DWM have a subnormal IQ, although some may have normal function.

Ultrasound findings. Sonographic survey may reveal extracranial anomalies that are also associated with DWM, including cardiac anomalies, polydactyly, facial clefts, and urinary tract anomalies.

Sonographic features of DWM include the following:

- A posterior fossa cyst that can vary considerably in size (Figure 37-24)
- Splaying of the cerebellar hemispheres as a result of the complete or partial agenesis of the cerebellar vermis
- An enlarged cisterna magna caused by the cerebellar vermis anomaly and posterior fossa cyst
- Ventriculomegaly (Figure 37-25)

The differential diagnosis should include arachnoid cyst, but the identification of the splayed cerebellar hemispheres may help to confirm DWM. Cerebellar hypoplasia should also be included when the cisterna magna is enlarged; however, confirming the small cerebellum may make this diagnosis.

HOLOPROSENCEPHALY

Holoprosencephaly encompasses a range of abnormalities resulting from abnormal cleavage of the prosencephalon (forebrain).[15] The incidence is 0.6 in 1000 live births, although the incidence in embryos has been much higher (1 in 250).[13] Cases of holoprosencephaly are sporadic, with a recurrence risk of 6%, although

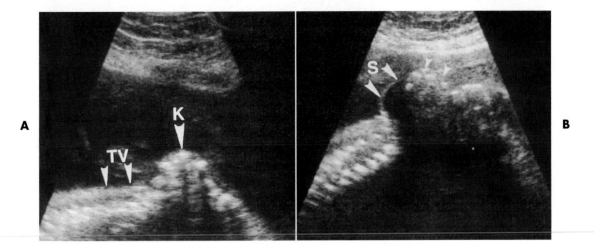

Figure 37-23 **A,** Meningomyelocele caused by a teratogen (valproic acid [Depakene]) in a 26-week fetus. Sagittal view showing thoracolumbar meningomyelocele with marked kyphus *(K)* of the spinal elements. *TV,* Thoracic vertebrae. **B,** In the same fetus a meningomyelocele sac *(S)* is observed outlining the marked disruption and malalignment of the vertebrae *(small* arrowheads). This mother was given valproic acid for a seizure disorder during the first trimester of pregnancy. Valproic acid is a known teratogen that may produce neural tube defects. Elevated levels of maternal serum alpha-fetoprotein prompted the fetal study. Coexisting anomalies included ventriculomegaly, small cranium, and a unilateral clubfoot.

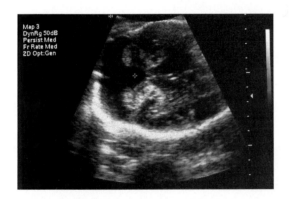

Figure 37-24 Dandy-Walker cyst. Note the splayed cerebellar hemispheres. (Courtesy Ginny Goreczky, Maternal Fetal Center, Florida Hospital, Orlando, Fla.)

there have also been genetic, teratogenic, and chromosomal associations.[21]

There are three forms of holoprosencephaly. The most severe form is classified as alobar, the intermediate form as semilobar, and the mildest form as lobar. Identification of the specific form depends on the degree of failed hemispheric division.

Alobar holoprosencephaly is characterized by a singular monoventricle, brain tissue that is small and may have a cup, ball, or pancake configuration (Figure 37-29), fusion of the thalamus, and absence of the interhemispheric fissure, cavum septum pellucidum, corpus callosum, optic tracts, and olfactory bulbs. Semilobar holoprosencephaly presents with a singular ventricular cavity with partial formation of the occipital horns, partial or complete fusion of the thalamus, a rudimentary falx and interhemispheric fissure, and absent corpus callosum, cavum septum pellucidum, and olfactory bulbs (Figure 37-26). In lobar holoprosencephaly there is almost complete division of the

ventricles with a corpus callosum that may be normal, hypoplastic, or absent, although the cavum septum pellucidum will still be absent.

The etiology of holoprosencephaly varies. It is usually sporadic but has been associated with chromosomal anomalies, most specifically trisomy 13, and there have been rare familial patterns transmitted in autosomal dominant and autosomal recessive forms. Multiple syndromes have also been associated with holoprosencephaly, including Meckel syndrome, Aicardi syndrome, Fryn's syndrome, and hydrolethalus syndrome. Teratogens reported to produce holoprosencephaly include alcohol, phenytoin, retinoic acid, maternal diabetes, and congenital infections.[21]

The prognosis for holoprosencephaly is considered uniformly poor. In its most severe forms, fetuses die at birth or shortly thereafter. In the least severe form, survival is possible, although usually with severe mental retardation.

Ultrasound findings. Sonographic features of holoprosencephaly include the following:

- A common C-shaped ventricle that may or may not be enlarged (Figure 37-27)
- Brain tissue with a horseshoe shape as it surrounds the monoventricle
- Fusion of the thalamus with absence of the third ventricle
- Absence of the interhemispheric fissure
- A dorsal sac with expansion of the monoventricle posteriorly
- Absence of the corpus callosum
- Absence of the cavum septum pellucidum

Holoprosencephaly is often associated with facial abnormalities, especially with the most severe forms (Figures 37-28 and 37-29). The facial anomalies identified include cyclopia, hypotelorism, an absent nose, a flattened nose with a single nostril, and a proboscis (Figures 37-30 and 37-31). Cebocephaly consists of the combination of hypotelorism with a normally placed nose with a single nos-

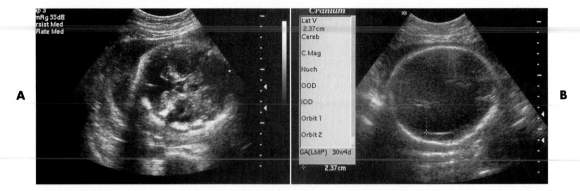

Figure 37-25 This patient had a history of elevated maternal serum alpha-fetoprotein. Follow-up in a maternal fetal center for a history of hydrocephalus revealed a Dandy-Walker malformation **(A)** and ventriculomegaly **(B).** The fetus was 30 weeks and 4 days of gestation with a head size typical of 36 weeks of gestation.

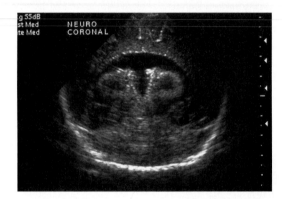

Figure 37-26 A neonatal ultrasound in a newborn revealed semilobar holoprosencephaly. There was no history of a prenatal ultrasound because of the normal course of the pregnancy. The infant only lived for a few weeks.

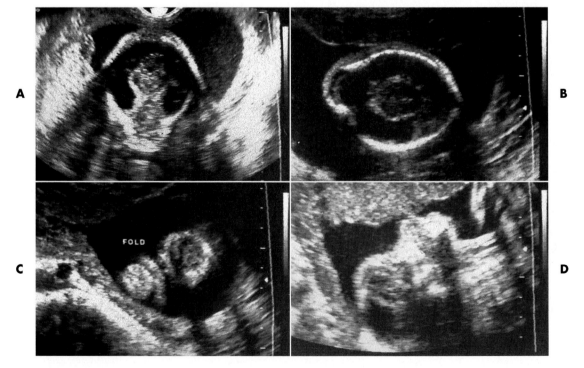

Figure 37-27 Holoprosencephaly. This patient had a history of six previous pregnancies, two of which were also affected by holoprosencephaly. This was an autosomal dominant form of holoprosencephaly. **A,** C-shaped monoventricle. **B,** An encephalocele was also noted. **C,** Imaging of the face revealed redundant skin folds at the level of the nose and hypotelorism. **D,** Note the abnormal-appearing profile.

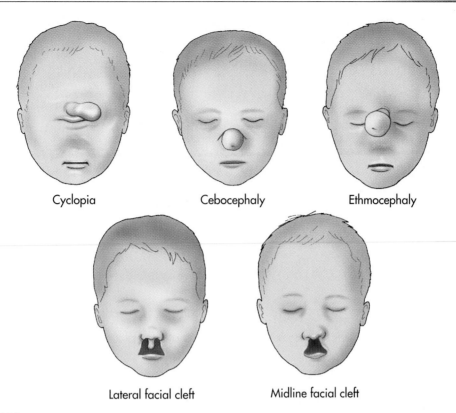

Cyclopia   Cebocephaly   Ethmocephaly

Lateral facial cleft   Midline facial cleft

Figure 37-28   Facial features of holoprosencephaly. These drawings illustrate the normal facial features in contrast with the variable facial features of holoprosencephaly. In cyclopia the proboscis projects from the lower forehead superior to one median orbit and the nose is absent. Ethmocephaly is very similar to cyclopia but has two narrowly placed orbits with a proboscis and absent nose. In cebocephaly a rudimentary nose with a single nostril and hypotelorism are present. Hypotelorism may occur with a median cleft lip or bilateral cleft lip.

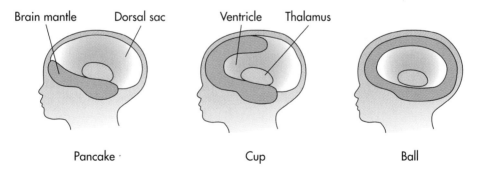

Brain mantle   Dorsal sac   Ventricle   Thalamus

Pancake   Cup   Ball

Figure 37-29   Diagram of three morphologic types of alobar holoprosencephaly (and semilobar holoprosencephaly) in sagittal view. In the pancake type the residual brain mantle is flattened at the base of the brain. The dorsal sac is correspondingly large. The cup type has more brain mantle present, but it does not cover the monoventricle. In the ball type the brain mantle completely covers the monoventricle, and a dorsal sac may or may not be present.

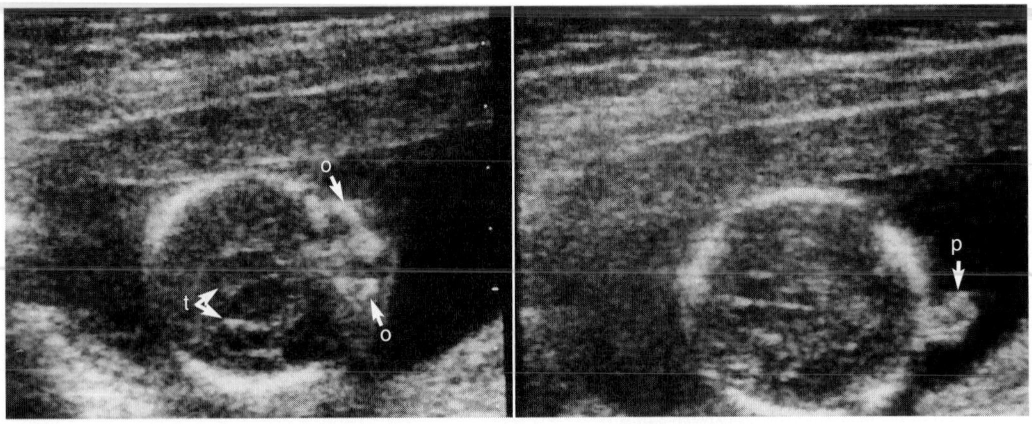

A

B

Figure 37-30 **A,** Transverse cross-section of the cranium in a 17-week fetus with holoprosencephaly. Fused thalami *(t)* and hypotelorism *(o)* are obvious. Measurements revealed abnormally closely spaced orbits (hypotelorism). **B,** In the same fetus a proboscis *(p)* is seen above the orbits, consistent with ethmocephaly.

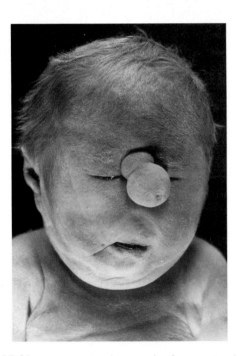

Figure 37-31 Postmortem photograph of a neonate with ethmocephaly. Note the proboscis and hypotelorism. The mouth appeared normal. A common ventricle and absent optic and ophthalmic nerves were found. The chromosomes were consistent with trisomy 13.

tril. Ethmocephaly consists of severe hypotelorism with a proboscis superior to the eyes. In addition, facial clefts may be present, with median or bilateral clefting most commonly observed.[21]

Other sonographic findings associated with holoprosencephaly include hydrocephaly, microcephaly, polyhydramnios, and intrauterine growth restriction (IUGR). In addition, renal cysts or dysplasia, omphalocele, cardiac defects, spina bifida, talipes, and gastrointestinal anomalies have been identified in the presence of holoprosencephaly. Chromosomal anomalies must also be considered if holoprosencephaly is present, especially trisomy 13.[18]

AGENESIS OF THE CORPUS CALLOSUM

The corpus callosum is a fibrous tract that connects the cerebral hemispheres and aids in learning and memory. Dysgenesis of the corpus callosum describes a range of complete to partial absence of the callosal fibers that cross the midline, forming a connection between the two hemispheres. The incidence is reported to be 1 to 3 in 1000 births.[20]

The corpus callosum begins to develop at 12 weeks of gestation and is not complete until 20 weeks. The etiology of agenesis of the corpus callosum is somewhat unclear but is thought to involve a vascular disruption or inflammatory lesion before 12 weeks.[1] Cases of agenesis of the corpus callosum, also known as callosal agenesis, are sporadic. It may be associated with other CNS malformations, and autosomal dominant, autosomal recessive, and X-linked syndromes have also been identified. Chromosomal anomalies that may accompany agenesis of the corpus callosum include trisomies 13 and 18.[1,18,20]

The prognosis for agenesis of the corpus callosum depends largely on the high incidence of associated anomalies, many of which carry a poor prognosis. As an isolated event, agenesis of the corpus callosum may be asymptomatic or associated with mental retardation (70%) and/or seizures (60%).[13]

Ultrasound findings. Sonographic features of agenesis of the corpus callosum include the following:

- Absence of the corpus callosum
- Elevation and dilation of the third ventricle (Figure 37-32)
- Widely separated lateral ventricular frontal horns with medial indentation of the medial walls
- Dilated occipital horns (colpocephaly), giving the lateral ventricles a teardrop shape
- Absence of the cavum septum pellucidum

Other sonographic findings associated with agenesis of the corpus callosum include other CNS anomalies such as

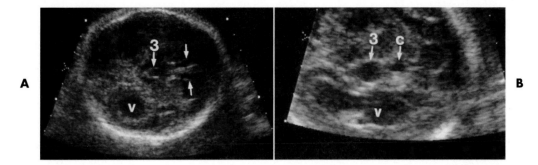

Figure 37-32   A, Agenesis of the corpus callosum in a 29-week fetus showing a dilated third ventricle *(3)* and a radial array pattern of the cerebral sulci *(arrows)*. *v,* Dilated ventricle (colpocephaly). **B,** In the same fetus an earlier scan at 25 weeks of gestation shows the dilated third ventricle *(3)* represented as an interhemispheric cyst displaced upward at the level of the lateral ventricles. A normal cavum septum pellucidum could not be recognized; instead, a circular area *(c)* was found.

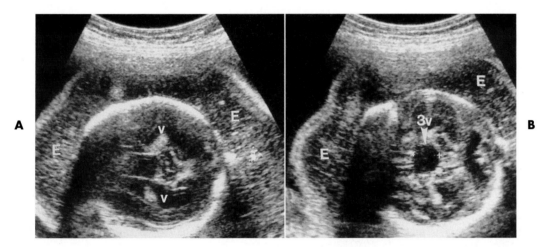

Figure 37-33   A, Ventricular view in a fetus with acquired aqueductal stenosis because of parvovirus infection. Dilation of the ventricular system *(v)* resulted from inflammation, causing obstruction to the flow of cerebrospinal fluid. The fetus was severely hydropic. Note the significant scalp edema *(E)*. **B,** In the same fetus, third ventricle *(3v)* dilation is demonstrated. Cordocentesis was performed to find a cause for the severe nonimmune hydrops, and parvovirus was detected within the fetal blood. The fetus died shortly after birth. *E,* Scalp edema.

holoprosencephaly, DWM, cranial lipoma, Arnold-Chiari malformation, septooptic dysplasia, hydrocephaly, encephalocele, porencephaly, microcephaly, and lissencephaly.[20,21] Other associated abnormalities associated with agenesis of the corpus callosum include cardiac malformations, diaphragmatic hernia, lung agenesis or dysplasia, and absent or dysplastic kidneys. Multiple chromosomal anomalies and syndromes have been linked with agenesis of the corpus callosum, including trisomies 13, 18, and 8, and Aicardi syndrome.[21]

AQUEDUCTAL STENOSIS

Aqueductal stenosis results from an obstruction, atresia, or stenosis of the aqueduct of Sylvius causing ventriculomegaly. The aqueduct of Sylvius connects the third and fourth ventricles, which explains the enlargement of the lateral ventricles and third ventricle in the presence of a normal fourth ventricle.

Aqueductal stenosis is usually a sporadic anomaly but may also result from intrauterine infections such as cytomegalovirus, rubella, and toxoplasmosis. Cranial masses and ventricular hemorrhage are also contributing factors of acquired obstruction. Primary aqueductal stenosis is usually X-linked and has an autosomal-recessive inheritance.[21]

The prognosis for aqueductal stenosis is considered poor and varies with associated anomalies. Approximately 90% of survivors have an IQ less than 70. Infants with X-linked aqueductal stenosis are profoundly mentally retarded.[21]

Ultrasound findings. Sonographic features of aqueductal stenosis include the following:

- Ventricular enlargement of the lateral ventricles, which may be severe (Figures 37-33 and 37-34)
- Third ventricular dilation.
- Flexion and adduction of the thumb (seen in the X-linked form)[21]

VEIN OF GALEN ANEURYSM

An aneurysm of the vein of Galen, also known as a vein of Galen malformation, is a rare arteriovenous malformation. The vein will be enlarged and communicate with normal-appearing arteries.

Vein of Galen aneurysm is considered a sporadic event and has a male predominance.[6] It is usually an isolated anomaly, although it has been associated with congenital heart defects, cystic hygromas, and hydrops.[21]

The prognosis for vein of Galen aneurysm is generally poor, especially when associated with hydrops and/or cardiac failure.[6,9] When symptoms present later in older children and young adults, the prognosis is generally good.[21]

Ultrasound findings. Sonographic features of vein of Galen aneurysm include the following:

- A cystic space that may be irregular in shape and is located midline and posterosuperior to the third ventricle
- Turbulent flow with Doppler evaluation

Other sonographic findings associated with vein of Galen aneurysm include fetal cardiomegaly and nonimmune hydrops. Ventriculomegaly with resultant macrocephaly may also develop.

The vein of Galen aneurysm may be confused with arachnoid cysts, which are very rare and may occur anywhere within the brain. Doppler evaluation of an arachnoid cyst will reveal no blood flow within the structure.

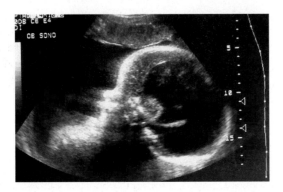

Figure 37-34   A sagittal image of a fetus with severe hydrocephaly that was thought to result from aqueductal stenosis.

Porencephalic cysts should also be listed in the differential diagnosis; however, these may be distinguished by the absence of blood flow and this cyst's communication with the ventricle.

CHOROID PLEXUS CYST

Choroid plexus cysts are round or ovoid anechoic structures found within the choroid plexus. These cysts are common and have been identified in approximately 1% of antenatal ultrasound examinations.[16,17] Choroid plexus cysts contain cerebrospinal fluid and cellular debris that has become trapped with the neuroepithelial folds.[22]

Choroid plexus cysts are usually isolated findings without association with other anomalies. Furthermore, they will often resolve by 22 to 26 weeks of gestation.[11] Choroid plexus cysts have been identified in association with aneuploidy, most commonly trisomies 18 and 21.[16,17]

Ultrasound findings. Sonographic features of choroid plexus cysts include the following:

- Cysts within the choroid plexus ranging in size from 0.3 to 2 cm
- Unilateral or bilateral cysts (Figures 37-35 and 37-36)
- Solitary or multiple
- Unilocular or multilocular
- Enlargement of the ventricle with large cyst

A careful sonographic survey for anomalies that might suggest aneuploidy should follow identification of a choroid plexus cyst to include nuchal fold measurement, meticulous survey of the heart, and a survey of the feet and hands to look for abnormal posturing and polydactyly. Amniocentesis for karyotyping may be offered, especially when other factors that may increase the risk for aneuploidy are considered, including maternal age, abnormal triple screen, and other ultrasound findings.

PORENCEPHALIC CYSTS

Porencephalic cysts, also known as porencephaly, are cysts filled with cerebrospinal fluid that communicate with the ventricular system or subarachnoid space. They may result from hemorrhage, infarction, delivery trauma, or inflam-

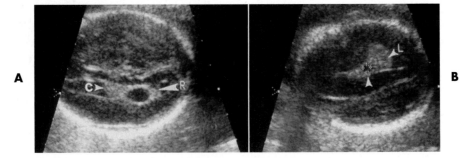

Figure 37-35   **A,** Bilateral choroid plexus cysts observed in a 21-week fetus. A 5-mm cyst *(R)* is visualized. *C,* Choroid plexus. **B,** In the same fetus a 2- to 3-mm cyst *(arrowhead)* is shown involving the left choroid plexus *(L).* Amniocentesis revealed a normal karyotype.

matory changes in the nervous system.[18] The affected brain parenchyma undergoes necrosis, brain tissue is resorbed, and a cystic lesion remains.

There are no known associated anomalies in fetuses with porencephalic cysts. Postnatal problems may include seizures, developmental delays, motor deficits, visual and sensory problems, and hydrocephalus.[18]

Ultrasound findings. The sonographic features of porencephalic cysts include the following:

• A cyst within the brain parenchyma without mass effect
• Communication of the cyst with the ventricle or subarachnoid space (Figure 37-37)
• Reduction in size of the affected hemisphere, which may cause a midline shift and contralateral ventricular enlargement

Porencephalic cysts may be confused with arachnoid cysts (Figure 37-40), although the lack of a mass effect seen with porencephaly may aid in differentiating the two.[18]

SCHIZENCEPHALY

Schizencephaly is a rare disorder characterized by clefts in the cerebral cortex. The clefts may be unilateral or bilateral, open-lip or closed-lip defects. Schizencephaly is thought to result from abnormal migration of neurons. These clefts can extend from the ventricle to the outer surface of the brain and are lined with abnormal gray matter.[19]

The etiology of schizencephaly remains unclear, although it has been linked with multiple assaults during pregnancy. Schizencephaly has been associated with congenital infections, drugs and other toxic exposures, vascular accidents, and metabolic abnormalities. There is also an association with aneuploidy.[19]

The prognosis for patients with schizencephaly varies, with mild to severe outcomes. Open-lip lesions and bilateral clefts carry a worse prognosis. Long-term effects include blindness; motor deficits, which may include spastic quadriparesis; hemiparesis; and hypotonia. Seizures, which may be uncontrollable, mental retardation, and language impairment are also possible. Hydrocephalus may be progressive and require shunt placement.[19]

Ultrasound findings. Sonographic features of schizencephaly include the following:

• A fluid-filled cleft in the cerebral cortex extending from the ventricle to the calvarium (Figure 37-38)
• Ventriculomegaly may be observed

Schizencephaly is associated with absence of the septum pellucidum and corpus callosum.[23] Septooptic dysplasia may also be present. Hydrocephaly can be seen when ventriculomegaly is present, but microcephaly has also been observed.

HYDRANENCEPHALY

Hydranencephaly is destruction of the cerebral hemispheres by occlusion of the internal carotid arteries. Brain parenchyma is destroyed and is replaced by cerebrospinal fluid. Because the posterior communicating arteries are preserved, the midbrain and cerebellum are present, and the basal ganglia, choroid plexus, and thalamus may also be spared.[13]

Hydranencephaly may also be associated with polyhydramnios. No coexisting structural or chromosomal anomalies are associated.

The etiology of hydranencephaly usually involves congenital infection or ischemia. Infections associated with hydranencephaly include cytomegalovirus and toxoplasmosis. Brain ischemia may result from maternal hypotension, twin to twin embolization, or vascular agenesis.[21] It is believed that hydranencephaly may occur later in pregnancy and that brain structures may initially be normal.[18] The assault to the brain by infection or ischemic event subsequently destroys normal brain tissue.[10]

The prognosis for hydranencephaly is grave, with death occurring at birth or shortly thereafter.[18]

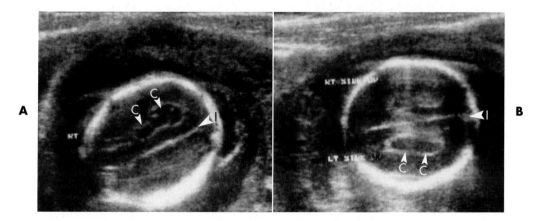

Figure 37-36 A, Bilateral choroid plexus cysts in trisomy 18. A 9-mm choroid plexus cyst is outlined in the proximal hemisphere *(C)*. *I,* Interhemispheric fissure. **B,** Similar cystic appearance of the distal choroid plexus *(C)*. Ventriculomegaly was present. Both choroid plexus cysts resolved by 26 weeks of gestation. A split-foot deformity ectrodactyly was also observed. *I,* Interhemispheric fissure.

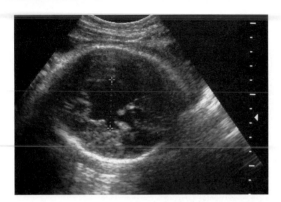

Figure 37-37 This patient was referred at 32 weeks of gestation to a fetal diagnostic center with a history of hydrocephalus seen on ultrasound examination. A porencephalic cyst was identified communicating with the lateral ventricle. Ventriculomegaly was also noted. The patient was counseled that this finding carried a poor prognosis.

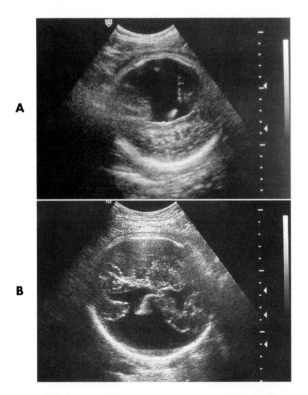

Figure 37-38 **A** and **B,** This patient came for an initial ultrasound at 32 weeks of gestation for late prenatal care. The ultrasound revealed hydrocephaly, and the patient was referred to a maternal-fetal center where the diagnosis of schizencephaly was made based on the cleft that extends to the calvarium. This diagnosis was confirmed at birth with computed tomography.

Ultrasound findings. Sonographic features of hydranencephaly include the following:

- Absence of normal brain tissue with almost complete replacement by cerebrospinal fluid (Figure 37-39)
- An absent or partially absent falx
- Presence of the midbrain, basal ganglia, and cerebellum

- The choroid plexus may be identified
- Macrocephaly may occur

Hydranencephaly may be confused with severe hydrocephaly, although the presence of an intact falx and surrounding rim of brain parenchyma may help to differentiate hydrocephaly from hydranencephaly. Holoprosencephaly with severe ventriculomegaly may also have a similar appearance. These three anomalies, however, have extremely poor outcomes.

VENTRICULOMEGALY (HYDROCEPHALUS)

Ventriculomegaly refers to dilation of the ventricles within the brain. Hydrocephalus occurs when ventriculomegaly is coupled with enlargement of the fetal head. The incidence of ventriculomegaly occurs in 0.5 to 1.8 per 1000 births.[7] Enlargement of the ventricles occurs with obstruction of cerebrospinal fluid flow. This obstruction may be caused by a ventricular defect such as aqueductal stenosis and is referred to as noncommunicating hydrocephalus. The obstruction may be outside of the ventricular system, such as with an arachnoid cyst (Figure 37-40), and is referred to as communicating hydrocephalus (Figure 37-41).[13] Rarely, ventriculomegaly results from an overproduction of cerebrospinal fluid by a choroid plexus papilloma.

Physiologically, when an obstruction occurs the ventricles dilate as the flow of cerebrospinal fluid is blocked. This increases the pressure within the ventricular system, which leads to ventricular expansion. Enlarged ventricles may exert pressure on the brain tissue, sometimes producing irreversible brain damage.

Hydrocephalus may be associated with an anomaly or the cause may remain unknown. Many of the abnormalities linked with ventricular dilation were discussed earlier in this chapter and include aqueductal stenosis, arachnoid cysts, and vein of Galen aneurysms. Common causes of ventriculomegaly include spina bifida and encephaloceles. Dandy-Walker Malformation, agenesis of the corpus callosum, lissencephaly, schizencephaly, and holoprosencephaly may also present with hydrocephalus. Intracranial neoplasm, such as a teratoma, may cause ventricular dilation. Ventriculomegaly may also be associated with musculoskeletal anomalies such as thanatophoric dysplasia and achondroplasia. Ventricular enlargement has also been linked to congenital infections such as toxoplasmosis and cytomegalovirus (Figure 37-42).[18]

Ventriculomegaly may be a manifestation of a syndrome or chromosomal abnormality. Mild ventriculomegaly has been associated with trisomy 21, and ventriculomegaly has also been identified in trisomies 13 and 18. Other syndromes associated with ventriculomegaly include Meckel-Gruber syndrome, Apert syndrome, Roberts' syndrome, hydrolethalus, Walker-Warburg, Smith-Lemli-Opitz syndrome, nasal-facial-digital syndrome, and Albers-Schonberg disease.[18]

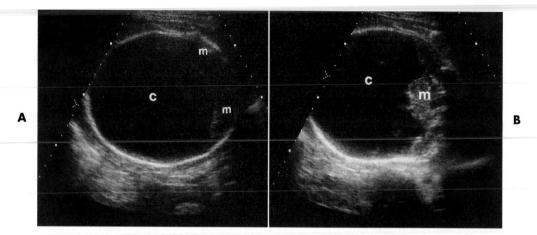

Figure 37-39   A, Hydranencephaly *(c)* in a fetus at 33 weeks of gestation showing massive collection of cerebrospinal fluid. Note the brain tissue in the occipital region *(m)*. **B,** In the same fetus, hydranencephaly *(c)* and the midbrain *(m)* are observed. Other anomalies included clubfoot and cardiac defects. In utero computed tomography scan confirmed the diagnosis of hydranencephaly. Macrocephaly (11-cm biparietal diameter) was found by cranial measurements. Cephalocentesis (decompression of the head) was performed to allow vaginal delivery.

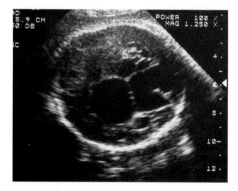

Figure 37-40   Multiple arachnoid cysts identified in this fetal head.

Fetal ventriculomegaly typically progresses from the occipital horns into the temporal and then to the frontal ventricular horns. Ventriculomegaly may be quantitated by measuring the ventricular atrium across the glomus of the choroid plexus. A ventricle is considered dilated when its diameter exceeds 10 mm. The proximal ventricle may be difficult to adequately image because of reverberation artifacts from the calvarium.[13] Transvaginal technique may be used to further clarify the defect when the fetus is in a vertex position.

The mortality for fetuses with hydrocephalus is high. Outcome depends largely on the presence and severity of associated anomalies. The prognosis for survivors is generally considered poor, with only half identified to have a normal intellect. Survivors may require ventricular shunting to improve survival and intellectual outcome.[13]

Ultrasound findings. Sonographic features of ventriculomegaly include the following:

- Lateral ventricular enlargement exceeding 10 mm (Figure 37-43)
- A "dangling choroid sign" as the gravity-dependent choroid plexus falls into the increased ventricular space (Figure 37-44)[13]

- Possible dilation of the third and fourth ventricles
- Fetal head enlargement when the biparietal and head circumference measurements exceed those for the established gestational age

The fetus should also be surveyed for associated anomalies, which are present in 80% of cases of ventriculomegaly.[13] Obstetric management may include amniocentesis to rule out chromosomal anomalies and laboratory tests to rule out congenital infections. In addition to numerous intracranial abnormalities associated with ventriculomegaly, the fetus should be surveyed for defects involving the face, heart, kidneys, abdominal wall, thorax, and limbs.

Severe hydrocephaly may be confused with hydranencephaly and holoprosencephaly. Documenting a complete falx and the presence of the choroid plexus in the lateral ventricles and a separate third and fourth ventricle may help to differentiate severe ventriculomegaly from other anomalies.

MICROCEPHALY

Microcephaly is an abnormally small head that falls 2 standard deviations below the mean.[21] It occurs because the brain is reduced in size. Isolated microcephaly occurs in 1 per 1000 births but is more commonly caused by an associated anomaly.[21]

Microcephaly may result from inheritance of either an autosomal-dominant or autosomal-recessive pattern. Microcephaly may also occur with chromosomal aberrations and various brain anomalies. Teratogens linked with microcephaly include congenital infections (rubella, toxoplasmosis, cytomegalovirus), maternal alcohol abuse, heroin addiction, mercury poisoning, maternal phenylketonuria, radiation, and hypoxia.[5,21]

The prognosis for fetuses with microcephaly depends somewhat on the etiology. About 85% of children with microcephaly are mentally retarded.[5]

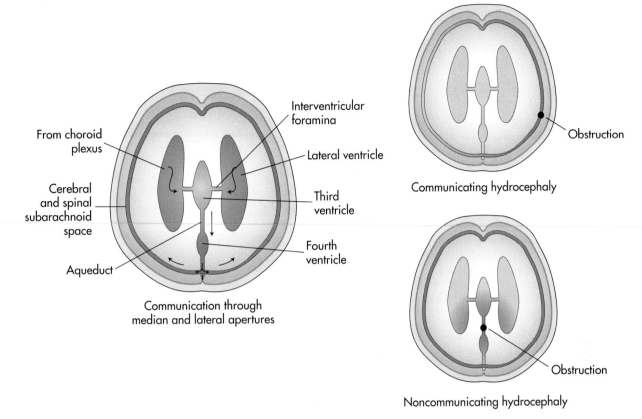

Figure 37-41 The course of the cerebrospinal fluid and its obstruction in hydrocephaly. Normally the cerebrospinal fluid from the choroid plexuses flows through the interventricular foramina to the third ventricle, aqueduct, fourth ventricle, median and lateral apertures, and spinal and cerebral subarachnoid space. It is then taken into the venous system (e.g., the cranial venous sinuses). Obstruction occurs within the ventricular system (e.g., at the aqueduct) in noncommunicating hydrocephaly (i.e., the ventricles and the subarachnoid space do not communicate). Obstruction occurs outside the ventricular system (e.g., in the cranial subarachnoid space) in communicating hydrocephaly (i.e., the ventricles and the subarachnoid space communicate).

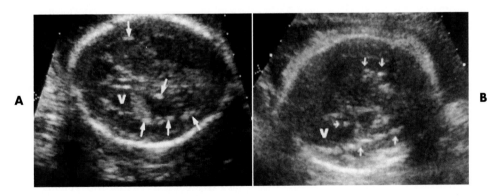

Figure 37-42 A, Periventricular calcifications *(arrows)* and ventriculomegaly *(v)* found in a 20-week fetus. An infectious etiology was suspected. All testing had proven negative. B, In the same fetus at 30 weeks of gestation, persistent periventricular calcifications *(arrows)* with ventriculomegaly *(v)* was observed. No other anomalies or complications were present.

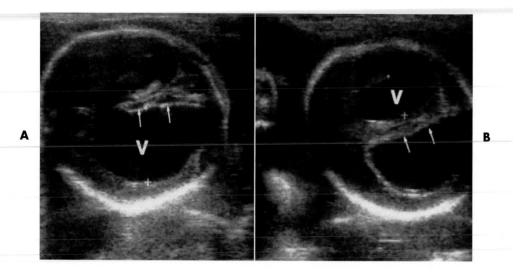

Figure 37-43 A, Ventriculomegaly observed in the distal cranial hemisphere in a 25-week twin fetus with severe growth restriction. The ventricle measured 28 mm in diameter. *Arrows,* Interhemispheric fissure. **B,** In the same fetus the proximal ventricle *(V)* is displayed measuring 17 mm in diameter. Note the asymmetry between the ventricles, suggesting a shift of the interhemispheric fissure *(arrows)* and porencephaly. The larger distal ventricle represents the actual porencephalic cyst, whereas the smaller ventricle has dilated in response to the infarction. Premature delivery occurred at 26 weeks of gestation because of chronic twin-twin transfusion syndrome in a monochorionic pregnancy. The twin, depicted in these figures, died shortly after birth. Autopsy confirmed the occurrence of the porencephalic event as an end result of the severe shunting of blood within the placental cotyledons.

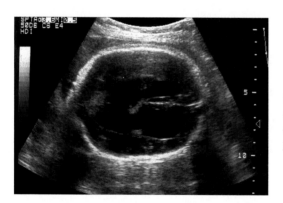

Figure 37-44 Ventriculomegaly caused by spina bifida. The anterior choroid plexus "dangles" into the posterior ventricle.

Ultrasound findings. Sonographic diagnosis of microcephaly depends on an accurate assessment of fetal age. Biparietal diameter, occipitofrontal diameter, and head circumference should be used when evaluating for microcephaly. In addition, ratios comparing the head perimeter to abdominal perimeter and the head perimeter to the femur length are also useful. Impaired cranial growth should coincide with appropriate growth of the abdominal circumference and femur length. Serial measurements for a fetus as risk for microcephalus should be performed at monthly intervals. Because microcephaly may manifest later in the pregnancy, diagnosis before 24 weeks of gestation may be impossible.

Sonographic features of microcephaly include the following:

• A small biparietal diameter (Figure 37-45)
• A small head circumference

• Abnormal head circumference/abdomen circumference and head circumference to femur length ratios

Other sonographic findings associated with microcephaly may include disorganized brain tissue and ventriculomegaly. A thorough search for evidence of an associated anomaly should ensue, including careful investigation of the fetal heart. Cerebral calcifications may be identified with congenital infections. A fetus with an encephalocele may have microcephaly because of the amount of brain tissue protruding outside the calvarium. Other cranial anomalies associated with microcephaly include porencephaly, agenesis of the corpus callosum, craniosynostosis, holoprosencephaly, lissencephaly, schizencephaly, macrogyria, microgyria, agyria, and Kleeblattschadel defect. Microcephaly has been associated with trisomies 13, 18, 21, and 22 and with triploidy. Numerous

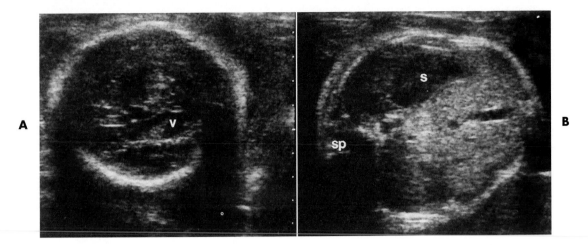

Figure 37-45 A, Microcephalus shown in a 32-week fetus with marked head to abdomen disproportion. Cranial diameters fell 3 to 5 standard deviations below the mean. Ventriculomegaly was observed. *v,* Lateral ventricle. **B,** In the same fetus the cross-section through the abdomen is shown. *s,* Stomach; *sp,* spine. There was a positive family history for autosomal-dominant congenital microcephalus.

syndromes have been linked with microcephaly, including Meckel-Gruber syndrome, Pena Shokeir, and Neu-Laxora syndrome.[18,21]

REVIEW QUESTIONS

1. Differentiate among anencephaly, acrania, and encephalocele and describe the sonographic features of each.
2. Describe ventriculomegaly.
3. What are the criteria for diagnosing ventriculomegaly?
4. What is a vein of Galen aneurysm and how would you distinguish it from an arachnoid cyst or porencephalic cyst?
5. Describe spina bifida and its sonographic features.

REFERENCES

1. Bennett GL and others: Agenesis of the corpus callosum: prenatal detection usually is not possible before 22 weeks of gestation, *Radiology* 199:447, 1996.
2. Callen PW: *Ultrasonography in obstetrics and gynecology,* ed 3, Philadelphia, 1994, WB Saunders.
3. Campbell J and others: Ultrasound screening for spina bifida: cranial and cerebellar signs in a high risk population, *Obstet Gynecol* 70:247, 1987.
4. Carlson BM: *Human embryology and developmental biology,* ed 2, St Louis, 1999, Mosby.
5. Chervenak FA and others: The diagnosis of fetal microcephaly, *Am J Obstet Gynecol* 149:512, 1984.
6. Chisholm CA and others: Aneurysm of the vein of Galen: prenatal diagnosis and perinatal management, *Am J Perinatol* 13:503, 1996.
7. Chung CS and others: Factors affecting risks of congenital malformations. I, Epidemiological analysis, *Birth Defects* 11:1, 1975.
8. Coniglio SJ and others: Developmental outcomes of children with myelomeningocele: prenatal predictors, *Am J Ostet Gynecol* 177:319, 1997.
9. Doren M and others: Prenatal sonographic diagnosis of a vein of Galen aneurysm: relevance of associated malformations for timing and mode of delivery, *Ultrasound Obstet Gynecol* 6:287, 1995.
10. Green MF and others: Hydranencephaly: US appearance during in utero evolution, *Radiology* 156:779, 1985.
11. Gupta JK and others: Clinical significance of fetal choroid plexus cysts, *Lancet* 346:724, 1995.
12. Hautman GD and others: Acrania, *J Ultrasound Med* 14:552, 1995.
13. Johnson SP and others: Ultrasound screening for anencephaly at 10-14 weeks of gestation, *Ultrasound Obstet* 9:14, 1997.
14. Main DM and others: Neural tube defects: issues in prenatal diagnosis and counseling, *Obstet Gynecol* 67:1, 1986.
15. Martin RA and others: Absence of the superior labial frenulum in holoprosencephaly: a new diagnostic sign, *J Pediatr* 133:151, 1998.
16. Montemagno R and others: Disappearance of fetal choroid plexus cysts during the second trimester in cases of chromosomal abnormality, *Br J Obstet Gynaecol* 102:752, 1995.
17. Morcos CL and others: The isolated choroid plexus cyst, *Obstet Gynecol* 92:232, 1998.
18. Nyberg DA, Mahony BS, Pretorius DH, editors: *Diagnostic ultrasound of fetal anomalies: text and atlas,* St Louis, 1990, Mosby.
19. Packard AM and others: Schizencephaly: correlations of clinical and radiologic features, *Neurology* 48:1427, 1997.
20. Ruge JR and others: Agenesis of the corpus callosum: female monozygotic triplets, *J Neurosurg* 85:152, 1996.
21. Saunders RC and others: *Structural fetal abnormalities,* St Louis, 1996, Mosby.
22. Shuangshoti S and others: Neuroepithelial (colloid) cysts, *Arch Pathol* 80:214, 1965.
23. Tegeler CH and others: *Neurosonology,* St Louis, 1996, Mosby.
24. Weissman A and others: Fetal acrania: five new cases and review of the literature, *J Clin Ultrasound* 25:511, 1997.

The Fetal Face and Neck

Sandra L. Hagen-Ansert

OBJECTIVES

- Describe the basic embryology of the face
- Evaluate the fetal face for normal and abnormal features
- Describe abnormalities of the orbits
- Evaluate for cleft lip and palate
- Describe abnormalities of the neck

EMBRYOLOGY

SONOGRAPHIC EVALUATION

ABNORMALITIES OF THE FACE
ABNORMALITIES OF THE FACIAL PROFILE
ABNORMALITIES OF THE ORBITS
ABNORMALITIES OF THE NOSE, MAXILLA, LIPS, AND PALATE
ABNORMALITIES OF THE ORAL CAVITY AND MANDIBLE
ABNORMALITIES OF THE NECK

REVIEW QUESTIONS

KEY TERMS

acrocephalopolysyndactyly - congenital anomaly characterized by a peaked head and webbed fingers and toes
anophthalmia - absent eyes
Beckwith-Wiedemann syndrome - group of disorders having in common the coexistence of an omphalocele, macroglossia, and visceromegaly
cephalocele - protrusion of the brain from the cranial cavity
craniosynostoses - premature closure of the cranial sutures
epignathus - teratoma located in the oropharynx
exophthalmia - abnormal protrusion of the eyeball
fetal cystic hygroma - malformation of the lymphatic system that leads to single or multiloculated lymph-filled cavities around the neck

holoprosencephaly - congenital defect caused by an extra chromosome which causes a deficiency in the forebrain
hypotelorism - eyes too close together
macroglossia - hypertrophied tongue
microcephaly - head smaller than the body
micronathia - small chin
microphthalmia - small eyes
nuchal lucency - increased thickness in the nuchal fold area in the back of the neck associated with trisomy 21
oculodentodigital dysplasia - underdevelopment of the eyes, fingers, and mouth
phenylketonuria (PKU) - hereditary disease caused by failure to oxidize an amino acid (phynyladlanine) to tyrosine, because of a defective enzyme; if PKU is not treated early, mental retardation can develop
strabismus - eye disorder in which optic axes cannot be directed to the same object
teratoma - solid tumor

Congenital anomalies of the face affect 1 in 600 births.[12,26] Cleft lip, hypotelorism and hypertelorism, and micrognathia are examples of facial problems that may be found by ultrasound during pregnancy (Table 38-1). As in other investigations, the detection of subtle facial malformations depends on scanner skill, the position of the fetus, the amount of amniotic fluid near the face, and ability to recognize facial pathology.

EMBRYOLOGY

In its 4th week the embryo has characteristic external features of the head and neck area in the form of a series of branchial arches, pouches, grooves and membranes. These structures are referred to as the branchial apparatus and bear a resemblance to gills.

There are six branchial arches; however, only the first four are visible externally (Figure 38-1, *A*). Each of the arches is separated by branchial grooves and is composed of a core of mesenchymal cells. The mesenchyme forms the cartilages, bones, muscles, and blood vessels.

The first branchial arch is also known as the mandibular arch that forms the jaw, zygomatic bone, ear, and tem-

TABLE 38-1	POTENTIAL FETAL MALFORMATIONS ASSOCIATED WITH MATERNAL DRUG OR CHEMICAL USE
Drug	**Fetal Malformations**
Acetaminophen overdose	Polyhydramnios
Acetazolamide	Sacrococcygeal teratoma
Acetylsalicylic acid	Intracranial hemorrhage, IUGR
Albuterol	Tachycardia
Alcohol (ethanol)	Microcephaly, micrognathia, cleft palate, short nose, hypoplastic philtrum, cardiac defects (VSD, ASD, double-outlet right ventricle, pulmonary atresia, dextrocardia, tetralogy of Fallot), IUGR, diaphragmatic hernia, pectus excavatum, radioulnar, synostosis, scoliosis, bifid xyphoid, NTDs
Amantadine	Cardiac defects (single ventricle with pulmonary atresia)
Aminopterin	NTDs, hydrocephalus, incomplete skull ossification, brachycephaly, micrognathia, clubfoot, syndactyly, hypoplasia of thumb and fibula, IUGR
Amitriptyline	Micrognathia, limb reduction, swelling of hands and feet, urinary retention
Amobarbital	NTDs, cardiac defects, severe limb deformities, congenital hip dislocation, polydactyly, clubfoot, cleft palate, ambiguous genitalia, soft tissue, deformity of neck
Antithyroid drugs	Goiter
Azathioprine	Cardiac defects (pulmonary valve stenosis), polydactyly
Betamethasone	Reduced head circumference
Bromides	Polydactyly, clubfoot, congenital hip dislocation
Busulfan	Pyloric stenosis, cleft palate, microphthalmia, IUGR
Caffeine	Musculoskeletal defects, hydronephrosis
Captopril	Leg reduction
Carbamazepine	NTDs, cardiac defects (atrial septal defect), nose hypoplasia, hypertelorism, cleft lip, congenital hip dislocation
Carbon monoxide	Cerebral atrophy, hydrocephalus, fetal demise
Chlordiazepoxide	Microcephaly, cardiac defects, duodenal atresia
Chloroquine	Hemihypertrophy
Chlorpheniramine	Hydrocephalus, polydactyly, congenital hip dislocation
Chlorpropamide	Microcephaly, dysmorphic hands and fingers
Clomiphene	NTDs, microcephaly, syndactyly, clubfoot, polydactyly, esophageal atresia
Cocaine	Spontaneous abortion, placental abruption, prematurity, IUGR, possible cardiac defects, skull defects, genitourinary anomalies
Codeine	Hydrocephalus, head defects, cleft palate, musculoskeletal defects, dislocated hip, pyloric stenosis, respiratory malformations
Cortisone	Hydrocephalus, cardiac defects, (VSD, coarctation of aorta), clubfoot, cleft lip
Coumadin	NTDs, cardiac defects, scoliosis, skeletal deformities, nasal hypoplasia, stippled epiphyses, chondrodysplasia punctata, short phalanges, toe defects, incomplete rotation of gut, IUGR, bleeding
Cyclophosphamide	Cardiac defects, cleft palate, flattened nasal bridge, four toes on each foot, syndactyly, hypoplastic midphalanx
Cytarabine	NTDs, cardiac defects, lobster claw hand, missing digits of feet, syndactyly
Daunorubicin	NTDs, cardiac defects, syndactyly
Dextroamphetamine	NTDs, cardiac defects, IUGR
Diazepam	NTDs, cardiac defects, absence of arm, syndactyly, absence of thumbs, cleft lip/palate
Diphenhydramine	Clubfoot, cleft palate
Disulfiram	Vertebral fusion, clubfoot, radial aplasia, phocomelia, tracheoesophageal fistula
Diuretics	Respiratory malformations
Estrogens	Cardiac defects, limb reduction
Ethosuximide	Hydrocephalus, short neck, oral cleft
Fluorouracil	Radial aplasia, absent thumbs, aplasia of esophagus and duodenum, hypoplasia of lungs
Fluphenazine	Poor ossification of frontal bone, cleft palate
Haloperidol	Limb deformities
Heparin	Bleeding
Imipramine	NTDs, cleft palate, renal cysts, diaphragmatic hernia
Indomethacin	Fetal demise, hemorrhage

TABLE 38-1	POTENTIAL FETAL MALFORMATIONS ASSOCIATED WITH MATERNAL DRUG OR CHEMICAL USE—cont'd	
Drug	**Fetal Malformations**
Isoniazid	NTDs
Lithium	NTDs, cardiac defects (VSD, Ebstein's anomaly, mitral atresia, dextrocardia)
Lysergic acid diethylamide (LSD)	NTDs, limb defects
Meclizine	Cardiac defects (hypoplastic left heart), respiratory defect
Meprobamate	Cadiac defects, limb defects
Methotrexate	Oxycephaly, absence of frontal bones, large fontanelles, micrognathia, long webbed fingers, low-set ears, IUGR, dextrocardia
Methyl mercury	Microcephaly, asymmetric head
Metronidazole	Midline facial defects
Nortriptyline	Limb reduction
Oral contraceptives	NTDs, cardiac defects, vertebral defects, limb reduction, IUGR, tracheoesophageal malformation
Paramethadione	Cardiac defects, IUGR
Phenobarbital	NTDs, digital anomalies, cleft palate, ileal atresia, IUGR, pulmonary hypoplasia
Phenothiazines	Microcephaly, syndactyly, clubfoot, omphalocele
Phenylephrine	Eye and ear abnormalities, syndactyly, clubfoot, hip dislocation, umbilical hernia
Phenylpropanolamine	Pectus excavatum, polydactyly, hip dislocation
Phenytoin (hydantoin)	Microcephaly, wide fontanelles, cardiac defects, IUGR, cleft/lip palate, hypertelorism, low-set ears, short neck, short nose, broad nasal bridge, hypoplastic distal phalanges, digital thumb, hip dislocation, rib-sternal abnormalities
Polychlorinated biphenyls	Spotted calcification in skull, fetal demise, IUGR
Primidone	Cardiac defects (VSD), webbed neck, small mandible
Procarbazine	Cerebral hemorrhage, oligodactyly
Progesterones	NTDs, hydrocephaly, cardiac defects (tetralogy of Fallot, truncus arteriosus, VSD), absent thumbs
Quinine	Hydrocephalus, cardiac defects, facial defects, vertebral anomalies, dysmelias
Retinoic acid (vitamin A)	Hydrocephalus, cerebral malformations, microcephaly, cardiac defects, limb deformities, fetal demise, cleft palate, rib abnormalities
Spermicides	Limb reduction
Sulfonamide	Limb hypoplasia, foot defects, urethral obstruction
Tetracycline	Limb hypoplasia, clubfoot
Thalidomide	Cardiac defects, spine defects, limb reduction (amelia), phocomelia, hypoplasia, duodenal stenosis or atresia, pyloric stenosis
Thioguanine	Missing digits
Tobacco	IUGR
Tolbutamide	Syndactyly, absent toes, accessory thumb
Toluene	IUGR, neonatal hyperchloremia acidosis, possible mental dysfunction, cardiac defects, dysmorphic facies
Trifluoperazine	Cardiac defects, phocomelia
Trimethadione	Microcephaly, low-set ears, broad nasal bridge, cardiac defects (ASD, VSD), IUGR, cleft lip and palate, esophageal atresia, malformed hands, clubfoot
Valproic acid	NTDs, microcephaly, wide fontanelle, cardiac defects, IUGR, cleft palate, hypoplastic nose, low-set ears, small mandible, depressed nasal bridge, polydactyly

From Nyberg DA, Mahoney BS, Pretorius DH: *Diagnostic ultrasound of fetal anomalies: text and atlas,* St. Louis, 1990, Mosby.
IUGR, intrauterine growth restriction; *ASD,* atrial septal defect; *NTD,* neural tube defects; *VSD,* ventricular septal defect.

poral bone (Figure 38-1, *B*). The second branchial arch contributes to the hyoid bone.

The branchial arches consist of mesenchymal tissue derived from intraembryonic mesoderm covered by ectoderm and containing transderm. Neural crest cells migrate into the branchial arches and proliferate, resulting in swellings that demarcate each arch. The neural crest cells develop the skeletal parts of the face and the mesoderm of each arch develops the musculature of the face and neck.

The maxillary prominences arise from the first branchial arch and grow cranially just under the eyes, and the mandibular prominence which grows inferiorly. The primitive mouth is an indentation on the surface of the ectoderm (referred to as the stomodeum) (Figure 38-2). By the 5th week of development, five prominences are identified: the frontal nasal prominence, forming the upper boundary of the stomodeum; the paired maxillary prominences of the first branchial arch, forming the lateral

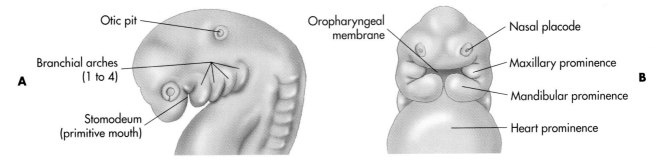

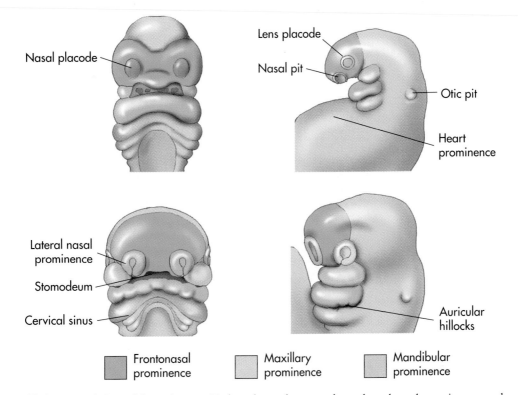

Figure 38-1   **A,** Lateral view of the embryo at 28 days shows 4 of the 6 branchial arches, otic pit, and stomodeum. **B,** Frontal view of the embryo at 24 days demonstrates the nasal placode, maxillary prominence, and mandibular prominence.

Figure 38-2   Frontal view of the embryo at 33 days shows the stomodeum, lateral nasal prominence, and cervical sinus.

boundaries of the stomodeum; and the paired mandibular prominences forming the caudal boundary.

The nasal pits are formed as the surface ectoderm thickens into the nasal placodes on each side of the frontal nasal prominence; as these placodes invaginate, the nasal pits are formed (Figure 38-3). Until 24 to 26 days of gestation, the stomodeum is separated from the pharynx by a membrane that ruptures by around 26 days, to place the primitive gut in communication with the amniotic cavity.[6]

The maxillary prominences grow medially between the 5th and 8th weeks. This growth compresses the medial nasal prominences together toward the midline. The two medial nasal prominences and the two maxillary prominences lateral to them fuse together to form the upper lip

(Figure 38-4). The medial nasal prominences form the medial aspect of the lip, which is the origin of the labial component of the lip, the upper incisor teeth, and the anterior aspect of the primary palate. The lateral nasal prominences form the alae of the nose. The maxillary prominences and lateral nasal prominences are separated by the nasolacrimal groove. The ectoderm in the floor of this groove forms the nasolacrimal duct and lacrimal sac.

The nose is formed in three parts. The bridge of the nose originates from the frontal prominence, the two medial nasal prominences form the crest and tip of the nose, and the lateral nasal prominences form the sides, or alae. The mandibular prominences merge at the end of the 4th to 5th week and form the lower lip, chin, and mandible.

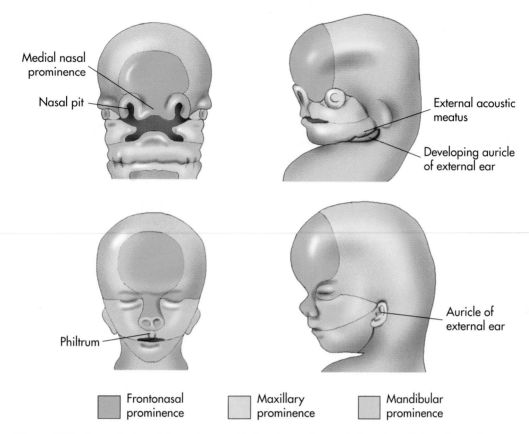

Figure 38-3 Frontal view of the embryo at 40 days shows the nasal pit and medial nasal prominence.

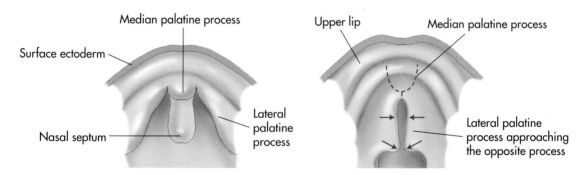

Figure 38-4 First trimester development of the roof of the mouth showing the formation of the upper lip and palate.

SONOGRAPHIC EVALUATION

Fetal facial evaluation is not routinely included in a basic fetal scan; however, when there is a family history of craniofacial malformation or when another congenital anomaly is found, the face should be screened for a coexisting facial malformation. Many fetuses with a facial defect also have chromosomal abnormalities. Extensive facial screening may be hindered by bone shadowing, poor fetal positioning, oligohydramnios, and maternal obesity. Facial anomalies often indicate a specific syndrome or condition (e.g., orbital fusion and a proboscis suggest alobar holoprosencephaly). The use of three-dimensional ultrasound reconstruction shows promise for outlining specific facial detail (Box 38-1).

Facial anomalies are heterogeneous and occur as isolated defects or as part of a syndrome. A family history of a facial anomaly (e.g., cleft lip) may prompt a targeted study, although recurrence risks are relatively low (less than 5%).

ABNORMALITIES OF THE FACE

ABNORMALITIES OF THE FACIAL PROFILE

Forehead. The fetal forehead may be appreciated by evaluation of the profile. This is achieved by a series of midsagittal scans through the face. The fetal forehead (frontal bone) appears as a curvilinear surface with differ-

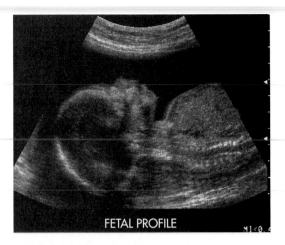

Figure 38-5 The fetal profile is well seen with amniotic fluid surrounding the face. This is a useful place to image the forehead, nose, lips, and chin.

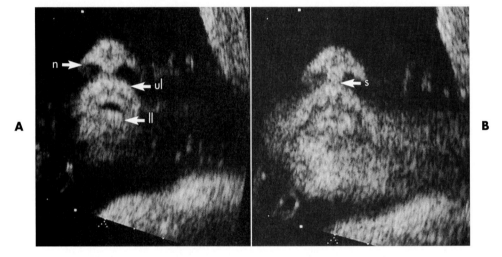

Figure 38-6 **A,** Axial view through the upper *(ul)* and lower lip *(ll)* in a fetus with an open mouth. Note the nares *(n)* and nasal septum. This is the view used to check for a cleft of the upper lip. **B,** In the same fetus, same anatomy viewed with a closed mouth. *s,* Nasal septum.

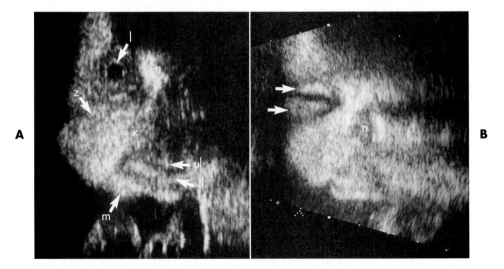

Figure 38-7 **A,** Coronal view showing facial features. Lens *(l),* zygomatic bone *(z),* maxilla *(x),* upper lip *(ul),* lower lip *(ll),* mandible *(m),* nasal bones *(n).* **B,** In the same fetus, in a more anterior coronal view, the upper and lower eyelids *(arrows)* and nose *(n)* are shown.

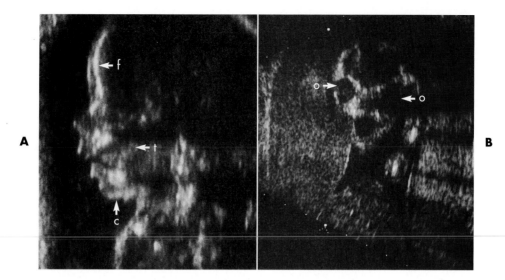

Figure 38-8   A, Sagittal view in a 23-week fetus, showing the contour of the face in profile. Note the smooth surface of the frontal bone *(f)* the appearance of the nose, upper and lower lips, tongue *(t)* and chin, *(c)*. **B,** Coronal facial view in an 18-week fetus, revealing a wide-open mouth. Note the nasal bones between the orbits *(o)*.

BOX 38-2   QUESTIONS THE SONOGRAPHER SHOULD ANSWER

- Are the orbits normally spaced?
- Are the nose and nasal bridge clearly imaged; is a proboscis or cebocephaly present?
- Are any periorbital masses apparent?
- Is the upper lip intact?
- Is the tongue normal size?
- Is the chin abnormally small?
- Are the ears normal size and position?

BOX 38-3   SONOGRAPHY OF THE FACIAL PROFILE

Use midsagittal scans through the face
- Appears as curvilinear surface with differentiation of forehead, nose, lips, and chin
- Clover-leaf skull: misshapened skull with clover leaf appearance
- Frontal bossing: Lemon-shaped skull or absent, depressed nasal bridge
- Strawberry-shaped cranium: Bulging of frontal bones
- Masses of nose and upper lip: Distortion of facial profile (look for cleft lip)

---

entiation of the forehead, nose, lips, and chin. This view allows diagnosis of anterior cephaloceles, which may arise from the frontal bone. Anterior cephaloceles may cause widely spaced orbits (hypertelorism) (Boxes 38-2 and 38-3).[23]

Off-axis encephaloceles have also been reported with amniotic band syndrome. This occurs when the amnion disrupts early in the embryonic period, leaving strains of tissue within the uterus that may lead to malformation of the fetus.[13]

Skull. *Clover-leaf* skull appears as an unusually misshapen skull with a clover-leaf appearance. Clover-leaf skull has been associated with skeletal dysplasias (dwarfism) and ventriculomegaly.[7,23] Any irregularities in the contour of the forehead should prompt the investigator to search for other malformations. Profile views of the fetal skull are also helpful in the study of fetuses at risk for thanatophoric dysplasia, achondroplasia, and osteopetrosis, in which a prominent forehead is characteristic.[51]

Frontal bossing may be observed in a fetus with a lemon-shaped skull (from spina bifida) or when there is an absent or depressed nasal bridge (found in achondroplasia,

chondrodysplasia punctata, and asphyxiating thoracic dysplasia). In a fetus with a strawberry-shaped cranium, there may be bulging of the frontal bones (Figure 38-9).

Frontonasal dysplasia is a median-cleft face syndrome consisting of a range of midline facial defects involving the eyes, forehead, and nose. Abnormalities include ocular hypertelorism, a variable bifid nose, broad nasal bridge, midline defect of the frontal bone, and extension of the frontal hairline to form a widow's peak.[14] The cause of frontonasal dysplasia is unknown, and the occurrence is sporadic.

By ultrasound, the primary finding is hypertelorism. If one cranial abnormality is found, the sonographer should carefully look for additional dysmorphic features.[14]

Nuchal Area. The association of first-trimester fetal nuchal lucency with aneuploidy is well established and is dependent on the size and extent of the nuchal abnormality.[22] Fetuses with diffuse fetal nuchal fluid and hydrops involving the fetal torso have a high prevalence of chromosomal anomalies and poor outcome.[22] In one study 44 fetuses between 9 and 14 weeks of gestation were identified as having an isolated nuchal lucency measuring 3 cm or more.[23] All patients with diffuse cystic hygromas, hydrops, or other abnormality were excluded from the study. Five fetuses had chromosomal abnormalities (trisomy 21). Three fetuses spontaneously aborted. Of the 36 fetuses 27 had normal karyotype by amniocentesis. Twenty patients showed resolution of the nuchal lucencies. The study concluded that the presence of an isolated nuchal lucency in the first trimester is associated with a 12.5% prevalence of chromosomal abnormalities and an increased risk of spontaneous miscarriage and premature delivery.

Nose and Upper Lip. Masses of the nose and upper lip may distort the facial profile and indicate a cleft lip (Figures 38-10 and 38-11).

The sonographer should look for nostril symmetry, nasal septum integrity, and continuity of upper lip to ex-

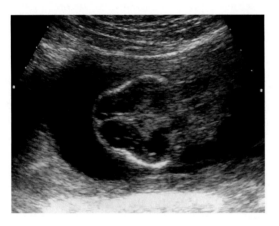

Figure 38-9 Axial view of the fetal head that demonstrates a "strawberry"-shaped cranium secondary to bulging of the frontal bones.

clude a cleft lip and palate. Tumors may disrupt facial contours, such as epignathus or a teratoma.

Tongue. Tongue protrusion may suggest macroglossia (enlarged tongue), a condition found in Beckwith-Wiedemann syndrome (congenital overgrowth of tissues).

Congenital **micrognathia** may be suspected when a small chin is observed.

Ear. Ear malformations are rarely predicted prenatally. Low-set ears may be appreciated in a longitudinal view when the placement of the ear appears lower than usual (e.g., as in clover-leaf skull). Ear malformation may be observed in Goldenhar's syndrome with anophthalmia (absent eye) and hemifacial microsomia.[20] Small ears (Robert's syndrome) and inadequate development of the ear (Nager acrofacial dystosis syndrome) may be observed prenatally.[19]

ABNORMALITIES OF THE ORBIT
Orbital architecture has become increasingly important in the evaluation of craniofacial anomalies. The anatomy of the orbits, their use in gestational age assessment, and their role in detecting ocular abnormalities have been investigated (Figure 38-12).[16,18]

The sonographer must document the presence of both eyes and assess the overall size of the eyes to exclude **microphthalmia** (small eyes) and **anophthalmia** (absent eyes). Masses of the orbit (periorbital) and of the eye (intraocular) may be excluded with careful scanning of the eyes. Periorbital masses, such as lacrimal duct cysts (dacryocystoceles), dermoids, and hemangiomas, have been reported.[20]

Transvaginal sonography has aided in early detection of ocular anomalies and other intracranial abnormalities. The

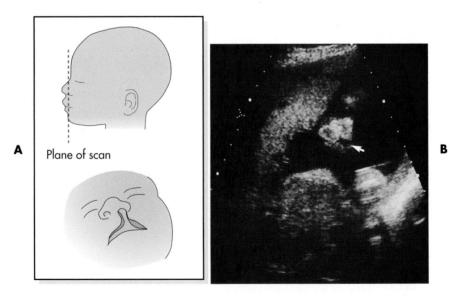

A   Plane of scan

B

Figure 38-10 **A,** Facial cleft. This drawing illustrates a plane of section that visualizes clefts of the upper lip. **B,** Axial view of upper lip *(arrow)* and nose suggesting a unilateral cleft of the lip in a 25-week fetus. There was a positive family history of cleft lip.

fetal eyes are evaluated on transvaginal sonography in a transverse section of the fetal skull at the orbital plane.[5] In addition, an oblique tangential section from the nasal bridge is used to detect the hypoechogenic circles lateral to the nose, in the anterior part of the orbits, representing the fetal lens. Using this method, ocular abnormalities, including strabismus, microphthalmia, divergence of lens, exophthalmia, and cataracts have been demonstrated.[5]

Orbital distance measurements are helpful in the diagnosis of fetal conditions in which hypotelorism or hypertelorism is a feature. Both of these conditions are associated with other anomalies, and often the orbital problem elucidates the type of cranial anomaly or genetic syndrome. An anatomic and biometric evaluation of the fetal orbits should be attempted in fetuses at risk for abnormal orbital distance.

Hypotelorism. Hypotelorism is a condition characterized by a decreased distance between the orbits (Figures 38-13 and 38-14). It is associated with several syndromes and other anomalies.[18,23] These conditions include holoprosencephaly, microcephaly, craniosynostoses, and phenylketonuria.

Hypotelorism may be seen in cyclopia by observing closely spaced orbits (see Figure 38-13) or eyes within a single orbit, and in ethmocephaly and cebocephaly (Figures 38-14 and 38-15).[18] Measurements of orbital width may identify fetuses with hypotelorism.

Hypertelorism. Hypertelorism is characterized by abnormally widely spaced orbits (Figure 38-16). Hypertelorism is found in several abnormal fetal conditions, genetic syndromes, and chromosomal anomalies. Fetuses

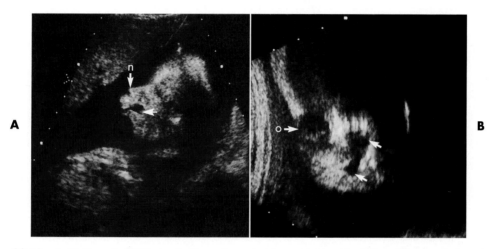

Figure 38-11 **A,** Unilateral cleft lip in the fetus shown in Figure 38-10, with clefting defect extending through the palate into the nasal cavity *(arrow)* in a sagittal plane in a 25-week fetus. Note the globular appearance of the tissue under the nose *(n)* (premaxillary protuberance). **B,** In the same fetus a coronal plane illustrates the extent of the clefting *(arrows).* Note the defect extending from the upper lip to the nasal cavity. Orbit *(o).*

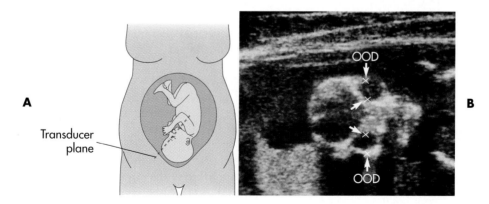

Figure 38-12 **A,** Frontal view demonstrating a fetus in a vertex presentation with the fetal cranium in an occipitotransverse position. The transducer is placed along the coronal plane (approximately 2 cm posterior to the glabella-alveolar line). **B,** Sonogram demonstrating the orbits in the coronal view. The outer orbital diameter *(OOD)* and inner orbital diameter, *IOD (angled arrows)* are viewed. The IOD is measured from the medial border of the orbit to the opposite medial border *(angled arrows).* The OOD is measured from the outermost lateral border of the orbit to the opposite lateral border.

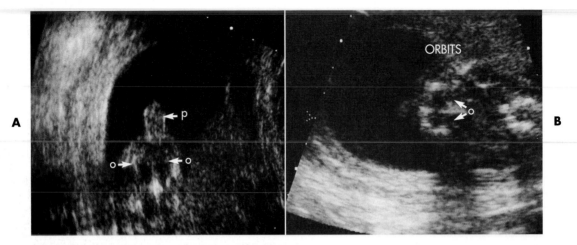

Figure 38-13 **A,** Proboscis *(p)* observed in a frontal facial view in a midline position above the closely spaced orbits *(o)* in a 20-week fetus with ethmocephaly. **B,** In the same fetus the orbits *(o)* are observed. A single eye was found with fused orbits. Trisomy 13 was found after delivery.

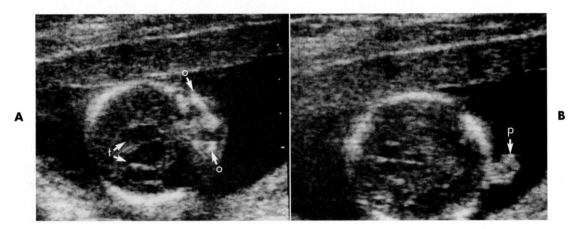

Figure 38-14 **A,** Transverse cross-section of the cranium in a 17-week fetus with holoprosencephaly. Fused thalami *(t)* and hypotelorism *(o)* are obvious. Measurements revealed abnormally closely spaced orbits (hypotelorism). **B,** In the same fetus a proboscis *(p)* is seen above the orbits, consistent with ethmocephaly.

exposed to phenytoin (Dilantin) during pregnancy may manifest signs of hypertelorism as part of the fetal phenytoin syndrome (microcephaly; growth abnormalities; cleft lip and/or palate; cardiac, genitourinary, central nervous system, and skeletal anomalies). In Pfeiffer's and Apert syndromes, hypertelorism and brachycephaly have been described as a result of abnormal closure of the cranial sutures (craniosynostosis).[23] In both syndromes, ventriculomegaly may be present. Other conditions that manifest with hypertelorism and premature suture closure include Crouzon syndrome, cephalosyndactyly, acrocephalopolysyndactyly, and oculodentodigital dysplasia.[23]

Fetal hypertelorism may be diagnosed by orbital distances that fall above normal ranges for gestational age.

Recognition of hypertelorism may provide evidence for a particular genetic syndrome or concurrent anomalies. Frontal cephaloceles may widen the space between the eyes. The reader is referred to comprehensive sources for a detailed list of conditions associated with hypertelorism.[20]

Frontonasal dysplasia (median cleft face syndrome) was diagnosed in a fetus with ventriculomegaly based on the sonographic findings of hypertelorism and cleft lip[10] (see Figure 38-16).

ABNORMALITIES OF THE NOSE, MAXILLA, LIPS, AND PALATE
The nose, maxilla, lips, and palate may be viewed by placing the transducer in a lateral coronal plane, sagittal profile plane, and in modified tangential maxillary view (inferior-superior projection) (see Figure 38-10).[4] In the lateral coronal view the integrity of the nasal structures in relationship to the orbital rings and maxillae is studied. In a profile plane the contour of the nose, upper and lower lips, and chin is observed. This is an important view in assessing the presence or absence of the nose, lips, and chin. Irregularities in nasal contour may indicate a particular syndrome. Tangential cuts, with the transducer angled inferiorly to superiorly through the maxilla, demonstrate the nasal septum, openings of the nostrils, and nares. In holo-

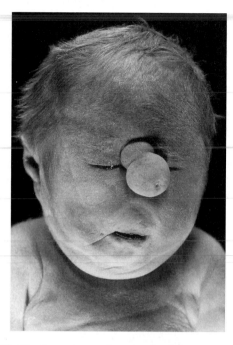

Figure 38-15   Postmortem photograph of a neonate with eth-mocephaly. Note the proboscis and hypotelorism. The mouth appeared normal. A common ventricle and absent optic and ophthalmic nerves were found. The chromosomes were consistent with trisomy 13.

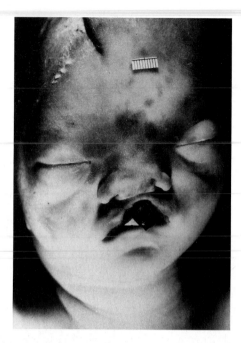

Figure 38-16   Postmortem photograph of neonate with median cleft face syndrome (frontonasal dysplasia). Note the hypertelorism and mass of the upper lip. Other abnormalities observed prenatally included severe ventriculomegaly with a shift of the interhemispheric fissure.

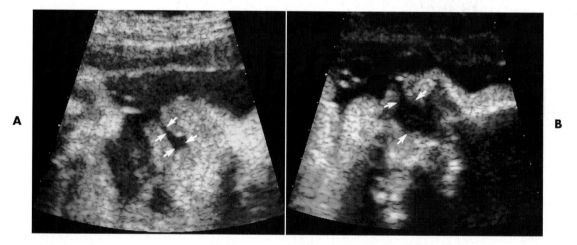

Figure 38-17   **A** and **B,** Facial profile of a fetus with a cleft lip and palate *(arrows).*

prosencephaly, nasal anomalies range from the presence of a proboscis to a single-nostril nose.

Evaluation of the nasal triad should assess (1) nostril symmetry, (2) nasal septum integrity, and (3) continuity of the upper lip to exclude cleft lip and palate. The sonographer should not mistake the normal nostrils or frenulum for a cleft. The maxilla marks the posterior border of the nose and is a landmark in assessing the fetus at risk for premaxillary protuberance as seen in Robert's syndrome.

Lip and Palate.   Cleft lip with or without cleft palate represents the most common congenital anomaly of the face (Figure 38-17).[2,24] Cleft lip occurs because of failure of fusion of the primary and secondary palate resulting in a clefting defect coursing anteriorly through the upper lip and alveolus. A cleft palate occurs when the lateral palatine processes fail to fuse in the midline. Cleft lip and palate occur together when both fusions are absent.[17,19]

A facial cleft may involve only the upper lip or may extend to involve the alveolus, posterior hard palate, and soft palate. Clefts may be unilateral or bilateral and may occur in isolation or in association with other anatomic and karyotype abnormalities.[2] Isolated posterior cleft palate is rec-

ognized as a distinct entity, quite separate from cleft lip alone or cleft lip and palate.

Clefts of the face may occur along various facial planes. Defects range from clefting of the lip alone to involvement of the hard and soft palate, which may extend into the nose and in rare cases to the inferior border of the orbit (Figure 38-18).[25] The frequency of cleft lip with or without a cleft palate shows ethnic variation. This disorder occurs in 1 per 600 births in Caucasians, in 1 per 3000 births in African Americans, in 1 per 350 births in Asians, and 1 in 150 to 1 in 250 births in Native Americans.[12,26]

Isolated cleft lip may occur as a unilateral or bilateral defect and when unilateral, commonly originates on the left side of the face. When there is a bilateral lesion, cleft palate is found in up to 85% of neonates. When unilateral, cleft palate may be seen in 70% of infants. Isolated cleft palate is a separate disorder from cleft lip associated with cleft palate. There are more than 200 facial cleft syndromes and counseling regarding recurrence is challenging.

The majority of cleft lip and/or palate occurrences are thought to have multiple causes.[25] Causes that may be prenatally detected include a familial predisposition for a cleft or chromosomal abnormalities (trisomies 13, 18, 21, triploidy, and translocations). Other prenatally detectable clefting conditions include acrocephalopolysyndactyly, amniotic band syndrome, anencephaly, congenital cardiac disease, diastrophic dysplasia, holoprosencephaly, Kniest dysplasia, spondyloepiphyseal dysplasia congenita, and Meckel-Gruber, Robert's, and multiple pterygium syndromes.[20] The combination of facial clefting, macroglossia, and an abnormally shaped mouth may suggest a syndrome.

A premaxillary protrusion or paranasal echogenic mass suggests the presence of a bilateral cleft lip and palate, even when sonographically only a unilateral defect is suspected. This paranasal mass of tissue corresponds to the abnormal anterior herniation of the hard palate and teeth caused by the defect.[21]

Sonographically, visualization of the hard and soft palates remains a diagnostic challenge because of considerable bony shadowing. The sonographer needs to use a systematic approach to examine the fetal face for clefts in the coronal and axial planes. Clinical investigation with three-dimensional ultrasound may contribute additional

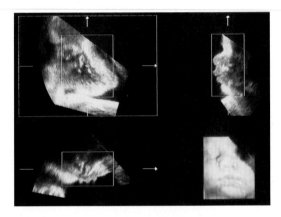

Figure 38-18 Three dimensional reconstruction of the fetal face in a 3 to 4 week fetus. The X, Y, and Z axis is aligned to reproduce the 3-dimensional image on the lower right.

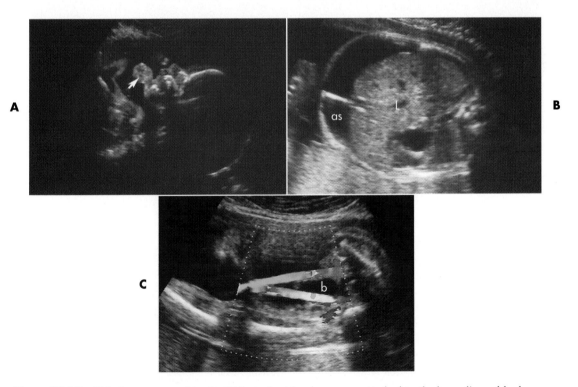

Figure 38-19 This fetus presented in the 26th week with a large mass attached to the lower lip and hydrops. **A,** Facial profile shows the solid mass *(arrow)* attached to the lower lip. **B,** Section across the fetal abdomen shows the fetal ascites *(as)* surrounding the liver *(L)*. **C,** Dilated hypogastric arteries *(color)* are shown on either side of the fetal bladder *(b)*.

information to image the palate and lip (Figure 38-19) (Box 38-4).

ABNORMALITIES OF THE ORAL CAVITY AND MANDIBLE

Oral Cavity. Few congenital malformations of the oral cavity exist. The normal fetus may exhibit various behavioral patterns, such as swallowing, protrusion and retrusion of the tongue, and hiccoughing. An abnormal positioning of the tongue may be indicative of a mass of the oral cavity, an obstructive process, or macroglossia (large tongue in Beckwith-Wiedemann syndrome).

The antenatal sonographic diagnosis of **epignathus** has been reported.[11] An epignathus is a teratoma located in the oropharynx (Figure 38-20). These masses may be highly complex and contain solid, cystic, or calcified components. In fetuses with epignathus, swallowing may be impaired, resulting in hydramnios. In these cases a small stomach may be present.

Mandible. A rare anomaly that causes a reduction of the chin (micrognathia) has been diagnosed. It is important to remember that hydramnios is a common feature with craniofacial malformations because of swallowing difficulties.

The fetal mandible (chin) may be observed in a profile view. The texture of the triangular-shaped mandible resembles that of the maxilla. Meticulous scanning should

ensue when a mass originates from the face. Attempts should be made to identify the origin of the mass to allow optimal counseling concerning prognosis, mode of delivery, and neonatal management.

ABNORMALITIES OF THE NECK

Congenital anomalies of the neck are rare but when present may represent life-threatening disorders. Neck masses are usually large and obvious because their presence causes distortion of the neck contour and adjacent structures. The most common neck mass is cystic hygroma colli (lymphatic obstruction). Rarer lesions include cervical meningomyelocele, hemangiomas, teratomas, goiter, sarcoma, and metastatic adenopathy.[20] Branchial cleft cysts (Figure 38-21) are prenatally detectable.

Clinically, a fetal neck mass is cause for concern. When a large tumor exists, delivery of the infant is complicated because the tumor may cause delivery dystocia (inability to deliver the trunk once the head has been delivered) and obstruction of the airway, which requires immediate intubation.

A goiter observed prenatally suggests that the mother may have hypothyroidism. When cystic hygroma is found (Figure 38-22), there is a high risk for Turner's syndrome (45,X). Other chromosomal defects are also associated with cystic hygroma (Figure 38-23). Cystic hygroma or lymphangiectasia may also result from heart failure (e.g., because of a cardiac malformation) (Figures 38-24 to 38-25).

Cystic Hygroma. **Fetal cystic hygroma** results from a malformation of the lymphatic system that leads to single or multiloculated lymph-filled cavities around the neck. Failure of the lymphatic system to properly connect with the venous system results in distension of the jugular lymph sacs and the accumulation of lymph in fetal tissues.[8, 27] This abnormal collection of lymph causes distension of the lymph cavities, causing fetal hydrops and even fetal death. Cystic hygromas are developmental defects of the lymphatic vessels. Normally the lymphatic vessels empty into two sacs lateral to the jugular veins (jugular lymph sacs). These sacs communicate with the venous sys-

---

> **BOX 38-4   SONOGRAPHIC FINDINGS OF CLEFT LIP AND PALATE**
>
> - Medial cleft lip: Caused by incomplete merging of the two medial nasal prominences in the midline
> - Oblique facial cleft: Failure of maxillary prominence to merge with the lateral nasal swelling, with exposure of the nasolacrimal duct
> - Complete bilateral cleft lip and palate: Large gap in upper lip on modified coronal view; nose is flattened and widened
> - Unilateral complete cleft lip and palate: Incomplete fusion of maxillary prominence to the medial prominence on one side; modified coronal view
> - Incomplete cleft: Nose is intact; modified coronal view of lip.

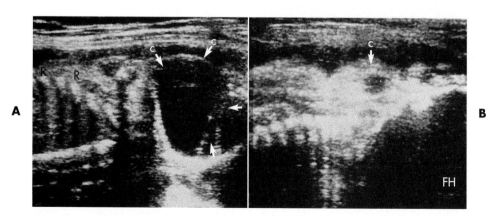

Figure 38-20   A, Brachial cleft cyst represented as a large unilateral septated cystic neck mass *(c, arrows).* R, Rib. **B,** In the same fetus the brachial cleft cyst *(c)* at term had almost completely resolved. The neonate had no complications after birth. *FH,* Fetal head.

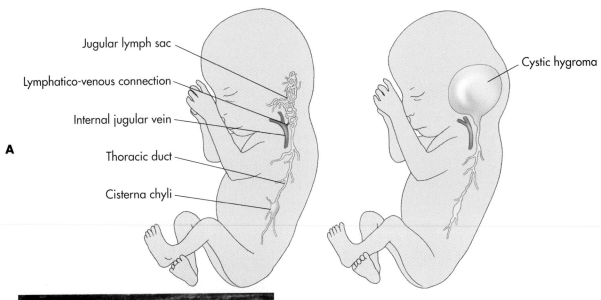

Jugular lymph sac
Lymphatico-venous connection
Internal jugular vein
Thoracic duct
Cisterna chyli

A

Cystic hygroma

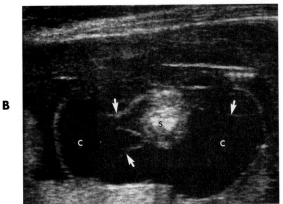

B

Figure 38-21 **A,** Lymphatic system in a normal fetus *(left)* with a patent connection between the jugular lymph sac and the internal jugular vein and a cystic hygroma and hydrops from a failed lymphaticovenous connection *(right).* **B,** Transverse neck view showing large posterolateral cystic masses *(c)* representing cystic hygromas in a fetus with Turner's syndrome. Note the multiple septations within the hygromas *(arrows).* s, Cervical spine. (**A** from Chervenak FA and others: *N Eng J Med* 309:822, 1985.)

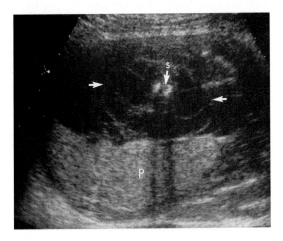

Figure 38-22 Cystic hygroma in a fetus with trisomy 21. Bilateral posterolateral cystic hygromas *(arrowheads)* identified at 19-weeks. *s,* Spine; *P,* placenta.

tem and form the right lymphatic duct and thoracic duct (see Figure 38-21).

Cystic hygromas may be small and regress because of alternative routes of lymph drainage. With this type of hygroma, webbing of the neck and swelling of the extremities may be appreciated after birth. These features are fre-

quently seen in neonates with Turner's syndrome. (45,X). These females are of short stature and are sterile. Cardiac and renal diseases are common. Cystic hygromas may present as isolated small cystic cavities with or without septations and may arise from the anterior, lateral, or posterior neck.[9] Small hygromas may be associated with other fetal anatomic defects.

Large fetal cystic hygromas have a typical sonographic appearance. Bilateral large cystic masses at the posterolateral borders of the neck may in severe cases surround the neck and head. Typically, a dense midline septum divides the hygroma, with septations noted within the dilated lymph sacs. Because of an accumulation of lymph in the fetal tissues, fetal hydrops results. Pericardial or pleural effusions, edema of thoracic and abdominal skin, ascites, and limb edema are common. Heart failure commonly results in intrauterine death.

A high incidence of large cystic hygromas have been demonstrated with Turner's syndrome.[8] Cystic hygromas are associated with other chromosomal anomalies. The prognosis for fetuses with cystic hygromas and hydrops is uniformly dismal. Because other fetal malformations are common, a careful study of fetal anatomy is necessary whenever a hygroma has been detected.

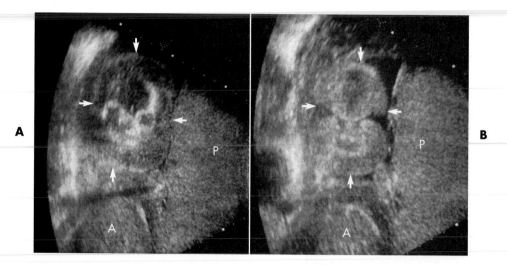

Figure 38-23 **A,** A coronal facial view shows significant facial edema *(arrows)* in a 22-week fetus with cystic hygromas (see Figure 38-25) and severe hydrops. Note the swelling of the scalp, cheeks, and chin. The placenta *(P)* appears hydropic. *A,* Abdomen. **B,** In the same fetus in a more frontal plane, soft-tissue swelling is evident. *A,* Abdomen. Amniocentesis revealed a normal karyotype.

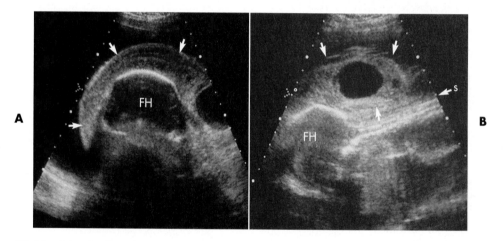

Figure 38-24 **A,** In the fetus shown in Figure 38-25, at 26 weeks of gestation, fetal movements were decreased, prompting ultrasound evaluation, which revealed a fetal demise. Note the helmetlike appearance of the scalp edema *(arrow)*. *FH,* Fetal head. **B,** In the same fetus, sagittal views revealed the posterolateral cystic hygroma *(arrow)* caused by lymphangiectasia from heart failure. *FH,* Fetal head; *s,* spine. Tetralogy of Fallot was revealed on autopsy.

The differential diagnosis for cystic hygroma includes meningomyelocele, encephalocele, nuchal edema, branchial cleft cyst, cystic teratoma, hemangiomas, and thyroglossal duct cysts.

A linear specular reflection has been routinely imaged along the back of the fetal neck in the late first trimester.[15] This normal finding should not be mistaken for a cystic hygroma in the first trimester. Typically, cystic hygromas appear as a multiseptated, thin-walled cystic masses near the fetal head or neck. Changes in configuration of the pseudomembrane occurring with fetal movements such as neck flexion and extension distinguish it from other sources of intrauterine membranes such as normal amnion, amniotic bands, and uterine synechiae.

The membrane seen in the first trimester appears hypoechoic because the underlying subcutaneous and muscular tissues are not well differentiated and contain few interfaces.

As the pregnancy progresses, the tissue becomes more complex with increased echogenicity.

Fetal Goiter. Reports of sonographically detected goiters are found in the literature.[3,28] A **fetal goiter** appears as a solid mass arising from the anterior fetal neck in the region of the fetal thyroid gland. A bilobed appearance may be visualized.[3] The esophagus may be obstructed by a goiter, resulting in hydramnios and a small or absent stomach. Follow-up studies of fetuses with goiter should include size

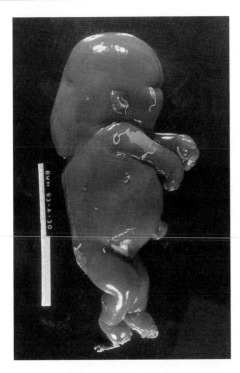

Figure 38-25 In the neonate shown in Figure 38-24, a side view shows the posterior lateral positioning of the cystic hygromas.

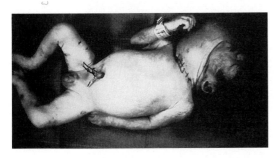

Figure 38-26 Large teratoma was found to arise from the posterior neck on this neonate. Multiple ultrasound studies demonstrated the mass to be complex in texture.

estimations, presence and size of fetal stomach, and amniotic fluid.

Teratoma. Neck **teratomas** are usually unilateral and may have complex sonographic (cystic, solid, echogenic) patterns similar to teratomas of other organs (Figure 38-26).[9,23]

The sonographer should evaluate a neck mass for the following characteristics:

- Position of mass (anterior, posterior, lateral, or midline)
- Unilateral or bilateral lesion
- Presence of nuchal ligament
- Doppler properties (hemangiomas have arterial and venous characteristics)
- Hydramnios is a common finding
- Heart failure and hydrops
- Coexisting anomalies
- Hyperextension, which may suggest neck mass or iniencephaly (fusion of occiput to spine)

The neck is often difficult to assess when amniotic fluid is decreased, when the fetus is in an unfavorable position, or when the neck is in close proximity to the placenta. Nonetheless, evaluation of the neck should be routinely attempted.

REVIEW QUESTIONS

1. Describe cleft lip and cleft palate. How are these conditions diagnosed prenatally?
2. Describe hypotelorism and hypertelorism?
3. Name conditions associated with hypotelorism and hypertelorism.
4. What facial anomalies are associated with holoprosencephaly?
5. What is cystic hygroma?
6. Describe the various sonographic presentations and conditions associated with cystic hygroma.

ACKNOWLEDGMENT

The author wishes to recognize the contribution of Kara Mayden Argo to this chapter of the fourth edition.

REFERENCES

1. Babcook CJ and others: Axial ultrasonographic imaging of the fetal maxilla for accurate characterization of facial clefts, *J Ultrasound Med* 16:619-625, 1997.
2. Barone CM and others: Sonographic detection of fetal goiter, an unusual cause of hydramnios, *J Ultrasound Med* 4:625, 1985.
3. Birnholz JC: Fetal portraiture helps to align ultrasound with traditional medicine, *Diagno Imaging* 1986, p 83.
4. Bronshtein M and others: First and second trimester diagnosis of fetal ocular defects and associated anomalies: report of eight cases, *Obstet Gynecol* 77:443-449, 1991.
5. Callen DW, editor: *Ultrasonography in obstetrics and gynecology,* ed 3, Philadelphia, 1995, WB Saunders.
6. Chervenak FA and others: Antenatal sonographic findings of thanatophoric dysplasia with cloverleaf skull, *Am J Obstet Gynecol* 146:948, 1983.
7. Chervenak FA and others: Fetal cystic hygroma: cause and natural history, *N Engl J Med* 309:822, 1983.
8. Chervenak FA and others: Antenatal sonographic diagnosis of epignathus, *J Ultrasound Med* 3:235, 1984.
9. Chervenak FA and others: Median cleft face syndrome: ultrasonic demonstration of cleft lip and hypertelorism, *Am J Obstet Gynecol* 149:94, 1984.
10. Chervenak FA and others: Diagnosis and management of fetal teratomas, *Obstet Gynecol* 66:666, 1985.
11. Chung CS and others: Factors affecting risks of congenital malformations. I. Epidemiological analysis, *Birth Defects* 11:1, 1975.
12. Finberg HJ and others: Craniofacial damage from amniotic band syndrome subsequent to pathologic chorioamniotic separation at 10 weeks gestation, *J Ultrasound Med* 15:665-668, 1996.
13. Frattarelli JL and others: Prenatal diagnosis of frontonasal dysplasia (Median cleft syndrome), *J Ultrasound Med* 15:81-83, 1996.

14. Hertzberg BS and others: Normal sonographic appearance of the fetal neck late in the first trimester: the pseudomembrane, *Radiology* 171:427-429, 1989.

15. Jeanty P and others: The binocular distance: a new parameter to estimated fetal age, *J Ultrasound Med* 3:241, 1984.

16. Kincaid K and others: Prenatal sonographic detection of cleft lip and palate, *J Diagn Med Sonogr* 6:309, 1989.

17. Mayden KL and others: Orbital diameters: a new parameter for prenatal diagnosis and dating, *Am J Obstet Gynecol* 144:289, 1982.

18. Moore KL, editor: *The developing human: clinically oriented embryology*, ed 4, Philadelphia, 1988, WB Saunders.

19. Nyberg DA, Mahony BS, Pretorius DH, editors: *Diagnostic ultrasound of fetal anomalies: text and atlas*, St Louis, 1990, Mosby.

20. Nyberg DA and others: Premaxillary protrusion: a sonographic clue to bilateral cleft lip and palate, *J Ultrasound Med* 12:331, 1993.

21. Reynders CS and others: First trimester isolated fetal nuchal lucency: significance and outcome, *J Ultrasound Med* 16:101-105, 1997.

22. Sanders RC: Ultrasonic assessment of the face and neck. In Sanders RC, editor: The principles and practice of ultrasonography in obstetrics and gynecology, Norwalk, Conn, 1985, Appleton-Century-Crofts.

23. Seeds JW and others: Techniques of early sonographic diagnosis of bilateral cleft lip and palate, *Obstet Gynecol* 62:2S, 1983.

24. Shafer WG and others: Developmental disturbances of oral and paraoral structures. In Shafer WG, editor: *A textbook of oral pathology*, ed 3. Philadelphia, 1974, WB Saunders.

25. Slavkin HC: Congenital craniofacial malformations: issues and perspectives, *J Prosthet Dent* 51:109, 1984.

26. van der Putte SC: Lymphatic malformation in human fetuses: a study of fetuses with Turner's syndrome or status: Bonnevie-Ullrich, *Virchows Arch [A] (Pathol Anat)* 376:233, 1977.

27. Weiner S and others: Antenatal diagnosis and treatment of a fetal goiter, *J Reprod Med* 24:39, 1980.

The Fetal Thorax

Sandra L. Hagen-Ansert

KEY TERMS

asphyxiating thoracic dystrophy - significantly narrow diameter of the chest in a fetus

bronchogenic cyst - most common lung cyst detected prenatally

bronchopulmonary sequestration - extra pulmonary tissue is present within the pleural lung sac (intralobar), or connected to the inferior border of the lung within its own pleural sac (extralobar)

congenital bronchial atresia - pulmonary anomaly which results from the focal obliteration of a segment of the bronchial lumen

cystic adenomatoid malformation (CAM) - abnormality in the formation of the bronchial tree with secondary overgrowth of mesenchymal tissue from arrested bronchial development

diaphragmatic hernia - opening in the pleuroperitoneal membrane that develops in the first trimester

foramen of Bochdalek - type of diaphragmatic defect that occurs posterior and lateral in the diaphragm; usually found in the left side

foramen of Morgagni - diaphragmatic hernia that occurs anterior and medial in the diaphragm that may communicate with the pericardial sac

lymphangiectasia - dilation of a lymph node

pleural effusion (hydrothorax) - accumulation of fluid within the thoracic cavity

pulmonary hypoplasia - small, underdeveloped lungs with resultant reduction in lung volume; secondary to prolonged oligohydramnios or as a consequence of a small thoracic cavity

The detection of thoracic defects is important, because many lesions may compromise fetal breathing and require surgery in the immediate neonatal period. Lung and diaphragm disorders are discussed in this section. Heart abnormalities may also cause devastating secondary compression effects (pulmonary hypoplasia) and are discussed in Chapter 40 (see also Table 38-1).

EMBRYOLOGY OF THE THORACIC CAVITY

One of the important determinants of whether the fetus can survive as a neonate in the air-filled, ex utero environment is the adequate biochemical and structural development and maturity of the lungs.[5] The adequacy of pulmonary development is probably the single most important determinant for fetal viability, and pulmonary immaturity is the

major reason why fetuses younger than 24 weeks of gestation are generally considered nonviable.

In early development, mesenchymal buds from the early trachea form and penetrate the masses destined to become the lungs.[5] The bronchi, bronchioles, alveolar ducts, and alveoli are developed through multiple divisions and budding. Between 16 and 20 weeks, the normal number of bronchi have formed. Between 16 and 24 weeks a dramatic increase in the number and complexity of air spaces, and vascular structures has occurred. After 24 weeks, another important developmental phenomenon occurs: progressive flattening of the epithelial cells lining the air spaces. This allows closer apposition of capillaries to the fluid-filled air space lumen and results in further development of the air-blood barrier, which is necessary for efficient gas exchange after birth.[5]

The breathing movements that occur before birth result in the aspiration of fluid into the lungs. The lungs at birth are about half filled with fluid derived from the amniotic cavity, tracheal glands, and lungs. The fluid in the lungs at birth clears by three routes: (1) through the mouth and nose, (2) into the pulmonary capillaries, and (3) into the lymphatics and the pulmonary vessels.[12]

NORMAL SONOGRAPHIC CHARACTERISTICS

The fetal thorax is examined by the sonographer in both the transverse and coronal or parasagittal planes. The nor-

---

mal shape of the thoracic cavity is symmetrically bell shaped, with the ribs forming the lateral margins, the clavicles forming the upper margins, and the diaphragm forming the lower margin. The lungs serve as the medial borders for the heart and inferior borders for the diaphragm. The diaphragm may be observed on real-time sonography as a smooth hypoechoic muscular margin between the fetal liver or spleen and the lungs (Box 39-1).

SIZE

The thorax is normally slightly smaller than the abdominal cavity (Figure 39-1). The ratio (thoracic circumference to abdominal circumference) has been reported to remain constant throughout pregnancy (0.94 ±0.05).[10] Extreme variations in thoracic size should signal the sonographer to look for other anomalies. In the presence of oligohydramnios, resultant pulmonary hypoplasia may be seen with a reduction in the overall thoracic size.

Chest circumference measurements are made in the transverse plane at the level of the four chamber view of the heart (Figure 39-2). In a fetus with a significant narrow diameter of the chest may have **asphyxiating thoracic dystrophy;** several syndromes may be associated with this finding, including thanatophoric dwarfism. The best ultrasonic determination for predicting pulmonary hypoplasia is the chest area (CA) minus the heart area (HA) times 100 divided by the chest area (CA)[17]:

$$\frac{CA - HA \times 100}{CA}$$

POSITION

The central portion of the thorax is occupied by the mediastinum with the majority of the heart positioned in the midline and left chest. The apex of the heart should be directed towards the spleen; the base of the heart lies horizontal to the diaphragm (Figure 39-3). The location of the heart is impor-

---

> BOX **SONOGRAPHY OF THE NORMAL FETAL**
> **39-1 CHEST**
>
> - Transverse, coronal, and/or parasagittal
> - *Evaluate chest:* Size, shape, symmetry
> - *Evaluate heart:* Position, size, rate, pericardial fluid
> - Evaluate pulmonary texture
> - Centrally positioned mediastinum

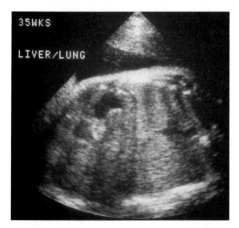

Figure 39-1 Longitudinal view of the fetal thorax and abdomen. The lungs are well seen above the diaphragm. Rib shadowing may be seen in the thoracic cavity. The stomach bubble is up indicating the left side of the fetus is closer to the maternal uterine wall.

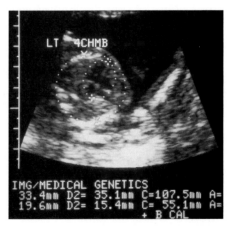

Figure 39-2 The ratio of the heart to the thorax is measured in a transverse view of the chest. The heart circumference normally measures at least one third of the thoracic circumference.

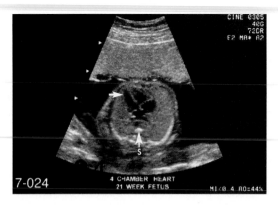

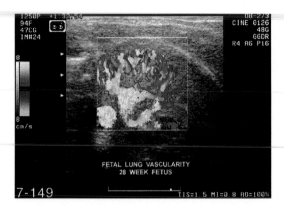

Figure 39-3 Transverse image of the chest shows the apex *(arrow)* of the heart pointing toward the left side of the abdomen. The axis is rotated 45 degrees from midline, which is normal. The spine *(s)* is seen at 6 o'clock, with the aorta just anterior to the spine.

Figure 39-5 Color Doppler image of fetal lung vascularity in a 24-week fetus.

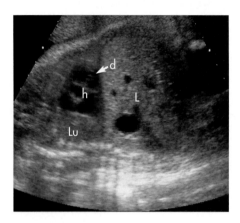

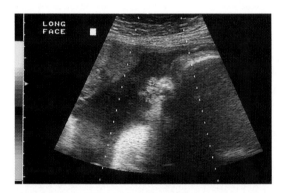

Figure 39-4 Longitudinal view of the fetal chest and abdomen shows the homogeneous, moderately echogenic texture of the lungs *(Lu)*, heart *(h)*, diaphragm *(d)*, and liver *(L)*.

Figure 39-6 Color Doppler image of the fetal breathing pattern seen through the movement of the nostrils.

tant to document in a routine sonographic examination as the detection of abnormal position may indicate the presence of a chest mass, pleural effusion, or cardiac malformation.

TEXTURE

The fetal lungs appear on sonography as homogeneous and of moderate echogenicity. Early in gestation, the lungs are similar to or slightly less echogenic than the liver (Figure 39-4), and as gestation progresses, there is a trend toward increased pulmonary echogenicity relative to the liver.[5] Overlying ribs and acoustic enhancement produced by blood in the heart are two important problems that may complicate the exact determination of echogenicity of the lungs. Color Doppler may be used to outline the vascular pattern within the lungs (Figure 39-5). Ultrasound cannot be used to assess lung maturity.

RESPIRATION

Fetal breathing becomes most prominent in the second and third trimesters. The mature fetus spends almost one third of its time breathing. Fetal breathing movements were considered to be present if characteristic seesaw

movements of the fetal chest or abdomen were sustained for at least 20 seconds. Fetal breathing movements were considered absent if no such fetal activity was noted during the 20-minute observation period.[1]

Color flow Doppler may be used to detect fetal breathing through the nostrils. The fetal facial profile should be obtained with the nose clearly demonstrated; as color is turned on, movement may be seen to flow from the nostrils (Figure 39-6).

The biophysical profile that is used by many obstetricians to assess fetal well-being, uses the respiration pattern as one factor in its scoring. Fetal respiration may vary in response to maternal activities and substance ingestion; it is stimulated by increased sugar doses and decreased by smoking.

ABNORMALITIES OF THE THORACIC CAVITY

ABNORMALITIES OF THE LUNGS

The sonographic evaluation of the fetal lungs is important in routine obstetric assessment and is essential in fetuses at high risk for lung masses. Normal fetal lung texture ap-

TABLE 39-1   FETAL THORACIC CIRCUMFERENCE MEASUREMENTS*

Gestational Age (week)	No.	Predictive Percentiles								
		2.5	5	10	25	50	75	90	95	97.5
16	6	5.9	6.4	7.0	8.0	9.1	10.3	11.3	11.9	12.4
17	22	6.8	7.3	7.9	8.9	10.0	11.2	12.2	12.8	13.3
18	31	7.7	8.2	8.8	9.8	11.0	12.1	13.1	13.7	14.2
19	21	8.6	9.1	9.7	10.7	11.9	13.0	14.0	14.6	15.1
20	20	9.5	10.0	10.6	11.7	12.9	13.9	15.0	15.5	16.0
21	30	10.4	11.0	11.6	12.6	13.7	14.8	15.8	16.4	16.9
22	18	11.3	11.9	12.5	13.5	14.6	15.7	16.7	17.3	17.8
23	21	12.2	12.8	13.4	14.4	15.5	16.6	17.6	18.2	18.8
24	27	13.2	13.7	14.3	15.3	16.4	17.5	18.5	19.1	19.7
25	20	14.1	14.6	15.2	16.2	17.3	18.4	19.4	20.0	20.6
26	25	15.0	15.5	16.1	17.1	18.2	19.3	20.3	21.0	21.5
27	24	15.9	16.4	17.0	18.0	19.1	20.2	21.3	21.9	22.4
28	24	16.8	17.3	17.9	18.9	20.0	21.2	22.2	22.8	23.3
29	24	17.7	18.2	18.8	19.8	21.0	22.1	23.1	23.7	24.2
30	27	18.6	19.1	19.7	20.7	21.9	23.0	24.0	24.6	25.1
31	24	19.5	20.0	20.6	21.6	22.8	23.9	24.9	25.5	26.0
32	28	20.4	20.9	21.5	22.6	23.7	24.8	25.8	26.4	26.9
33	27	21.3	21.8	22.5	23.5	24.6	25.7	26.7	27.3	27.8
34	25	22.2	22.8	23.4	24.4	25.5	26.6	27.6	28.2	28.7
35	20	23.1	23.7	24.3	25.3	26.4	27.5	28.5	29.1	29.6
36	23	24.0	24.6	25.2	26.2	27.3	28.4	29.4	30.0	30.6
37	22	24.9	25.5	26.1	27.1	28.2	29.3	30.3	30.9	31.5
38	21	25.9	26.4	27.0	28.0	29.1	30.2	31.2	31.9	32.4
39	7	26.8	27.3	27.9	28.9	30.0	31.1	32.2	32.8	33.3
40	6	27.7	28.2	28.8	29.8	30.9	32.1	33.1	33.7	34.2

From Chitkara and others: *Am J Obstet Gynecol* 156:1069, 1987.

*Measurements in centimeters.

pears homogeneous. The lungs serve as medial borders for the heart and inferior borders for the diaphragm. The peripheral boundaries are the chest walls. The mediastinum is difficult to clearly define.

To exclude masses, a thorough investigation of lung texture and homogenicity is necessary. Lung masses are separate from the heart and are located above the level of the diaphragm. Lesions of the lungs may be cystic, solid, or complex. Fetal echocardiography is beneficial in excluding cardiac involvement, and evaluation of an intact diaphragm is necessary to exclude diaphragmatic hernia. Abnormalities in cardiac rhythm and fetal hydrops may be present in fetuses with lung masses because of compression of venous return and cardiac failure. Pleural effusions are commonly found in conjunction with lung masses.

The lungs will not grow or develop properly when there is a small uterine cavity resulting from severe oligohydramnios, when the chest cavity is abnormally small, when the balance between tracheal and airway pressure and fluid volume is inadequate, or when the fetus is unable to practice breathing movements.[13]

A mass within the thoracic cavity may have detrimental effects on lung development. The heart and mediastinal structures may be displaced from the normal position and the lung may be compressed and destroyed. These effects may lead to pulmonary hypoplasia.

When evaluating the fetus for a lung mass, the sonographer should check for normal heart position and axis and measure the thoracic circumference. When the heart position and axis vary from normal, a mass should be suspected.

Cardiac axis may be evaluated in a four-chamber heart view (see Chapter 27) by estimating the angle at which the intraventricular septum cross-sects the spine at the anterior chest wall (see Figure 39-3). The normal cardiac axis ranges from 22 to 75 degrees (average is 45 degrees). Deviation from the normal axis may suggest the presence of an intrathoracic mass. Measurements of thoracic circumference may aid in estimating the size of the thoracic cavity and may predict an abnormally small chest cavity and secondary pulmonary hypoplasia. Nomograms for thoracic circumference size are available (Table 39-1).

Pulmonary Hypoplasia. Pulmonary hypoplasia (reduction in lung volume resulting in small, inadequately developed lungs) most commonly occurs from prolonged oligohydramnios or secondary to a small thoracic cavity as a result of a structural or chromosomal abnormality.

Pulmonary hypoplasia may also occur when there is an extreme reduction in amniotic fluid volume. Kidney abnormalities (bilateral renal agenesis, bilateral multicystic kidney disease, severe renal obstruction [e.g., posterior urethral valve syndrome], unilateral renal agenesis with contralateral multicystic kidney development or severe obstruction, and infantile polycystic kidney disease) result in lethal pulmonary hypoplasia. Pulmonary hypoplasia may also occur in fetuses with severe intrauterine growth restriction and early rupture of the membranes.

Masses within the thoracic cavity, including pleural effusion, diaphragmatic hernia (and eventration), cystic adenomatoid malformation of the lung, bronchopulmonary sequestration, and other large cysts and tumors of the lung and thorax may lead to pulmonary hypoplasia. Cardiac defects, some skeletal dysplasias, central nervous system disorders, and chromosomal trisomies (13, 18, and 21) may manifest with pulmonary hypoplasia. A small percentage of infants have pulmonary hypoplasia without any fetal or uterine problem.

Unilateral pulmonary agenesis or hypoplasia is a rare anomaly that is often associated with other fetal malformations.[2] An absent lung should be considered in the differential diagnosis of every fetus with a mediastinal shift and apparent chest mass—especially when it is seen in conjunction with other defects, such as esophageal abnormalities.[2]

The prognosis for infants with pulmonary hypoplasia is grave, with 80% dying after birth. The severity of pulmonary hypoplasia depends on when pulmonary hypoplasia occurred during pregnancy, its severity, and duration (Box 39-2).

Ultrasound findings. The sonographer may be able to check for pulmonary hypoplasia by measuring the thoracic circumference at the level of the four-chamber heart view, excluding the skin and subcutaneous tissues.[6,13] A thoracic circumference below the 5th percentile suggests the possibility of pulmonary hypoplasia. The sonographer should understand that this measurement may not be helpful in

conditions in which there is an intrathoracic mass that compresses lung tissue and yet the thoracic circumference remains normal (diaphragmatic hernia, pleural effusion, and cystic adenomatoid malformations). The sonographer should also look for small echogenic lungs as they lie lateral to the cardiac chambers.

Cystic Lung Masses. Lung cysts are echo-free masses that replace normal lung parenchyma (Figure 39-7). Lung cysts may vary in size, ranging from small isolated lesions to large cystic masses that cause marked shifts of intrathoracic structures. Simple cysts may be surgically excised after delivery (Box 39-3).

Bronchogenic cysts. **Bronchogenic cysts** represent the most common lung cyst detected prenatally.[11] Bronchogenic cysts occur as a result of abnormal budding of the foregut and lack any communication with the trachea or bronchial tree. They typically occur within the mediastinum or lung; infrequently they are inferior to the diaphragm.

Ultrasound findings. Sonographically, bronchogenic cysts appear as small circumscribed masses without evidence of a mediastinal shift or heart failure (see Figure 39-7 and 39-8). Amniotic fluid volume is within a normal range.

Pleural Effusion. **Pleural effusions** (hydrothorax) (see Figure 39-7) are accumulations of fluid within the pleural cavity that may appear as isolated lesions or secondary to multiple fetal anomalies. The most common reason for a pleural effusion is chylothorax occurring as a right-side unilateral collection of fluid secondary to a malformed thoracic duct. Hydramnios often accompanies chylothorax resulting from esophageal compression.

Pleural effusions may result from immune (e.g., Rh disease) or nonimmune causes or from congestive heart failure. Effusions may also occur in fetuses with chromosomal abnormalities (e.g., trisomy 21) or in the fetus with a cardiac mass. Other reasons for pleural effusions include **lymphangiectasia,** cystic adenomatoid malformations, bronchopulmonary sequestration, diaphragmatic hernia, hamartoma, atresia of the pulmonary vein, or other unknown causes.

Ultrasound findings. Sonographically, pleural effusions appear as echo-free peripheral masses on one or both sides of the fetal heart (Figure 39-9). The effusions conform to the thoracic cavity and often compress lung tissue. Compression of lung parenchyma may cause pulmonary hypoplasia, which often represents a life-threatening consequence for the neonate (Figure 39-10).

The presence of a pleural effusion may cause a shift of mediastinal structures, compression of the heart, and inversion of the diaphragm. The shape of the lung appears normal in the presence of a pleural effusion.

Once a pleural effusion has been discovered, a careful search for lung, cardiac, and diaphragmatic lesions should be attempted. Likewise, evaluation for signs of hydrops

---

BOX 39-2 PULMONARY HYPOPLASIA

- Reduction in lung volume resulting in small, inadequately developed lungs
- Occurs from prolonged oligohydramnios or secondary to small thoracic cavity
- Look for chromosome anomalies, renal anomalies, intrauterine growth restriction, premature rupture of membranes, masses within thoracic cavity

---

BOX 39-3 CYSTIC LUNG MASSES

- *Bronchogenic cysts:* Most common; unilocular or multilocular cysts usually within mediastinum or lung; normal amniotic fluid
- *Pleural effusions:* Hydramnios accompanies chylothorax (esophageal compression); may result from immune or nonimmune causes or congestive heart failure; may occur with cardiac mass; lymphangiectasia, CAM, sequestration, hernia; compression of lung tissue; shift of mediastinal structures

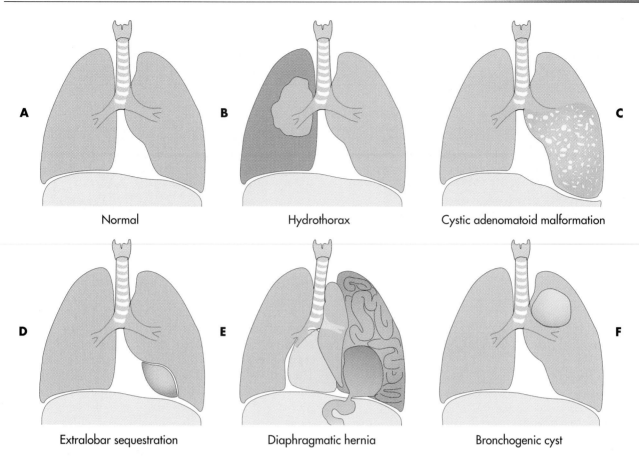

Figure 39-7   Schematic drawings of thoracic masses and mass effect. **A,** Normal thorax. The lungs have convex margins anterolaterally. **B,** Hydrothorax. Anechoic pleural fluid displaces the lungs away from the chest wall and compresses the lungs. **C,** Cystic adenomatoid malformation. An intrapulmonary mass of variable echogenicity may shift the mediastinum and create hydrops. **D,** Bronchopulmonary extralobar sequestration. A spherical or triangular echogenic mass is evident in the inferior portion of the thorax or upper abdomen. **E,** Diaphragmatic hernia. A complex mass (usually on the left-side) creates mediastinal shift. Peristalsing bowel in the thorax provides convincing evidence of the diagnosis. Displaced stomach or scaphoid abdomen is an ancillary finding. **F,** Bronchogenic cyst. A simple cyst near the mediastinum or centrally in the lung may produce mediastinal shift, if it causes bronchial compression.

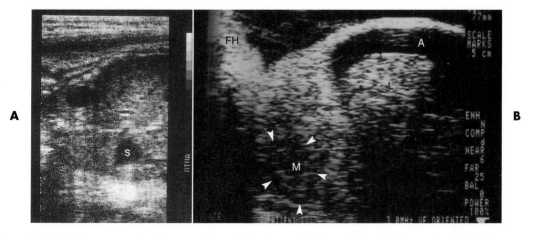

Figure 39-8   A, Longitudinal section of chest revealing small cystic mass in the lung. Note the relationship of the stomach *(s)* to the cyst. A benign bronchogenic cyst was found after birth. **B,** Longitudinal scan showing bulky noncystic mass *(M)* in thorax consistent with cystic adenomatoid malformation (type 3). Abdominal ascites *(A)* is present. *L,* Liver; *FH,* fetal head.   (From Mayden KL and others: *Am J Obstet Gynecol* 148:349, 1984.)

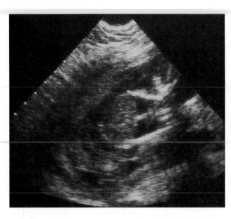

Figure 39-9 Bilateral pleural effusions in a 23-week fetus.

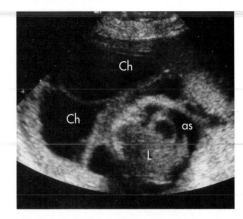

Figure 39-10 Tranverse scan of a 26-week fetus with a huge cystic hygroma *(Ch)* and fetal hydrops. Ascites *(as)* may be seen surrounding the fetal liver *(L)*. The sonographer should also look for the presence of pleural and pericardial effusion.

BOX **SONOGRAPHIC FINDINGS**
39-4 IN SEQUESTRATION

- Echogenic solid mass resembling lung tissue
- Rarely occurs below diaphragm
- Associated with hydrops and polyhydramnios, diaphragmatic hernia, gastrointestinal anomalies
- Normal intraabdominal anatomy
- Intralobar has good outcome; extralobar has poorer outcome (associated anomalies and hydrops)

(ascites, scalp edema, and tissue edema) should be undertaken. Correlation with clinical parameters is warranted to exclude immunologic causes of pleural effusions.

The mortality rate for the infant with a pleural effusion approaches 50%; the prognosis is poorer with associated hydrops. When the pleural effusion is large, lung development is impaired, which may result in pulmonary hypoplasia. Some advocate draining a large pleural collection (thoracentesis) by placing a thoracoamniotic shunt within the pleural space. This is an attempt to allow for lung growth when it is performed during the second trimester of pregnancy. Thoracentesis may be performed to determine whether the lung has the ability to reexpand once the fluid is removed, thus excluding pulmonary hypoplasia, lessening the effects of hydramnios, and obtaining a fetal karyotype using lymphocytes from the aspirated lung fluid.[14]

Solid Lung Masses. Solid tumors of the fetal lungs have been reported by ultrasound, appearing as echodense masses in the lung tissue.[8,11] Bronchopulmonary sequestration and certain types of cystic adenomatoid malformations (CAM) appear as solid lung masses (see Figures 39-7 and 39-8) (Box 39-4).

In a study of 25 cases of echogenic or complex fetal lung masses seen on sonography and suspected of being CAM or sequestrations of the lung, many fetuses with lung masses showed improvement of the sonographic findings in utero and many of the infants were not symptomatic at birth.[3] In this study the majority of the masses were diagnosed at 22 weeks of gestation or earlier. The lesions occurred with almost equal frequencies in both lungs. Survival correlated with the type of lesion, as well as with the presence or absence of hydrops. In the patients with CAM the survival data did not significantly differ between type 1 and type 3 lesions. A higher risk of congenital abnormalities was found with type 2 CAM. Fetuses with a mild cardiac shift had a better survival rate. Polyhydramnios with the lung lesion had a poorer perinatal outcome. The group concluded that when a lung mass is identified sonographically, an attempt should be made to identify the type of lesion, determine the degree of mediastinal shift, and estimate the amniotic fluid volume.

Brochopulmonary sequestration. In **bronchopulmonary sequestration,** extra pulmonary tissue is present within the pleural lung sac (intralobar) or is connected to the inferior border of the lung within its own pleural sac (extralobar).[8,15] This probably develops from a separate outpouching of the foregut or by separation of a segment of the developing lung from the tracheobronchial tree.[15] This extra lung tissue is nonfunctional and receives its blood supply from systemic circulation. The arterial supply is usually from the thoracic aorta, with venous drainage into the vena cava.

Ultrasound findings. Sonographically, an echo-dense solid mass resembling lung tissue is observed, usually in the lower lobe of the lung (Figure 39-11). The majority of extralobar defects occur on the left side and rarely below the diaphragm. Intralobar lesions are spherical, and extralobar sequestration appears as a cone-shaped or triangular mass. These lesions may resemble a cystic adenomatoid (type II) malformation. Color Doppler may aid the sonographer in viewing this anomalous circulation. A hypoplastic lung may be observed on the affected side. Hydrops is a frequent finding. Other associated anomalies are diaphrag-

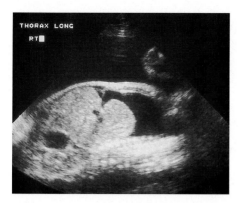

Figure 39-11   Longitudinal scan of the 23-week fetus with a right-side pulmonary sequestration. The echo-dense mass is well seen in the lower lobe of the thoracic cavity. A large pleural effusion surrounds the mass.

matic hernia and gastrointestinal and lung anomalies (pulmonary hypoplasia).

The prognosis for intralobar sequestration is very favorable, whereas extralobar sequestration carries a poor prognosis because of associated anomalies and hydrops.

Laryngeal atresia may be diagnosed when bilateral lung enlargement is observed (Figure 39-12).

Cystic adenomatoid malformation. **Cystic adenomatoid malformation (CAM)** is an abnormality in the formation of the bronchial tree with secondary overgrowth of mesenchymal tissue from arrested bronchial development (see Figures 39-7 and 39-8). Three forms of cystic adenomatoid malformations have been described.[16] In type I, one or several large cysts replace normal lung tissue (single or multiple cysts measuring more than 2 cm and up to 10 cm) (Figure 39-13); type II lesions consist of multiple small cysts (less than 1 cm) (Figure 39-14).[16] Type II lesions are associated with fetal and/or chromosomal abnormalities in 25% of cases. These anomalies may include renal agenesis, pulmonary anomalies, and diaphragmatic hernia. Type III malformations are characterized as bulky, large, noncystic lesions appearing as echo-dense masses of the entire lung lobe (Figure 39-15).[8,11] When there is a shift of the mediastinal structures, lung compression may occur and hydrops may develop. Hydramnios may be observed secondary to esophageal compression, preventing normal fetal swallowing.

Differentiation of the type of cystic adenomatoid malformations is imperative, because prognosis varies depending on the type of lesion. Type I lesions have favorable outcomes, whereas type II and III lesions have poor prognoses.[16]

Ultrasound findings. When a cystic or solid lung mass has been identified, the sonographer should attempt to do the following:

- Determine the number and size(s) of cystic structures
- Check for presence or absence of a mediastinal shift
- Identify and assess the size of the lungs
- Look for fetal hydrops
- Exclude cardiac masses
- Search for other fetal anomalies

Based on these findings, an appropriate prognosis and management plan may be instituted (Box 39-5).

A review of the spontaneous improvement of these thoracic masses in utero indicates the following[4]:

- Sonographically detected fetal chest masses may result in pathologically proved thoracic-derived lesions or may resolve, some without sequelae
- These mass lesion may change in size and echogenicity
- Sonograms of fetuses with CAM may be normal in the first and second trimester and only later show abnormalities on ultrasound
- The outcomes for the fetuses vary, with 9 out of 14 surviving and 5 out of 14 resulting in perinatal demise or termination of pregnancy
- The presence of polyhydramnios, hydrops, or marked cardiac deviation predicts poor outcome more accurately than the lesion type.

Congenital bronchial atresia. **Congenital bronchial atresia** is a pulmonary anomaly that results from the focal obliteration of a segment of the bronchial lumen. It is found most commonly in the left upper lobe and appears on ultrasound as an echogenic pulmonary mass lesion.

Complex Lung Masses. The internal components of complex lung masses are cystic and solid and appear heterogeneous. At times, compressed adjacent thoracic organs further complicate determination of the type of lesion (pleural effusion surrounding lungs and heart). Congenital dilation of the bronchial tree may have both cystic and solid characteristics.[11]

ABNORMALITIES OF THE DIAPHRAGM

The diaphragm is an important muscle separating the thoracic cavity from the abdomen. The diaphragm is specifically studied in fetuses at risk for congenital defects of the diaphragm or when atypical structures are found in the fetal chest. In the normal fetus the diaphragm should appear as a curvilinear structure coursing anteriorly to posteriorly (Figure 39-16). The fetal stomach and liver should be identified caudal to the diaphragm with the lungs and heart positioned cephalad. Failure to recognize these normal relationships should prompt the sonographer to search for diaphragmatic defects.

Diaphragmatic Hernia. **Diaphragmatic hernia,** a sporadic defect occurring in 1 per 2000 to 1 in 5000 births is an opening in the pleuroperitoneal membrane, which divides the pleural cavity from the peritoneal cavity.[13] This defect probably develops between the 6th and 10th week of gestation, when the gut is returning from the yolk sac and the diaphragm is developing.

The diaphragmatic hernia permits the abdominal organs to enter the fetal chest (see Figures 39-7 and 39-17 to 39-19). The most common type of diaphragmatic defect (over 90% of defects) occurs posteriorly and laterally in the diaphragm (herniation through **foramen of Bochdalek**).[7] These hernias are usually found on the left

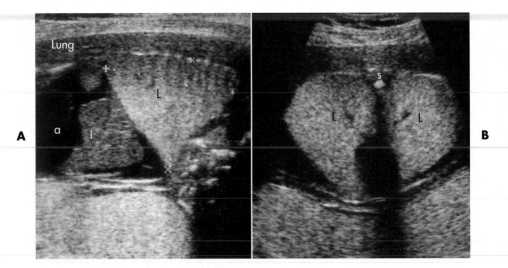

Figure 39-12   **A,** Echogenic lung (*L, in calipers*) in a 21-week fetus with severe hydrops. The opposite lung appeared similar in texture. Oligohydramnios and episodes of bradycardia were evident. *a,* Ascites; *l,* liver. **B,** In the same fetus, both echogenic lungs *(L)* are viewed. Laryngeal or tracheal agenesis was suspected. It is believed that excess lung fluid is manufactured by the abnormal lung. *s,* Spine.

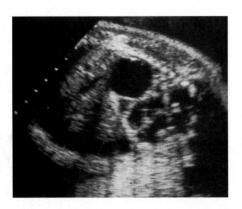

Figure 39-13   Type I cystic adenomatoid malformation showing multiple large cystic areas replacing normal lung tissue.

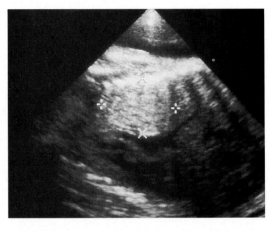

Figure 39-14   Type II cystic adenomatoid malformation shows multiple cystic areas under 1 cm in size. The mass is echogenic at the base of the thoracic cavity.

BOX | **SONOGRAPHIC FINDINGS IN CYSTIC**
39-5 | **ADENOMATOID MALFORMATIONS**

- *Type I:* Single or multiple large cysts >2 cm in diameter; good prognosis after resection of affected lung
- *Type II:* Multiple small cysts <1 cm in diameter, echogenic; high incidence of other congenital anomalies (renal, gastrointestinal)
- *Type III:* Large, bulky, non-cystic lesions producing mediastinal shift; poor prognosis
- Usually only one lobe is affected
- Associated polyhydramnios and anasarca have poor prognosis

---

side of the diaphragm, and left-sided organs (stomach, spleen, and portions of the liver) enter the chest through the opening. The abnormally positioned abdominal organs shift the heart and mediastinal structures to the right side of the chest. Usually the stomach is in the

chest near the heart, instead of below the diaphragm. The sonographer should look for peristalsis or displacement of the liver (Box 39-6).

Defects on the right side of the diaphragm allow the right-side abdominal viscera (liver, gallbladder, intestines) to enter the chest. As a consequence of herniated abdominal organs, the lungs are compressed and may become hypoplastic.

Ultrasound findings. On ultrasound examination, the sonographer will see the liver in the chest, with the heart deviated to the left. The stomach alignment will be abnormal and moved to the right. Color may help to trace the portal vasculature in the liver as it lies within the chest cavity. At birth, respiration may be severely compromised, which may result in death of the newborn.[9]

Diaphragmatic hernias may occur anteriorly and medially in the diaphragm (through **foramen of Morgagni**) and

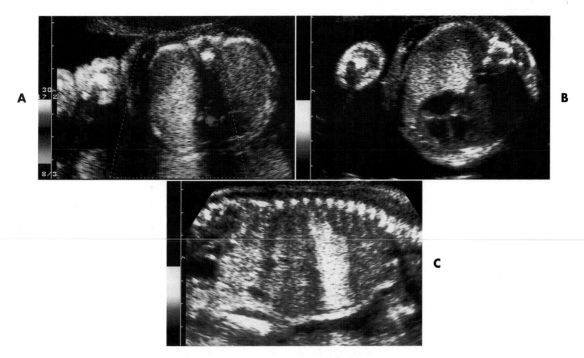

Figure 39-15 A fetus is found at 32 weeks to have asymmetry in the lung tissue, which turned out to be type III cystic adenomatoid malformation. This echogenic mass affected the right lung. **A,** Gray-scale transverse scan comparing both textures of the lung. The right lobe is clearly more echogenic. **B,** B-Color display of the cystic adenomatoid malformation as it slightly displaced the cardiac axis. **C,** Longitudinal B-Color scan of the echo-dense mass just above the diaphragm in the thoracic cavity.

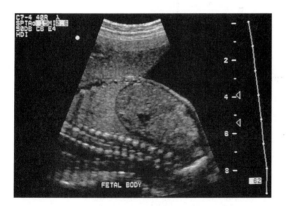

Figure 39-16 Longitudinal scan of the diaphragm as it separates the thoracic from the abdominal cavities.

BOX 39-6	SONOGRAPHIC CRITERIA SUGGESTIVE OF A DIAPHRAGMATIC HERNIA

- Shift of the heart and mediastinal structures (right shift in left-side defects; left shift in right-side defects)
- Mass within the thoracic cavity (liver, stomach, spleen, and large bowel in left-side defects; liver, gallbladder, intestines in right-side defects)
- Small abdominal circumference resulting from herniated abdominal structures.
- Obvious diaphragm defect
- Hydramnios
- Over 50% have structural anomalies or chromosomal abnormalities.
- Structural defects include cardiovascular (tetralogy of Fallot and others), genitourinary (renal agenesis, cystic dysplasia, and ureteropelvic junction obstruction), central nervous system (holoprosencephaly, hydrocephalus, and spinal anomalies), clubbed feet, hemivertebrae and absent ribs, genital (ambiguous genitalia and others), and gastrointestinal (imperforate anus, annular pancreas, and absence of the gallbladder)*
- Growth restriction suggests associated anomalies
- The abdominal circumference below the 5th percentile and liver in the chest indicate poor prognosis†

*Data from Nyberg DA, Mahony BS, Pretorius DH, editors: *Diagnostic ultrasound of fetal anomalies: text and atlas,* St Louis, 1990, Mosby.

†Data from Teixeira J and others: Abdominal circumference in fetuses with congenital diaphragmatic hernia: correlation with hernia content and pregnancy outcome, *J Ultrasound Med* 16:407, 1997.

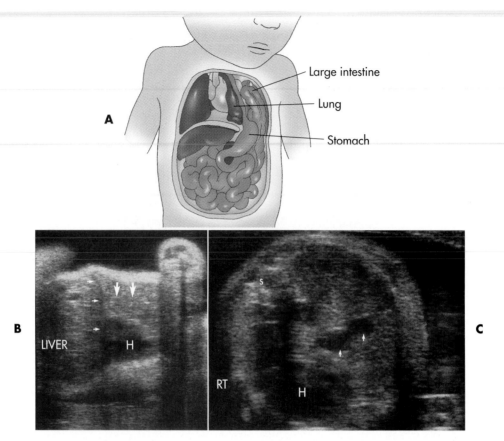

Figure 39-17 **A,** Schema demonstrating hernia of intestinal loops and part of the stomach into left pleural cavity. The heart and mediastinum are pushed to the right while the left lung is compressed. **B,** Sagittal view in a fetus with a diaphragmatic hernia. The heart *(H)* is displaced to the right side of fetal thorax by herniated bowel *(large arrows)*. *Small arrows,* Diaphragm. **C,** Transverse section in same patient showing the herniated stomach *(arrows)* at the level of the heart *(H)*. *s,* Spine.

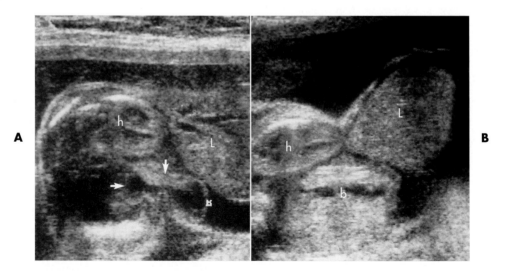

Figure 39-18 **A,** Diaphragmatic hernia in association with omphalocele shown in a 28-week fetus. Displacement of the heart, *h,* to the right chest is demonstrated. Herniated bowel *(arrowheads)* with peristalsis demonstrated by real-time imaging confirmed the diagnosis. *L,* Lung. **B,** In the same fetus the liver *(L)* is shown in close proximity to the heart *(h)* and bowel *(b)* because of the absent diaphragm.